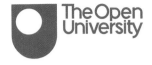

Living with Diabetes

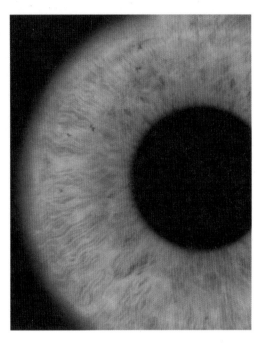

This publication forms part of an Open University course SK120 *Diabetes care*. Details of this and other Open University courses can be obtained from the Student Registration and Enquiry Service, The Open University, PO Box 197, Milton Keynes, MK7 6BJ, United Kingdom: tel. +44 (0)870 333 4340, email general-enquiries@open.ac.uk

Alternatively, you may visit the Open University website at http://www.open.ac.uk where you can learn more about the wide range of courses and packs offered at all levels by The Open University.

To purchase a selection of Open University course materials visit http://www.ouw.co.uk, or contact Open University Worldwide, Michael Young Building, Walton Hall, Milton Keynes MK7 6AA, United Kingdom for a brochure. tel. +44 (0)1908 858785; fax +44 (0)1908 858787; email ouwenq@open.ac.uk

The Open University
Walton Hall, Milton Keynes
MK7 6AA

First published 2005.

Edited, designed and typeset by The Open University.

Printed and bound in the United Kingdom by CPI, Glasgow.

ISBN 0 7492 6982 0

1.1

THE SK120 COURSE TEAM

Course Team Chair and Academic Editor

Duncan Banks, Department of Biological Sciences, Faculty of Science

Course Managers

Tracy Finnegan, Faculty of Science

Simone Pitman, Department of Chemistry, Faculty of Science

Course Team Assistant

Dawn Partner, Department of Biological Sciences, Faculty of Science

Course Team Author

Cathy Lloyd, Faculty of Health and Social Care (co-author and academic adviser Chapters 1–10)

Academic Readers

Duncan Banks, Department of Biological Sciences, Faculty of Science

Robin Harding, Science Staff Tutor, Scotland

Cathy Lloyd, Faculty of Health and Social Care

Hilary MacQueen, Department of Biological Sciences, Faculty of Science

External Course Assessor

Professor Trisha Greenhalgh OBE, Department of Primary Care and Population Sciences, University College London Medical School

Media Project Manager

Rafael Hidalgo

Editors

Rebecca Graham

Gillian Riley

Bina Sharma

Design

Sarah Hofton

Jenny Nockles

Illustration

Sara Hack

DVD-ROM Production

Jason Jarratt

Video Production

Martin Chiverton, Producer

John Foakes, Sound

Derek Firmin, Camera

Mike Ford, Photographer

Owen Horn, Producer/Director

Mike Levers, Photographer

Dave Muscroft, Photographer

Course Website

Ewan Salter

Picture Researcher

Lydia K. Eaton

Rights Executive

Sarah Gammon

Martin Keeling

Indexer

Jane Henley

Consultants

Neil Baker, Ipswich Hospital NHS Trust (co-author Chapter 6)

Jackie Bryan, Homerton School of Health Studies (co-author Chapters 1, 5, 6)

Janet Cox, University of Luton (co-author Chapters 1, 5, 6)

Sue Cradock, Portsmouth Hospitals NHS Trust and Portsmouth City PCT (co-author Chapter 9)

Jill Hill, Heart of England NHS Trust (co-author Chapters 1, 3, 5, 6, 7)

Renee Page, Nottingham City Hospital NHS Trust (author Chapters 2 and 4)

Chas Skinner, University of Southampton (author Chapter 8, co-author Chapter 9)

Julie Smith, Homerton School of Health Studies (co-author Chapters 3 and 7, project liaison, developmental testing, Associate Lecturer recruitment)

Rosemary Walker, In Balance Healthcare, UK (author Chapter 10, revision Chapters 1–10)

Other Contributors

The Course Team would like to thank the following people for their involvement in the production of SK120:

Critical readers: Vickie Arrowsmith, Elizabeth Bradley, Carole Hewitt, Peter Lees, Gail Nixon.

Video participants and production: Janice Brown, Kerri Ellis, Toby Mart, Jonathan Roland.

Developmental Testers: Keith Beechener, Safia Begum, Janice Brown, Mick Crammer, Kreshnik Doli, Kerri Ellis, Tahmina Kauser, Fatima Khanom, Jane Masters, Mike McGuire, Naheed Mirza, Nighat Zaidi.

Thanks are also due to Shanaz Mughal (competency adviser and pilot study coordinator, Birmingham), Florence Brown (diabetes project), Jo Hood (diabetes project manager).

CONTENTS

CHAPTER 1 INTRODUCTION TO DIABETES CARE | 1
Learning Outcomes | 1
1.1 Introduction | 1
1.2 The impact of diabetes | 2
1.3 The diabetes team | 6
1.4 Team work | 10
1.5 Communication in teams | 11
1.6 Informed consent | 16
1.7 Record keeping | 16
1.8 Confidentiality | 17
1.9 Safety | 19
1.10 Summary of Chapter 1 | 25
Questions for Chapter 1 | 26
References | 27

CHAPTER 2 WHAT IS DIABETES? | 29
Learning Outcomes | 29
2.1 Introduction | 29
2.2 What is diabetes? | 30
2.3 Parts of the body and hormones involved in diabetes | 31
2.4 How to diagnose diabetes | 40
2.5 Classification of diabetes | 43
2.6 Genes and risk | 49
2.7 Summary of Chapter 2 | 52
Questions for Chapter 2 | 52
References | 53

CHAPTER 3 AWARENESS OF CARE | 55
Learning Outcomes | 55
3.1 Introduction | 55
3.2 Who provides care? | 55
3.3 A framework for care | 61
3.4 Ways of delivering care | 66
3.5 Summary of Chapter 3 | 70
Questions for Chapter 3 | 70
References | 71

CHAPTER 4   MEDICAL MANAGEMENT   73

Learning Outcomes   73
4.1   Introduction   73
4.2   Managing diabetes   73
4.3   Diagnosis   74
4.4   Aims of medical management   76
4.5   Blood-glucose-lowering therapies   77
4.6   Complementary therapies and diabetes   95
4.7   Medical management of pregnancy and diabetes   96
4.8   Other therapies for people with diabetes   97
4.9   How do you know if things are well controlled?   99
4.10 Risk reduction   100
4.11 Summary of Chapter 4   100
Questions for Chapter 4   101
References   101

CHAPTER 5   MONITORING RISK FACTORS FOR DIABETES
COMPLICATIONS   103

Learning Outcomes   103
5.1   Introduction   103
5.2   Assessing diabetes complication risk factors   103
5.3   Monitoring blood glucose levels   108
5.4   Monitoring ketone levels   117
5.5   Monitoring lipid levels   118
5.6   Blood pressure monitoring   119
5.7   Calculating body mass index   122
5.8   Making sense of the measurements   123
5.9   Summary of Chapter 5   124
Questions for Chapter 5   124
References   125

CHAPTER 6   SCREENING FOR COMPLICATIONS OF
DIABETES   127

Learning Outcomes   127
6.1   Introduction   127
6.2   Becoming aware of the complications of diabetes   127
6.3   The types of complication associated with diabetes   130

6.4	Diabetes and eye disease	130
6.5	Diabetes and renal disease	137
6.6	Diabetic neuropathy	140
6.7	Care of feet in people with diabetes	144
6.8	Cardiovascular disease	147
6.9	Summary of Chapter 6	150
	Questions for Chapter 6	151
	References	151

CHAPTER 7 HYPERGLYCAEMIA AND HYPOGLYCAEMIA: LIVING ON THE EDGE? — 153

	Learning Outcomes	153
7.1	Introduction	153
7.2	Hyperglycaemia	153
7.3	Hypoglycaemia	161
7.4	Summary of Chapter 7	169
	Questions for Chapter 7	171
	References	171

CHAPTER 8 PSYCHOSOCIAL ASPECTS OF DIABETES — 173

	Learning Outcomes	173
8.1	Introduction	173
8.2	How people think about diabetes – beliefs	177
8.3	Emotions	190
8.4	Depression and diabetes	196
8.5	Summary of Chapter 8	200
	Questions for Chapter 8	200
	References	200

CHAPTER 9 EDUCATION FOR EFFECTIVE SELF-MANAGEMENT — 203

	Learning Outcomes	203
9.1	Introduction	203
9.2	Empowerment, compliance and concordance – what's in a word?	207
9.3	The challenge of dietary management	214
9.4	Medication taking and adjustment	219
9.5	Self-monitoring	220

9.6	Emotions: awareness and management	221
9.7	Communication skills and the consultation	223
9.8	Qualities of effective communication	227
9.9	Summary of Chapter 9	229
Questions for Chapter 9		230
References		230

CHAPTER 10 LIVING WITH DIABETES — 233

Learning Outcomes		233
10.1	Introduction	233
10.2	Culture	234
10.3	Driving	236
10.4	Insurance	238
10.5	Employment	240
10.6	Family	242
10.7	Sex, relationships and diabetes	243
10.8	The demands of treatment	243
10.9	Pregnancy	245
10.10	Lifestyle and diabetes	247
10.11	Living with long-term complications of diabetes	249
10.12	Living with someone who has diabetes	251
10.13	Summary of Chapter 10	251
Questions for Chapter 10		252
References		253

ANSWERS TO QUESTIONS — 255

ACKNOWLEDGEMENTS — 268

INDEX — 270

CHAPTER 1

INTRODUCTION TO DIABETES CARE

Learning Outcomes

When you have completed this chapter you should be able to:

1.1 Define and use, or recognise definitions and applications of, each of the terms printed in **bold** in the text.

1.2 Describe the possible impact of diabetes on an individual and their family.

1.3 List the members of the diabetes team and state the contribution each makes to the management of diabetes.

1.4 Identify ways in which members of the diabetes team work together to ensure that safe, appropriate care and advice are given to an individual with diabetes.

1.5 Describe how good communication can enhance the care of people with diabetes.

1.6 Identify different ways by which information about the person with diabetes may be obtained and recorded.

1.7 State the meaning of confidentiality and its implications for the family and working environment of the person with diabetes.

1.8 Outline the principles of risk assessment and of working in a safe environment.

1.1 Introduction

Welcome to the first chapter of the course *Diabetes care*; we hope you find studying with us a valuable experience. This course is designed to inform people from a variety of backgrounds about diabetes and its management. You might be hoping to learn more about diabetes because you plan to have a career in the health services, or you may be caring for someone with this condition, or you may have diabetes yourself. In Chapter 2 you will learn more about what diabetes is, but we wanted to start this book with an overview of some of the key issues in diabetes and its management. You will begin by thinking about the diagnosis of diabetes before considering the individuals who make up the team of people who care for those with diabetes. Following this you will consider in more detail the issues in team work and the importance of good communication when working in a team, before moving on to matters around safety and risk.

You will come across the term 'patient' in many places in this chapter and the others that follow. But people are not always patients, so we have tried to use the term 'patient' only when we are talking about situations within health care (the general practice or hospital clinic, for example). When we are referring to situations outside the health care services (at home or in the community) we talk more about the person with diabetes. Of course the term 'diabetes' will appear many, many times and as you probably know there are several types of diabetes.

'Diabetes' will be used to refer to general issues that cover all types of diabetes mellitus; when there needs to be an example from a specific type of diabetes, the text will indicate this. But for now, if you haven't already done so, start by reading the Learning Outcomes at the beginning of this chapter.

1.2 The impact of diabetes

'About eight years ago, somebody dumped a big, awkward parcel in my arms, and told me that I had to carry it … until the end of my life. No warning, no explanation, and no escape route. I didn't see who did it to me, and I didn't even know what was in the parcel.'

(Anon)

You will read more about this person in Chapter 8, but for now we will think about the 'parcel' they describe. The parcel in the above quote is diabetes – a condition which is now described as an epidemic, as it is becoming increasingly common not just in this country but throughout the world. The World Health Organization (WHO) estimated that in 2002 there were 177 million people in the world with diabetes, an increase of 42 million from 1995 (WHO, 2002). Diabetes UK, the charity that supports both people with diabetes and much of the research into diabetes, suggested that in the UK in 2004 there were 1.8 million people who were known to have diabetes (Diabetes UK, 2004a). However, they believe that there are at least another million people who have diabetes but who have not yet been diagnosed, usually because they have no obvious symptoms.

It does not matter where you live or work, you will come across people with diabetes. The person quoted above found it very difficult to live with diabetes, but many others in similar circumstances live life to the full and find it causes them few problems. You may think of people like Steve Redgrave, the Olympic rower, who has certainly not been limited by his diabetes. However, some people do find living with diabetes difficult and it can be costly in personal, financial and social terms. Some people find that diabetes can affect their job prospects, mortgage, what vehicle they can drive, and their relationships. This is before taking into account the problems caused when diabetes is poorly controlled.

'I always had me injection but I had high blood glucose all the time, so I was always in moods and violent … so I never really did well at school. I always wanted to concentrate and that … but with diabetes and high blood glucose and parents [splitting up] and everything, I never did well, no.'

(Mark, who has Type 1 diabetes)

'You do become a different person with diabetes. [You] get mood swings and tempers. I sometimes think of my poor children having a mum like a dragon.'

(Jane, who has Type 1 diabetes)

'I have been diagnosed only months. They advised me to control food intake, so I am taking a meal only once in a day.'

(Sunita, who has Type 2 diabetes)

(Adapted from Hiscock et al., 2001)

These quotes are taken from a research study in which people with diabetes were asked about their experience of diabetes and the services provided to help them. You can see from these statements the impact that diabetes has had on their lives. (Type 1 and Type 2 diabetes will be explained in Chapter 2.) It has affected their emotional state, their ability to concentrate and work, their families and their eating pattern – though Sunita, quoted above, had misunderstood the advice she was given. (You will learn more about diet and diabetes in Chapter 4.) Two of the people suffered from mood swings and this affected their relationships with those around them, including other members of their immediate family. The family may also be involved in delivering care to the person with diabetes; for example, ensuring that the person receives the correct diet.

However, the diagnosis of diabetes does not have to be negative. Some people find it a relief to know what is wrong with them and, once diagnosed, find that the treatment makes them feel much better.

Activity 1.1   A short introduction to diabetes

Suggested study time 30 minutes

This activity offers you a short introduction to diabetes. It will help you to become more familiar with some of the terms used, and will prepare you to complete the other activities in this chapter. All of the information in this activity will be covered in much more detail in later chapters, particularly Chapters 2 and 4.

Read Offprint 1.1 in the *Offprint Booklet*. This extract is taken from pages 2–4 of Diabetes UK's *Understanding diabetes* (Diabetes UK, 2004a). As you read the extract, make brief notes about the different types of diabetes and who they affect. Also, note down the most common symptoms of diabetes.

Did you find any differences between what you thought before you read the extract and what you now know?

Comment

You have read that the main types of diabetes are Type 1 and Type 2. Type 1 occurs when people do not make any natural insulin at all. In Type 2 diabetes, people still make insulin of their own but either there is not enough of it or it does not work properly, or both. Because insulin is a hormone that regulates the level of glucose in the blood, if it is not there or is not working properly, the blood glucose level becomes too high – a key sign of diabetes.

The symptoms of diabetes are related to a high level of blood glucose. They include passing a lot of urine, especially at night, and being very thirsty. These symptoms occur because the body tries to remove the excess glucose via the urine, and passing a lot of urine causes dehydration and thirst. Tiredness occurs because the glucose stays in the blood and cannot be used for energy production by muscles. Wounds heal slowly (also mentioned in the extract) because the high level of glucose in the blood slows down the healing process.

The extract also includes a list of things that do not cause diabetes. These may have been among your thoughts before undertaking this activity – they are common myths.

Diabetes does not only affect the individual and their family. It also has cost implications for the National Health Service (NHS): diabetes care in the UK accounts for about 10% of the NHS budget. A study called CODE-2 UK, which looked into the costs of diabetes, estimated that the average annual cost of NHS care for a person with diabetes was about £1500 (Bottomley et al., 1999). This cost includes medication, monitoring and treatment for complications of diabetes. The complications of diabetes can be blindness, kidney failure, amputation, stroke and heart attack. (You will learn more about these, and the reasons they occur, in Chapters 5 and 6.) It is expected that the cost to the NHS will increase in the future as the number of people with diabetes increases. There is therefore a need to prevent diabetes wherever possible, and to manage it effectively in order to minimise complications.

Everyone with diabetes should have the same quality of care, and opportunities to get the help they need to manage their diabetes themselves. Unfortunately, this is not always the case, as was illustrated by the Audit Commission report, *Testing Times: A Review of Diabetes Services in England and Wales* (Audit Commission, 2000). This report showed that there was a huge variation across the country as to how easy it was for people with diabetes to access help, whether from the hospital or from their GP, both during and outside normal working hours. Certain people found it particularly difficult. These included people living in residential homes and those who did not speak English. The report also showed that even when people were given help and advice it could be inconsistent and confusing, as shown by the following comments taken from the report.

'I wish there was someone I could speak to when I don't feel well in the weekend.' (p. 39)

'I do not read English or Urdu. Therefore my care information should be in another format, like an audio tape in mother tongue language.' (p. 37)

'I have nobody to contact after hours and sometimes feel very alone with this.' (p. 40)

'Two district nurses said my tablets would make me lose weight, but the diabetes nurse said different, said the tablets make you fat. It is this kind of information which makes you not want to bother. You don't know which advice to believe.' (p. 43)

(Audit Commission, 2000)

In response to the Audit Commission's report, the government published the **National Service Framework** for Diabetes (Department of Health, 2001a). National Service Frameworks (NSF) are government plans to ensure equality in the delivery of a high-quality service. The NSF for diabetes set a 10-year target for the delivery of 12 standards of care for diabetes (see Table 1.1). You can read these standards in detail, as well as some examples of good practice, on the Department of Health website, which you can access from the course website. (The NSF for diabetes document is also on the course DVD-ROM.)

Table 1.1 NSF standards of care for diabetes.

Standard number	Title of standard
1	Prevention of Type 2 diabetes
2	Identification of people with diabetes
3	Empowering people with diabetes
4	Clinical care of adults with diabetes
5 and 6	Clinical care of children and young people with diabetes
7	Management of diabetic emergencies
8	Care of people with diabetes during admission to hospital
9	Diabetes and pregnancy
10, 11 and 12	Detection and management of long-term complications

As you can see, the 12 standards are very comprehensive, and cover all aspects of care that someone with diabetes may expect throughout their life.

Diabetes is a lifelong condition. It can affect people of any age, from young babies to the very old. If a young child is diagnosed he or she will have to live with this for the rest of their life. The person with diabetes lives with it 24 hours a day, on holiday, during exams, when having a baby, on Christmas Day or during Ramadan. The events and pressures of everyday life will affect how well that person copes with controlling the condition; sometimes it will be relatively easy, sometimes the diabetes is ignored or put aside in favour of more pressing concerns.

Activity 1.2 Effects of diabetes

Suggested study time 10 minutes

People with diabetes may have to take tablets regularly, inject themselves with insulin, test their blood or urine and eat meals at regular times. If you have diabetes yourself, note down at least three ways in which having diabetes affects your lifestyle. If you do not have diabetes, try to imagine what it would be like and then write down three ways in which you think it might affect you.

Comment

There is no correct answer to this activity, but here are some things that you may have mentioned in your answer.

You might feel that you would have to plan things in advance and, indeed, many people with diabetes complain that they are unable to do things on the spur of the moment. It would depend on how regular your lifestyle is – some people lead a very orderly life, whilst others like to have a more flexible routine. Even if you have a very organised lifestyle there are always emergency situations that you cannot plan for in advance. If, for example, you have diabetes and you need to take your child to the accident and emergency department at the hospital, you may have problems getting something to eat at the right time. However, many people manage the demands of diabetes very well and feel that diabetes has had very little effect on their lifestyle.

Given that diabetes can impact on so many areas of life, and can lead to many different physical and psychological effects, it follows that a 'team' approach to diabetes care is the most appropriate, with the person with diabetes being at the centre of that team.

1.3 The diabetes team

There are many people involved in enabling the person with diabetes to live with the condition, and to manage it effectively. These people, together with the person with diabetes, make up the diabetes team. Many members of this team are health care professionals who are based in GP surgeries or hospitals. However, other people may also be part of the team. For example, in Case Study 1.1, Sheila (Tom's primary carer) is one of the most important members of the diabetes team.

Case Study 1.1

Tom has Type 2 diabetes and has recently had a stroke, which has left him with a severe weakness down his right side and has made him forgetful. Sheila manages his daily diabetes care for him. She checks his blood glucose (often called blood sugar) each day by using a blood glucose meter. She prepares and injects insulin twice daily, and adjusts the dose according to his blood glucose results. Sheila is constantly alert for signs of low blood glucose, and knows how to treat this with a sugary drink and biscuits. She knows that Tom needs three regular meals each day and a bedtime snack. Every 6 months she drives him to the hospital diabetes clinic, where she and Tom discuss his diabetes control with the diabetes nurse and consultant, who advise them as necessary.

As you read in Case Study 1.1, because of Tom's physical difficulties and memory problems Sheila bears much of the responsibility for managing his diabetes. However, the most important member of the diabetes team is the person with diabetes, and, in a situation like Tom's, the main carer at home. The person with diabetes should form the centre or focus for the other members of the team, as the person who has to live with the condition. They need to give feedback to the team about how they are coping with the condition, and how well the treatments are working. Other members of the team are there to advise, assist, educate, and give feedback on diabetes control, to help the person with diabetes enjoy a good quality of life and avoid developing complications from their diabetes.

The aim of the team supporting the person with diabetes is to enable them to manage the condition as successfully as possible, within the limitations and difficulties of their everyday life. It is important, therefore, that the care is not imposed on the person but negotiated with them, so they can fit their diabetes management into their everyday life. The health care professionals making up each individual's diabetes team vary according to where their diabetes care is delivered (at their local GP surgery, health centre or in a hospital diabetes clinic) and the type of diabetes and whether there are diabetes complications present. You think about this further in Activity 1.3.

Activity 1.3 The diabetes team

Suggested study time 45 minutes

Read the two stories in Case Study 1.2 and then, for each, list the members of the diabetes team involved with the two people with diabetes. Note down what you think each team member does and then read the comment below.

Comment

You will have seen that the teams caring for the two people in Case Study 1.2 are considerably different and each is made up of a variety of different health care professionals. Teams such as these are often described as **multidisciplinary teams**, since they bring together people with differing expertise.

Case Study 1.2

Asha

Asha, aged 48, has had Type 2 diabetes for five years, which she controls with two tablets a day. Her diabetes care is based at her local health centre where she sees her GP and practice nurse twice a year. She has a diabetes eye check every year with her local accredited optometrist, and when she collects her monthly supply of diabetes tablets from the local pharmacist she sometimes asks him questions about the treatment.

Whitfield

Whitfield, aged 73, has had Type 2 diabetes for 15 years. He is on twice-daily insulin, and is overseen by the diabetes team at the hospital. At the clinic he is usually seen by the consultant diabetologist, dietitian and diabetes specialist nurse. He has blood samples taken by the clinic phlebotomist, and eye screening performed by the retinal screening technician. As he has a diabetic foot ulcer, he sees the podiatrist weekly at the diabetes foot clinic. He also sees the orthotist to be measured regularly for specially made shoes to relieve pressure on the foot ulcer. He has just been referred to the psychologist, as he has recently been feeling very depressed about his diabetes.

Each member of a diabetes team has a specific role.

Diabetes specialist nurses (DSN) work in both the hospital and community and educate the person with diabetes so that they are able to manage their condition as independently as possible. This education includes giving the person advice on:

- how to monitor their urine or blood glucose so that they can check if their diabetes is well controlled
- how to prepare and give insulin injections
- when to take their medication and how to identify and treat side-effects.

The DSNs aim to enable the person with diabetes understand what diabetes is and how they can make healthy choices in their everyday life to keep their diabetes well controlled. They can be contacted for advice if the person feels unwell or is concerned about some aspect of their care.

The **dietitian** encourages the person with diabetes to eat healthily and to organise their diet to avoid swings in their blood glucose level. The dietitian also gives advice on reducing the risks of diabetic complications by cutting down on foods that can contribute to this. (You will read more about diet and diabetes in Chapter 4.)

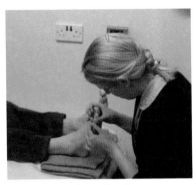

Figure 1.1 A podiatrist examining feet in a clinic.

The **diabetologist** is the senior doctor in the diabetes team, who usually works with a team of more junior doctors. Diabetologists are concerned with the detection and correction of risk factors leading to damage to blood vessels and nerves (this will be discussed in Chapter 5) and the early detection and treatment of complications (discussed in Chapter 6). They may also make referrals to other members of the team.

The **podiatrist** (Figure 1.1) identifies factors that can increase a person's risk of diabetic foot disease and gives advice on ways of preventing foot problems. The podiatrist treats foot problems at an early stage in order to prevent more serious damage and has expertise in the use of the most suitable dressings for foot ulcers.

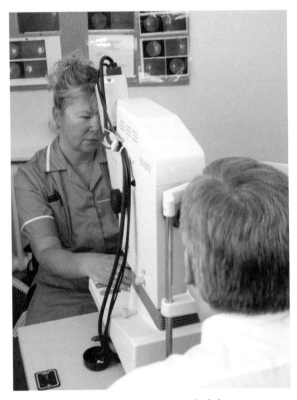

The **retinal screening technician** (Figure 1.2) takes photographs of the retina at the back of the eye. The pictures are then assessed or 'graded' by the technician or a doctor to see if there is evidence of damage. This screening is essential in the prevention of one of the most feared of all diabetic complications, blindness (discussed further in Chapter 6).

The **phlebotomist** (Figure 1.3) takes blood samples that are then sent to the hospital laboratory to be analysed. The tests required are usually decided by the doctor or DSN, and are discussed later in Chapter 5. People with diabetes have blood samples taken at least once a year, before their annual review; some people need them more frequently. An efficient phlebotomist who is able to obtain an adequate sample quickly and with minimum discomfort becomes a very important member of the diabetes team to the person with diabetes!

Figure 1.2 Retinal screening technician photographing the back of the eye with a digital camera.

The **diabetes clinic staff** ensure the journey through the clinic process is as efficient and comfortable as possible. The reception staff ensure the patient's personal details are correct and that their notes are available. Health care assistants or diabetes care technicians record results from routine tests such as blood pressure and weight, so that they are available for the diabetes team to use in assessing the patient and making decisions about treatments or referrals to other members of the team. **Asian link workers** are often available to assist clinic staff and patients, especially when communication is difficult or when there are specific diabetes education needs.

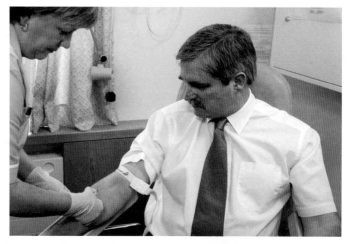

Figure 1.3 A phlebotomist taking a blood sample.

The **practice nurse** is a registered nurse who works in a GP surgery and may run diabetes (and other) clinics in the surgery.

The **general practitioner (GP)** is the doctor in the **primary care** team. Primary care includes health centres and GP surgeries. Sometimes the care of a person with diabetes is shared between the hospital and the GP in the primary care team. However, some GPs manage the care of the person with diabetes and only refer the person to the hospital team if there is a specific problem.

The **optometrist** assesses the health and function of the eyes.

The **orthotist** measures feet and designs suitable footwear, for example to relieve pressure on a foot ulcer.

The **pharmacist** dispenses drugs and, if requested, can give advice to individuals regarding these drugs.

The **psychologist** provides counselling and support for people with particular emotional and psychological needs.

The **diabetes care technician (DCT)** is an important new member of the team in some parts of the UK, who will become increasingly involved in carrying out some of the routine tests and screening procedures required by the person with diabetes. The DCT will have a significant role in liaising with other member of the team to ensure high-quality care for people with diabetes.

There are also many 'invisible' members of the team. For example, the blood and urine samples requested by the doctors are analysed in the hospital laboratory by clinical technicians, who also ensure the results are returned to the appropriate people. They alert the doctor quickly if a result requires urgent action.

As you have seen, not all diabetes teams are based in hospitals. There is a trend for much of the routine diabetes care to be managed by GPs and practice nurses in local health centres and surgeries. There is often a dietitian and podiatrist available to provide specialist advice. Some aspects of diabetes management may be too complex or specialised for the GP to deal with, but may not require hospital treatment. People with such complications may be referred to community diabetes teams, who visit or are based in a local health centre or community clinics.

1.4 Team work

With so many people involved in diabetes care you have probably realised the importance of the team working together effectively. The whole purpose of the existence of the team is the person with diabetes. All members contribute to enabling this person to live with their diabetes. The contribution of the different team members will vary throughout the person's life. For example, when first starting insulin treatment, the person with diabetes may find the most valuable person at that time is the DSN. If a few years later they are struggling with their weight, they may spend more time with the dietitian.

Teams are only effective if each member values the others and recognises the contribution each makes to the management of the care of the individual with diabetes. This includes the team in the community (primary care) and in the hospital (**secondary care**). Everyone is working to the same goal of maintaining the health and well-being of the person with diabetes. Working together requires clear communication between all involved, including the person with diabetes.

Work through Activity 1.4 to consider the aspects of communication between members of a team in more depth.

Activity 1.4 Communication within the team

Suggested study time 15 minutes

Gordon McCarthy has been given a form by his GP for a blood glucose test. He attends the hospital to have the blood sample taken. Make a list of all the people who might be involved before the final test result reaches Mr McCarthy. Also, make a note of what types of communication might be used.

Comment

You may have included the doctor explaining to Mr McCarthy about the need for the test and writing a blood sample request form; Mr McCarthy takes this to the phlebotomist who reads the instructions so that the correct sample is taken. The porter then takes the sample to the laboratory and the technician reads the form so the correct tests are carried out on the sample. The data are then processed on the laboratory computer and stored, the results being posted to the doctor via the hospital postal system or added to Mr McCarthy's electronic record. If the results are urgent or abnormal, the technician may telephone or bleep the doctor. Mr McCarthy may ring up for his results or be given them at his next appointment.

You can see that there are numerous communication processes involved in even a simple procedure such as a blood test. These include verbal, written, and electronic processes using a variety of vehicles such as referral and request forms, telephone, computer records and email. Often team members communicate informally with each other, for example to discuss a patient they have seen at a clinic. Alternatively this may be done formally, for example at a case conference where all the members involved in the care of an individual meet to discuss future plans with that individual. Good communication between the team members is crucial to the well-being of the person with diabetes. If messages are missed or misunderstood, problems can arise.

> 'Every time I change my prescription, the diabetic doctor gives me a pink slip with changes on to give to my GP. Last time the GP read it wrong and gave me 5 ml needles instead of 8 ml so I got insulin lumps. If those two had just spoken on the phone, it would have avoided all the pain and trouble I went through.'
>
> (Hiscock et al., 2001, p. 27)

1.5 Communication in teams

1.5.1   The importance of communication

We have already noted that the team works in partnership with the person with diabetes, who is central to the whole diabetes management process. Communication between the individual and the team is therefore crucial. If the advice given to the person with diabetes is misunderstood or ignored, then the best outcome for the person with diabetes will not be achieved. The person with diabetes may not be listened to and so the advice given may be inappropriate. In these cases it is likely that the person with diabetes and the professional will end up feeling frustrated.

As already discussed, communication can be achieved through a range of processes. However, when communicating face to face with a person there are many different elements to the communication process and the skills used. We all use these skills all the time and so are not even aware of them, but they can either hinder or enhance communication between two parties. The way you communicate with a person can have a big impact on them. Being ignored can make them feel angry or unimportant, but a friendly approach can make them feel valued and feel that you are interested in them.

1.5.2   Non-verbal communication

Non-verbal communication is a key aspect of communication and is often more important than what is said. Non-verbal communication relates to our body language and facial expressions. We show we are interested in a person by:

* looking at them and making eye contact
* smiling at them
* showing that we are listening to them by responding appropriately, for example, nodding or making noises of agreement
* copying their body language – a process known as mirroring
* leaning towards them
* touch may be used sometimes, for example, if someone is upset you might hold their hand.

There are many other aspects of non-verbal communication that you may be able to identify. However, it is important to remember that the meaning of non-verbal communication can vary between cultures. In some cultures it is a sign of respect to look at a person when talking to them, but in others, a person shows respect by not looking directly at the person. This shows how non-verbal communication can be misunderstood.

1.5.3   Listening and questioning

Listening is another important aspect of communication and it is as important to listen carefully to what the person is telling you (or leaving out) as it is to talk to them. You can obtain information by asking questions and sometimes you may need to check that you have understood what you have been told by asking further questions or repeating what the person has said. Carry out Activity 1.5 to think further about communication skills.

Activity 1.5 Communication in the clinic

Suggested study time 15 minutes

The way you ask questions is important and affects what a person does or does not tell you. Read through the following encounter and think how you would have felt if you were Mr Meek. What did you notice about the communication skills used here?

Jane Critical (the diabetes care technician): Hello, Mr Meek. How are you?

Mr Meek (a gentleman with diabetes, sounding rather upset): Well, I …

Jane Critical (briskly): I need to check your blood glucose today and take your blood pressure. Have you got your record with you?

Mr Meek: Well, no. I'm afraid …

Jane Critical: That really is a nuisance you know. How can we keep an eye on you and make sure everything is normal if you don't bring along your records to the clinic? Well, never mind, I'll do a blood test for you here before you see the nurse. But first I'll just take your blood pressure. Have you had this done before? I expect you know all about this, don't you? So if that is OK with you just take off your coat and roll up your sleeve.

Comment

You probably thought that Mr Meek did not get a lot of time to say anything. Jane did ask him some questions but she did not give him time to answer. She also answered her own question and assumed that he did know all about his blood pressure measurement. Jane sounded very critical of Mr Meek, and asking a lot of questions very rapidly, as Jane did, can make people feel that they are being interrogated. So Mr Meek may well have felt intimidated, that he was a nuisance for not bringing in his record and that he was just a patient to be dealt with rather than an individual with specific needs. This may have made him feel angry, or he may even have decided not to come back again.

As we look at the encounter described in Activity 1.5, we can see different types of question being used. The first question Jane asked was an **open question** (How are you?). This encourages the person to answer fully. For example, Mr Meek might have wanted to tell Jane that he had lost his job, the cat had died last week, he had a bad cold, and had overslept and had to rush out to the clinic, consequently forgetting his record. However, Jane gave him no time to answer. Open questions often begin with 'How' or start with phrases like 'Can you tell me more about …'. **Closed questions** only give the opportunity to answer yes or no. They are useful if you want to obtain very specific information but they do not encourage the person to talk. **Leading questions** suggest the answer to the person and may mean they tell you what they think you want to hear rather than the truth.

In the encounter in Activity 1.5 Jane had her own plan of what she needed to do and say. Consequently she did not give Mr Meek time to speak, or listen when he tried to say something. It is also very easy to appear to listen to someone and then realise that you have no idea what they just said. So when listening you need to concentrate and if you are not certain what the person meant, ask them to explain further. This process is known as **active listening**.

Communication is a two-way process. As well as thinking about your own communication skills you need to think about what the other person is saying, both through their words and their body language. Returning to our interview with Jane Critical and Mr Meek, Jane might have noticed that Mr Meek was frowning or biting his lip. These are examples of non-verbal communication and might indicate that the person is worried or apprehensive. The tone of voice can also indicate how we are feeling. You may have noted that in the scenario given above it was stated that Mr Meek 'sounded' upset. Picking up these clues and following them up would have enabled Jane to find out precisely what Mr Meek was feeling and then she could have given the appropriate advice or support.

1.5.4 Negotiation

In the encounter between Jane and Mr Meek we have already noted that Jane needed to measure his blood glucose and blood pressure. She may also have had time constraints such as another person being booked in to see her in a few minutes time. She, therefore, had her own agenda for the consultation. Mr Meek may have had other concerns such as a problem with his foot which he wanted to discuss. He may, therefore, have come to this consultation with a completely different agenda. According to Middleton (2000) communication skills are the key to arriving at a mutually agreed and accepted plan when two people have different agendas (illustrated in Figure 1.4 overleaf). Jane clearly stated her requirements for the consultation but she did not allow time for Mr Meek to do this. In this situation Mr Meek would have had to be assertive and state that he had some questions to ask or a particular problem he wished to discuss.

Good communication is likely to mean that both Jane and Mr Meek will feel that they have achieved what was needed, and they are therefore both likely to go away from the consultation feeling positive. If there is no effective communication between Jane and Mr Meek, at least one of them will leave feeling dissatisfied.

Figure 1.4 Good communication – the key to a mutual understanding of treatment.

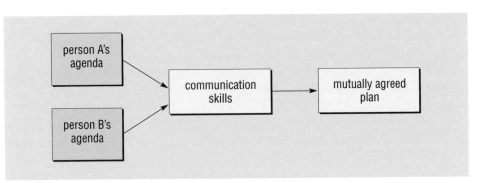

1.5.5 Communication barriers

Communication can be hindered by the emotional state of the people involved. A person with poorly controlled diabetes may appear aggressive or find it difficult to concentrate. Many people find that just visiting the GP's surgery or hospital can make them very anxious. Anyone may, of course, just be having a bad day! Emotions such as anger or anxiety may adversely affect communication. If the person to whom you are talking appears disinterested or responds abruptly, it is important to stay calm and focused on what you want to achieve. Becoming angry in response tends to be counter-productive and the problem often escalates.

Communication can be very difficult if the two people involved do not speak the same language. An interpreter may be available in the clinic, or the person with diabetes may bring a relative or friend along who is able to interpret. This can be very helpful, provided that the interpreter has translated correctly. Privacy and confidentiality issues may also arise when an interpreter is used. Many people find it hard to admit they have a problem with, for example, impotence or incontinence, either of which may occur with diabetes. It may be even harder to explain to someone else who then tells the doctor on your behalf. If it were a family member or friend who was acting as interpreter they would become party to some very personal information. Equally if there was an official interpreter the person might feel reluctant to tell them anything personal, especially if they were of the opposite sex. Sometimes people (usually women) are employed as Asian link workers and part of their job is to be an interpreter which overcomes some of the difficulties described, in some sections of the UK Asian population at least.

There are many other potential barriers to communication, some examples of which are given below.

Social and linguistic barriers:

- cultural differences in interpretation of non-verbal messages – what is polite behaviour in one culture may be very rude in another culture
- dialects and accents
- inability to read information
- use of jargon by the professionals.

Psychological barriers:

- shyness
- anxiety
- denial – the person may not want to hear what they are being told.

Physical problems:

- deafness
- visual problems
- speech impediments, for example a stammer.

Environmental factors:

- lack of privacy
- noisy environment
- lack of time.

Visual problems, in particular, can cause difficulties with communication since we do not just receive information by listening with our ears; non-verbal or body language communication is important in receiving messages from others, as we discussed above. It is therefore much easier when we can see the person to whom we are talking.

The potential barriers given above, and many other difficulties, create challenges in communication but it is important to find ways of overcoming these problems. Some of them are easy to overcome but others are more complex – as you consider in Activity 1.6.

Activity 1.6 Overcoming communication barriers

Suggested study time 20 minutes

Read through the list of communication barriers again and identify which ones may be relevant to you if you were to attend a consultation with a doctor. Make some notes on the ways you think they could be overcome.

Comment

There are many ideas you could have thought about but some suggestions are given here.

- If you feel you never have time to discuss your concerns you might want to bring a list of questions to the consultation or to use the available time well by asking important questions first.

- If you get very anxious and find it difficult to remember what you are told, you could have a friend with you or you could write down key points.

- If you have hearing difficulties you could ask for written information and make sure that you can see the face and lips of the person speaking to you.

- If you do not understand something that is said to you, you should ask if it can be repeated or rephrased.

- Most language barriers can be overcome by using interpreters and having leaflets with key information in the relevant language.

1.6 Informed consent

Before any procedure is carried out, the person with diabetes should give their consent. Sometimes consent is obtained formally by the patient signing a consent form. In some clinics this formal consent is required before the insertion of eye drops to dilate the pupils of the eyes prior to an eye screening examination (discussed in Chapter 6), since there is a small risk attached to this procedure. In most situations in the diabetes clinic, consent is obtained informally by verbally asking the patient's permission. Sometimes this agreement may be unspoken. For example, if the patient were to roll up their sleeve and hold out their arm when told that the health worker wanted to check their blood pressure, this would be deemed to be consent, as their actions imply agreement to the procedure. However, people do have the right to refuse any treatment or procedure and this must be respected. Sometimes people may refuse because they are frightened or unclear about what is going to happen to them. In these cases further explanation may be all that is required and they then may agree to the treatment. If the person continues to refuse, then this must be accepted, as nothing should be done to a person against their wishes (Department of Health, 2001b). The person in charge of the clinic would need to know about this situation so that they could offer suitable support and guidance.

Consent should also be informed. It is not enough that a person agrees; they should understand what is going to happen and whether there are any risks attached.

Some people may want a detailed explanation before they agree to anything, while other people are quite happy to agree following a very simple explanation. Every person has the right to as much information as they want before agreeing to a procedure. However, if a procedure or treatment does pose a specific risk then the person needs to be aware of this before they give consent. In practice, to protect both the patient and staff, formal written consent is usually obtained for procedures that have a higher risk attached, such as surgery. The procedure therefore needs to be explained by someone who has a full understanding of what is involved and who can answer specific questions from the patient. Written consent must be kept with the records for each patient. Accurate record keeping, in all aspects of patient care, is an important issue to which we now turn.

1.7 Record keeping

1.7.1 Importance of record keeping

The Department of Health (1999) states that:

> 'Records are a valuable resource because of the information they contain. That information is only usable if it is correctly recorded in the first place, is regularly up-dated, and is easily accessible when it is needed. Information is essential to the delivery of high quality evidence-based health care on a day-to-day basis ...'

> (Department of Health, 1999, paragraph 1.2)

We discussed earlier that the effectiveness of a team relies on good communication between members of that team. Effective record keeping is an essential part of this process. Written records must be accurate, concise, clear and legible so everyone can read the information the records are conveying. If the information is misinterpreted it can have serious consequences for the person with diabetes. For example, you may recall from Section 1.4 that someone was given the wrong sized needles as a result of the prescriber misreading the record. The person with diabetes may miss an appointment because they could not read the date properly or medication may be altered unnecessarily because a blood glucose result was recorded incorrectly. It is also very important that any abnormal results are brought to the attention of a senior member of the team. Diabetes clinics are busy places, and abnormal results may be overlooked if they are just recorded in the patient's notes. This can lead to early warning signs being missed.

Patient records, in whatever form, are legal documents. They are a record of care given (or omitted) and may be used as evidence if litigation or a complaint is brought by the person or their family. Usually by the time this happens, time has passed, some of the people involved may have moved on, and it is impossible to remember exactly what was done or told to the person concerned. Having a clear and accurate record of the care given is crucial. Everybody in the diabetes team therefore has a responsibility to ensure they maintain clear and accurate records for the safety of both the patient and the other members of the team.

1.7.2   Types of record

Information about patients may be kept in the form of written or computer records held by the multidisciplinary team. In the future it is likely that more records will be stored electronically, as this is part of government strategy for the NHS (NHS Executive, 1998). In some centres, patients may hold their own records (or part of their own records) and bring them along to the clinic each time they have an appointment. Patient-held records have the advantage that they are with the person, and nothing is hidden from the person concerned. When these patient-held records are used by all the health professionals involved in the care of the person, it should avoid conflicting advice and duplication of investigations (Diabetes UK, 2004b). It is important that the patient keeps their records safe, prevents them from being defaced or damaged and brings them to the clinic each time, otherwise the same problems of miscommunication may arise.

1.8 Confidentiality

One of the key issues with any form of record is that of **confidentiality**. Anyone working in the NHS has a duty of confidentiality to patients.

'In general, any personal information given or received in confidence for one purpose may not be used for a different purpose or passed to anyone else without the consent of the provider of the information.'

(Department of Health, 1999, paragraph 4.2)

Patients give health care personnel considerable amounts of information about themselves. So consideration needs to be given as to how information in records (written or electronic) is kept secure so that no unauthorised person has access to it. There are legal constraints in relation to this, and the Data Protection Act 1998 established a set of principles with which users of computerised personal information must comply. Each individual in the health service takes responsibility for ensuring that they treat patient information as confidential at all times. Provision should be made for patients to see their own records. The Freedom of Information Act 2000, that was activated within the NHS in October 2003, seeks to balance the right to confidentiality with the right to information.

Confidentiality needs to be maintained both for personal information in records and for information about a patient received verbally. It is a complex issue, however, and Activity 1.7 will help you to think about the extent of confidentiality; when can information be shared and with whom?

Activity 1.7 Confidentiality issues

Suggested study time 30 minutes

Think about the following questions and write some brief notes on how you think confidentiality applies.

(a) Who should be told if a person with diabetes has developed a foot ulcer?

(b) Should all members of the diabetes care team know if a person with diabetes is experiencing a very difficult family situation?

(c) A person with diabetes discloses that they are still driving when they have been advised not to drive. Should the diabetes team member report this?

Comment

(a) Confidentiality does not mean that relevant information cannot be shared within the team that is caring for the person. Unless information about the foot ulcer is passed to the other team members, appropriate care will not be given. However, the way this information is shared needs to be considered. An explanation could be given to the person about the need to share this information and permission sought to do this. If consent is given, confidentiality is not broken. However, it is important that this information is only given to those in the diabetes team. Family and friends of the patient should not be told, unless the patient has requested this, so where and how the information is passed on to other team members needs to be considered. Only the team members should be able to read the notes or hear the information. Notes should not be left lying around and discussions about patients should take place in private, not in the waiting room. In *Essence of Care*, a government publication, the importance of privacy has been emphasised and staff have been tasked with the responsibility of ensuring that they look at ways of maintaining privacy and confidentiality for clients (Department of Health, 2001c, 2003).

(b) If people are going through very difficult circumstances, it may affect their ability to manage their diabetes and so it is important that the team is made aware of this. Unless the person wants the team to know all the details, it would be sufficient for them to know that the patient is under significant additional stress due to family circumstances.

(c) There are some situations in which a person with diabetes may not be able to drive as they may be a risk to themselves or other people. (This is usually when they have hypoglycaemic unawareness – further details will be given in Chapter 7.) In these circumstances a person is advised to inform the Driver and Vehicle Licensing Agency (DVLA) who decides if they are allowed to drive or not. If the person fails to inform the DVLA and continues to drive, the doctor must inform the DVLA of the situation. In this case the need to maintain confidentiality is overridden by the need to ensure the safety of the person and the public.

1.9 Safety

1.9.1   Safe treatment

Safety is an important issue for everyone in health care. Any mistakes made may be very serious for the patient. If a test is carried out incorrectly the results will not be correct, but judgements will be made on the basis of this information and treatment may be changed. So a person may be given too much or too little of a drug, or early signs of complications may be missed resulting in the person developing problems that could have been prevented. You may have seen or heard in the media of incidents where mistakes have been made (for example, Figure 1.5).

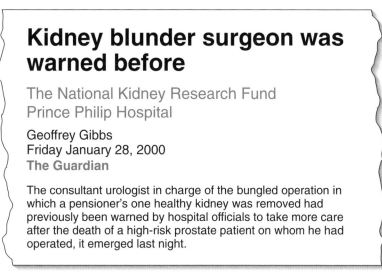

Kidney blunder surgeon was warned before

The National Kidney Research Fund
Prince Philip Hospital

Geoffrey Gibbs
Friday January 28, 2000
The Guardian

The consultant urologist in charge of the bungled operation in which a pensioner's one healthy kidney was removed had previously been warned by hospital officials to take more care after the death of a high-risk prostate patient on whom he had operated, it emerged last night.

Figure 1.5 As the headlines sometimes show, medical mishaps can occur.

These are extreme and fortunately rare events but hearing about them is very worrying for patients. Staff too are concerned to do the best they can for patients. In order to reduce risks various requirements have been set down for health care staff by the Department of Health.

- Mistakes and near-miss events must be recorded and reported to the National Patient Safety Agency. This agency analyses these events so that where systems lead to errors they can be identified and changes made.

- Where equipment and devices fail to work properly, this must be reported so the problems can be identified and corrected.

- Staff should not carry out procedures unless they have been trained and recognised as competent.

- Diabetes care is changing rapidly and new developments bring the need for training in the use of new equipment and procedures.

- Ongoing development and training is required, even if the person is competent in the procedures currently carried out in their place of work.

The advent of new knowledge and treatments means that the advice and information given to the person with diabetes changes over time. This does not mean that the original advice was necessarily wrong; it may have been correct at the time it was given, but new research has shown that different advice is now needed. An example of this is the change in dietary advice for people with diabetes. Recently the need for a healthy diet with reduced sugar has been emphasised. Currently the glycaemic index of different foods has been recognised as important and the DAFNE (Dose Adjustment for Normal Eating) methods for self-management are being used in some centres to help people manage their diabetes and diet. More information about diet is given in Chapter 4. In some situations the person may have read about, or found on the internet, information about a new treatment or advice which is different from that which they are receiving. Sometimes this new development is still only at the experimental stage and until it has been fully tested and proven safe, it will not be available for widespread use. At other times there may be two equally valid types of treatment or there may be particular reasons why a certain treatment is not suitable for that individual. Since the person with diabetes is the key member of the team they should be free to question the treatment they are receiving.

1.9.2 Risk assessment

Safety is not, however, only maintained by ensuring staff are trained and have up-to-date knowledge and skills. The environment in which health care is given, such as the clinic, should be free from hazards. One of the ways of ensuring a safe environment is through a process of **risk assessment**. In this process the working environment and practices are reviewed regularly to identify any areas of risk to clients or staff and necessary changes are made to minimise the risks. The Health and Safety at Work Act 1974 also makes it clear that it is the responsibility of both the employer and the employee (in this case individual members of the diabetes team) to maintain safety. This means that if a fire door was blocked, a floor was wet and slippery, or equipment was stored in such a way as to represent a hazard, the diabetes team member would be expected to take appropriate action to remove or minimise the risk.

1.9.3   Risk of infection

One area of risk that is much less obvious but which can be a major problem to both patients and staff is that of infection. Clinics tend to be held in confined spaces, and are usually crowded with people. Transfer of infection from one individual to another can easily occur in this environment and this is known as **cross infection**. In these circumstances there are three main ways in which infection can spread.

1 **Airborne spread**: This is a particular problem if a person has a cold or chest infection. They may cough and sneeze (Figure 1.6) and the bacteria or viruses from one person are spread in the atmosphere through droplets. Another person can inhale these and may develop the same illness. This does not mean that the person with diabetes who has a cold or minor infection should not attend the clinic. The infection may make their diabetes control unstable and they may, therefore, need to see the doctor or nurse urgently to review their treatment. Good hygiene can minimise the risk of spreading infection; for example, tissues should be disposed of in appropriate bins and hands washed.

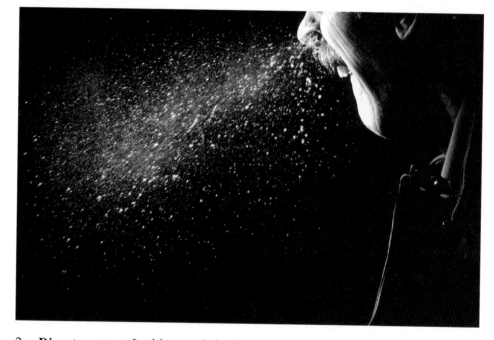

Figure 1.6 When we cough or sneeze, millions of bacteria are released into the air surrounding us.

2 **Direct contact**: In this case infection spreads directly from one person to another, often via hand contact. Failure of the diabetes team member to wash their hands before caring for a patient could result in the spread of infection. This could occur, even if the diabetes workers did not have an infection themselves, since every one of us carries bacteria on our hands. These bacteria, known as **normal flora**, are usually harmless but if they get into a wound of someone who has reduced immunity they can cause infection. The way to prevent this transfer is through good hand hygiene. The diabetes team member should wash their hands thoroughly with soap and water or use an alcohol rub (Figure 1.7), depending on the local policy, before seeing patients. Although hand washing cannot remove all bacteria it will remove the majority of them.

Figure 1.7 An alcohol rub can be used to help prevent the spread of infection.

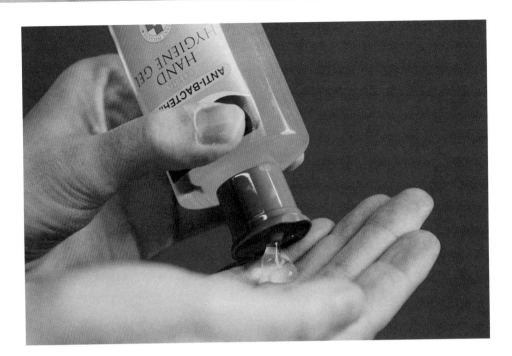

Infection could spread not only from the diabetes worker to the person with diabetes but also from the person with diabetes to the worker. This is a particular risk if there is contact with body fluids such as blood or urine, since certain diseases are transmitted in the body fluids. In order to prevent this, the diabetes care worker should wear disposable plastic gloves and ensure that any small cuts or infections on their hands are covered up with a waterproof plaster when dressing wounds or handling body fluids such as blood or urine.

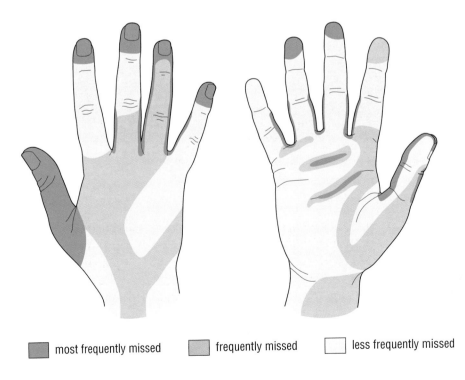

Figure 1.8 Care must be taken during hand washing to make sure that areas are not missed.

most frequently missed   frequently missed   less frequently missed

3   **Indirect contact**: Infection can be passed from one party to another via a third party or via equipment. If the diabetes worker is with a person who has an infection, and then goes to another person without washing their hands, bacteria could then be taken on the worker's hands to the next person (Figure 1.8). This is another reason why appropriate hand hygiene by diabetes staff is so important. Good hand hygiene usually removes all the transient bacteria which have just been picked up and so stops the spread of infection.

Infection can be spread by other means, and people can also infect themselves (Figure 1.9). Many people who have diabetes have to inject themselves with insulin or test a sample of their own blood. Failure to wash their hands before carrying out a finger prick test or re-using equipment which is only meant to be used once could result in an infection. The risk of this is quite low since the bacteria that the patient is exposed to are their own, and do not usually cause them any problems. The risk of infection is much greater when the person is exposed to bacteria to which they have not developed immunity, as may happen in the clinic.

Figure 1.9 Chain of infection.

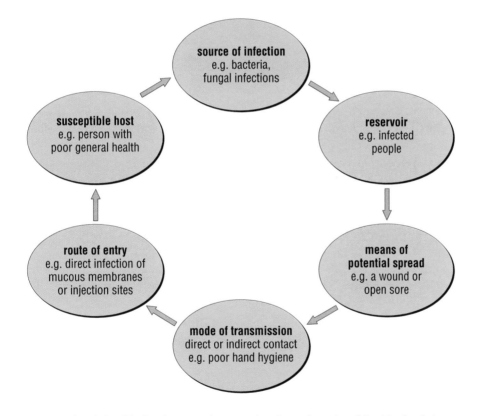

To reduce the risk of infection, equipment that breaches the skin (the body's normal defence against infection), for example when dressing a wound or taking a blood sample, should be sterile. Equipment supplied by the manufacturers is sterilised and sealed in a package or container, and providing the packaging remains undamaged and has not passed the expiry date, the equipment will remain sterile. Some sterile equipment, such as plasters, can be bought at a chemist or supermarket. Other sterile equipment, such as injection needles and certain wound dressings, are only available on prescription, or in the clinic or hospital. Whatever type of sterile equipment it is, even if only a plaster, the packaging should be checked to ensure it is intact and that the expiry date has not been reached. If the packaging has been damaged the contents are no longer sterile and should not be used. After opening the pack nothing that will come into contact with the wound or enter the person should be touched. For example, a plaster should be held by the sterile strips (Figure 1.10), and the point of a needle should not be touched. Once opened, the sterile equipment should be used straight away, otherwise the equipment may become contaminated. This technique, which ensures that only sterile equipment touches a wound, is known as an **aseptic technique**.

Figure 1.10 A plaster should be held by the sterile strips to avoid it becoming contaminated.

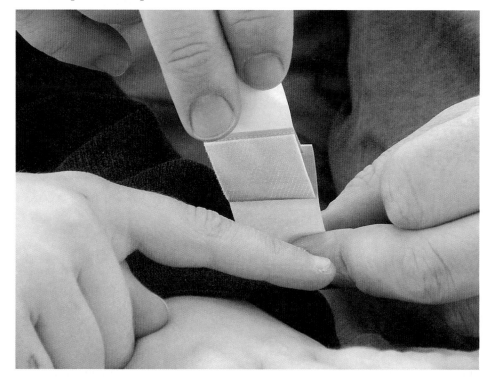

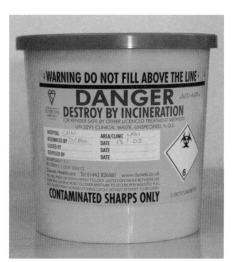

Figure 1.11 A sharps disposal box.

Care should be taken when handling equipment such as needles or lancets. Once opened they should not be re-sheathed. There are many aids available which have been designed to break off used needles from syringes to minimise the risk of **needle stick injuries**. These occur when a person is stabbed accidentally by a used needle or lancet. Infections such as hepatitis B and HIV can be carried in the blood, and can be transferred to other people indirectly via a needle stick injury. **Sharps disposal boxes** (such as in Figure 1.11) should be available for the collection and storage of used needles, lancets, broken glass, etc. to prevent anyone accidentally injuring themselves on a contaminated device. People with diabetes who use lancets or needles at home are given advice on how to dispose of them safely. Some areas provide a sharps box for use at home which is collected by the local authority. In other places the person with diabetes is asked to store the used sharps in a container such as a glass jar or empty bleach bottle with a secure lid, and then to take this to the GP surgery for disposal when full. This reduces the risk of needle stick injury and possible infection to family members and refuse collectors.

The risk of indirect infection from material that has been contaminated by blood or bacteria can be minimised by ensuring that this material is disposed of safely. In the clinic, this type of waste material is put in a colour-coded bag so that it can be identified and incinerated.

1.9.4   Safety and drugs

All drugs, including eye drops, need to be stored correctly and safely. This is not only to ensure that the drug retains its potency, it is also to ensure that no one else is put at risk. For example, if eye drops were left lying around in the clinic a child might pick them up and swallow them. At home, tablets can be picked up and eaten by young children who may think they are sweets. The storage of medicines, in clinics or hospitals, is governed by legislation. Other agents, such as chemical cleaners and disinfectants, could also be dangerous and legislation again gives clear guidance on the need to store safely any substance which could be a hazard to health (COSHH, 1994). Legislation does not cover storage at home and the person with diabetes can keep their drugs and equipment where they choose. However, common sense dictates that this should be out of the reach of children and that storage should be according to the manufacturer's guidelines, for example unopened insulin vials should be stored in a fridge, preferably one that can be locked.

1.10   Summary of Chapter 1

You have now come to the end of the first chapter on diabetes care. In this chapter you have seen that diabetes is a very common long-term medical condition, which has to be managed effectively by the person with diabetes, on a daily basis. The multidisciplinary diabetes team's role, whether in primary care (GP practice) or secondary care (hospital), is to inform, support and advise that person. This can only be achieved effectively by good communication between team members and the person with diabetes, in a safe environment. 'Safe' includes all aspects of the home and working environment, including physical protection from injury and infection, privacy and confidentiality when sharing information, and the participation in agreed, tested procedures performed by trained and sufficiently qualified staff, as well as the adoption of suitable aseptic techniques and disposal of sharps and contaminated materials to avoid cross-infection. Many of the issues highlighted in this chapter are addressed in those following, the first of which is a more detailed look at the physical nature of diabetes.

Questions for Chapter 1

Question 1.1 (Learning Outcome 1.2)

Mr Patel is a 55-year-old gentleman who is married with three children. He works as a taxi driver. He has been feeling very tired and lethargic recently and has just been told that he has Type 2 diabetes. One of his cousins has diabetes and some time ago had his leg amputated as a result of this. How do you think that Mr Patel may react to being told he has diabetes?

Question 1.2 (Learning Outcomes 1.1, 1.3 and 1.4)

Mr Patel was seen by his GP who advised him and his wife to see the practice nurse for advice. At the first appointment the practice nurse referred the Patels to the diabetes clinic to attend a group session for information, advice and support. At this session the diabetes specialist nurse, dietitian and podiatrist were all present. During the session it was also mentioned to Mr and Mrs Patel that, once a year, he would be sent an appointment for the eye clinic to see the retinal screening technician.

What is the function of the different diabetes team members named here?

Question 1.3 (Learning Outcome 1.4)

List three ways in which good team work can be achieved in diabetes care.

Question 1.4 (Learning Outcome 1.5)

What are the benefits of good communication in diabetes care?

Question 1.5 (Learning Outcome 1.6)

Describe three different ways by which the practice nurse or Mr Patel might obtain further information about his diabetes and his particular situation.

Question 1.6 (Learning Outcomes 1.1 and 1.6)

Look back at the interview between Jane Critical and Mr Meek (Activity 1.5). Identify the open, closed and leading questions here.

Question 1.7 (Learning Outcomes 1.1 and 1.7)

What does confidentiality mean in patient care? Give an example.

Question 1.8 (Learning Outcomes 1.4 and 1.8)

State three ways in which staff in diabetes care can ensure that they provide care for patients that is safe and effective.

Question 1.9 (Learning Outcome 1.8)

Why is it important to prevent needle stick injuries? Name two ways in which this can be done.

References

Audit Commission (2000) *Testing Times: A Review of Diabetes Services in England and Wales*, London, Audit Commission (12 April 2000) [online] Available from: www.audit-commission.gov.uk/reports (Accessed April 2005).

Bottomley, J., Lawlar, D. and Baxter, H. (1999) *CODE-2 UK: The Current Costs of Type 2 Diabetes in the UK*, ISPOR (International Society for Pharmacoeconomics and Outcomes Research, Edinburgh), November 1999 (poster).

COSHH (1994) Control of Substances Hazardous to Health, London, Her Majesty's Stationary Office.

Data Protection Act (1998) London, Her Majesty's Stationary Office.

Department of Health (1999) *For the Record – managing records in NHS trusts and health authorities*, London, Department of Health [online] Available from: http://www.dh.gov.uk/PolicyAndGuidance/OrganisationPolicy/RecordsManagement/fs/en (Accessed April 2005).

Department of Health (2001a) *National Service Frameworks for Diabetes, Standards*, London, Department of Health [online] Available from: http://www.dh.gov.uk/assetRoot/04/05/89/38/04058938.pdf (Accessed April 2005).

Department of Health (2001b) *Reference Guide to Consent for Examination or Treatment*, London, Department of Health [online] Available from: http://www.dh.gov.uk/PublicationsAndStatistics/Publications/PublicationsPolicyAndGuidance/PublicationsPolicyAndGuidanceArticle/fs/en?CONTENT_ID=4006757&chk=snmdw8 (Accessed April 2005).

Department of Health (2001c, 2003) *The Essence of Care – patient-focused benchmarking for health care practitioners*, London, Department of Health [online] Available from: http://www.dh.gov.uk/PublicationsAndStatistics/Publications/PublicationsPolicyAndGuidance/PublicationsPolicyAndGuidanceArticle/fs/en?CONTENT_ID=4005475&chk=A0A4iz (Accessed April 2005).

Diabetes UK (2004a) *Understanding diabetes* [online] Available from: http://www.diabetes.org.uk/diabetes/under.htm (Accessed April 2005).

Diabetes UK (2004b) *Good practice in diabetes care. Patient-held records and care planning* [online] Available from: www.diabetes.org.uk/good_practice/patient/index.html (Accessed April 2005).

Freedom of Information Act (2000) London, Her Majesty's Stationary Office.

Health and Safety at Work Act (1974) London, Her Majesty's Stationary Office.

Hiscock, J., Legard, R. and Snape, D. (2001) *Listening to Diabetes Service Users: Qualitative findings for the National Service Framework*, London, Department of Health [online] Available from: http://www.dh.gov.uk/PublicationsAndStatistics/Publications/PublicationsPolicyAndGuidance/PublicationsPolicyAndGuidanceArticle/fs/en?CONTENT_ID=4008645&chk=RIZ5wk (Accessed April 2005).

Middleton, J. (2000) *The Team Guide to Communication*, Abingdon, Radcliffe Medical Press.

NHS Executive (1998) *Information for Health: an information strategy for the modern NHS*, NHS Executive [online] Available from: http://www.dh.gov.uk/ PublicationsAndStatistics/LettersAndCirculars/HealthServiceCirculars/ HealthServiceCircularsArticle/fs/en?CONTENT_ID=4005016&chk=ZW8zFD (Accessed April 2005).

WHO (2002) *The Cost of Diabetes*. Fact sheet, no. 236, Geneva, World Health Organization.

CHAPTER 2

WHAT IS DIABETES?

Learning Outcomes

When you have completed this chapter you should be able to:

2.1 Define and use, or recognise definitions and applications of, each of the terms printed in **bold** in the text.

2.2 Explain how diabetes is diagnosed.

2.3 Describe the different types of diabetes and their possible causes.

2.4 Describe some of the structures and chemical changes involved in glucose regulation within the body.

2.5 Discuss the factors that make people prone to developing diabetes, including genetic aspects.

2.1 Introduction

So far you have been thinking about diabetes and its impact on the individual and their family. You have also been considering confidentiality and communication between the person with diabetes and the health care professionals involved in their care. This chapter moves on to introduce the parts of the body and processes involved in the development of diabetes. Type 1 and Type 2 diabetes are similar but distinct conditions and, for doctors, it is not always easy to decide which type of diabetes someone has. Does this matter, and is one type of diabetes worse than the other? There are many misconceptions about diabetes among health care professionals and the population in general. We hope this chapter will help you to explore and clarify your ideas about diabetes, starting with Activity 2.1.

Activity 2.1 Defining diabetes

Suggested study time 20 minutes

Read Case Study 2.1 and then think about the following questions. If you were Princess Rodgers' GP how would you explain diabetes to her? Make notes about how you would define diabetes. Do you know of different types of diabetes? Is one form more serious than another? If so, why?

Keep your notes safely so you can use them to compare what you think now with your understanding later in this chapter.

Comment

Princess Rodgers will be experiencing many emotions while being told about her diabetes, so it is important that the GP explains clearly to make sure she takes it in. He might need to go over his explanation more than once. It is important to spend time thinking about how you would define diabetes if you were asked to explain it to somebody, as this will help you to identify areas that you are uncertain about. It will also help you to understand that others will also have uncertainties about what diabetes is. There are many people like Mrs Rodgers who have misconceptions about the condition.

Case Study 2.1

Mrs Princess Rodgers was born in Jamaica but has lived in England for the last 50 years. She is now 55 years old and visited her GP last week seeking treatment for thrush. She returns a week later because it is no better. At her original visit the GP took the opportunity to take a number of blood tests, including a test for her blood glucose. On her return visit Mrs Rodgers is told that one of the tests has indicated that she has diabetes.

Mrs Rodgers suddenly feels very guilty about the four teaspoons of sugar she puts in her tea and is sure that that is why her diabetes has occurred. She is no longer listening to the GP but thinking about stopping the sugar, as she is sure this will cure her diabetes. She decides that she must have the mild kind like her granny who lived to be 84 years old.

2.2 What is diabetes?

Diabetes mellitus is a condition in which the glucose level in the blood is higher than it should be. The word 'diabetes' comes from the Greek word for 'siphon'. A siphon is a way of removing liquid, and diabetes is used to describe disorders that remove liquid from the body, resulting in excessive thirst and the production of large amounts of urine. There are two forms of diabetes, diabetes mellitus and diabetes insipidus, of which diabetes mellitus is the more common. The word 'mellitus' comes from the Latin word for 'honeyed'. Diabetes mellitus, therefore, describes a condition that produces 'sweet urine'. This production of sweet urine occurs as a result of a high blood **glucose** level. Glucose is a type of simple sugar that is a building block of more complex sugars called **carbohydrates**. Diabetes mellitus has been known for thousands of years, having been described by the Ancient Egyptians and the Romans. Over the years more and more has been discovered about diabetes mellitus, and the way it is diagnosed has been refined.

Diabetes insipidus is a different condition that will not be discussed in any detail. It is a very rare condition caused by the lack of a hormone needed to concentrate urine. This hormone is produced in the brain. Diabetes insipidus shares the name diabetes as it also results in the production of large quantities of urine, but has nothing to do with how the body manages glucose.

This course is aimed at developing an understanding of diabetes mellitus. Throughout the course the term diabetes will be used to describe diabetes mellitus, unless otherwise indicated.

2.3 Parts of the body and hormones involved in diabetes

Glucose is used as a fuel within the body. In people without diabetes, the blood glucose levels are kept within very narrow limits. The body does not allow them to become too high or too low. Several parts of the body are involved in this process. Some are large, for example the liver, and some are very small, such as the **cells** within the pancreas. Cells are small building blocks of the body and cannot be seen with the naked eye. In the human body there are many different types of cell doing many different tasks.

Hormones are signalling substances produced by cells that start or stop body processes. There are many different hormones acting all over the body. Insulin is an example of a hormone that is produced by the pancreas. Other examples that you may have heard of include thyroid hormone, testosterone and oestrogen. Hormones that are released into the blood and are taken around the body to where they work are called endocrine hormones and are produced by **endocrine glands**. Thyroid hormone, testosterone and oestrogen are examples of endocrine hormones and the thyroid gland, testes and ovaries are the endocrine glands that produce them. You may have heard the term endocrinologist used to describe the doctor looking after patients with hormone disorders.

2.3.1 Pancreas

The **pancreas** is a structure (an organ) that lies towards the back of the abdomen, the part of the body between the chest and the pelvis (hips). The abdomen contains the stomach, liver, spleen, pancreas, intestines and other structures. The pancreas is near the liver and the spleen (Figure 2.1).

The pancreas produces many substances, including the endocrine hormones insulin and glucagon. The cells that produce these hormones are situated in the pancreas within the islets of Langerhans (Figure 2.2). The islets comprise, amongst others, alpha and beta cells. The beta (β) cells produce insulin. The alpha (α) cells produce glucagon.

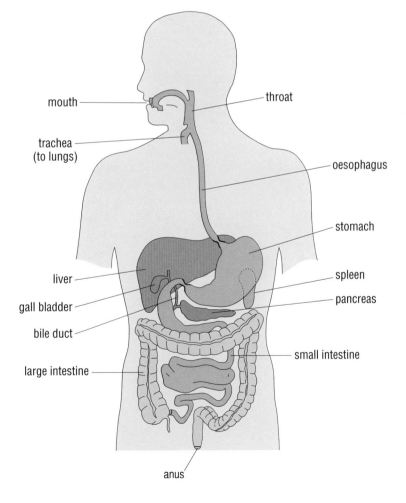

Figure 2.1 Diagram showing the location of the liver, stomach and pancreas within the abdomen. You do not need to remember the names of all the other structures shown: they are included for completeness.

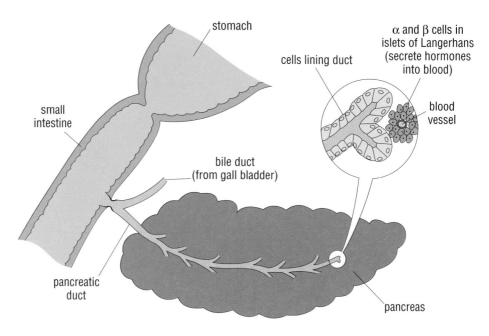

Figure 2.2 Diagram showing the α and β cells in the islets of Langerhans in the pancreas (not to scale).

If the pancreas is severely damaged or removed for some reason then no insulin is produced in the body and diabetes results.

2.3.2 Gut

The gut, or digestive tract, is where the food we eat is broken down (digested) and absorbed into the blood. The key food groups are fats, carbohydrates and proteins; vitamins and minerals are also required for a healthy diet and of course we need water too.

Examples of foods that are mainly protein are meat, fish, pulses and soya products. Fats, including butter and oil, are found in a range of foods, such as cheese and cream. Carbohydrates are found in bread, potatoes, rice and pasta, as well as within sugary foods and drinks. Vitamins and minerals are found in many foods, especially fruit and vegetables.

Within the gut, chemicals known as enzymes break down food into smaller components. Fats are broken down into fatty acids, carbohydrates into glucose, and proteins into amino acids. These smaller components can then be absorbed through the wall of the small intestine and transported in the blood to various parts of the body to provide energy or to be used as building blocks for growth (Figure 2.3). The level of glucose in the blood is altered by what and how much we eat.

● Which do you think will result in more glucose in the gut: a carbohydrate-rich meal, or a protein-rich meal?

○ If you eat a meal that is mainly carbohydrate you will produce more glucose in the gut to be absorbed than if you eat a meal that is mainly protein.

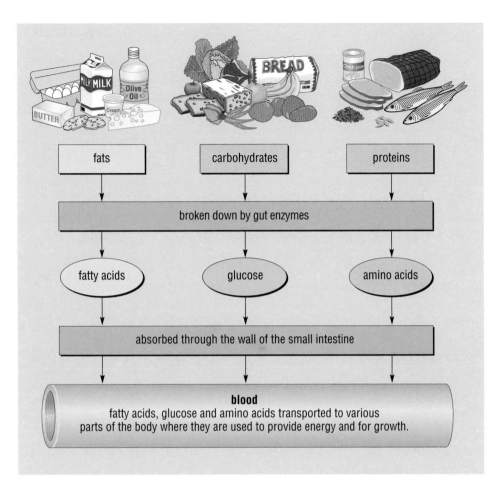

Figure 2.3 Diagram showing how food is broken down into smaller units within the gut and then absorbed into the blood through the wall of the small intestine.

When you read food labels you will find that some foods list sugars as glucose or fructose. Fructose is a building-block sugar, like glucose. Unlike complex carbohydrates, these simple sugars do not need breaking down as they are already in the required small units and so can be absorbed easily and quickly.

The speed with which food is broken down and absorbed depends on the combinations of food eaten at any particular time. People with diabetes often notice that eating a mixed meal that includes protein, fat and carbohydrate has a different effect on their blood glucose levels compared with a meal that consists of carbohydrate alone (see Section 4.5). Try Activity 2.2 below in order to think about this further.

Activity 2.2 The effect of drinking a sugary drink

Suggested study time 5 minutes

Make brief notes on the effect that a drink containing a lot of sugar such as glucose might have on the blood glucose level of an individual without diabetes. Examples of high-sugar drinks that you may know are Lucozade® and non-diet Coca-Cola®.

Comment

In people without diabetes the blood glucose levels are kept tightly controlled. Before a meal the blood glucose level is between 4 and 7 mmol/l. (Pronounced milly-moles per leeter, **mmol/l** is a unit of measurement, often used for substances within the blood. It represents the amount of substance per litre of blood.) After a meal the blood glucose usually peaks at less than 11 mmol/l. Drinking a sugary drink causes glucose to enter the blood quickly as it does not need to be broken down in the gut. The glucose makes the pancreas produce insulin, which will control the blood glucose level. We will see later how this is done. Without diabetes the level of blood glucose usually remains less than 11 mmol/l and drops back to its baseline level of about 4–7 mmol/l within a couple of hours.

In people who are diagnosed with diabetes, the term **hypoglycaemia** refers to the condition where the blood glucose level falls below 4 mmol/l and **hyperglycaemia** to the condition where the blood glucose level rises above 11 mmol/l.

2.3.3 Liver

The liver lies towards the right of the abdomen, as you saw in Figure 2.1. It is a large and important organ in the body, with many functions. It is important in helping control glucose levels, which it does by storing glucose. To do this it changes glucose into **glycogen**, a substance made of chains of glucose units stuck together. You can think of glycogen as a storage form of glucose. If there is plenty of glucose in the blood, the body makes glycogen to use later, at times when glucose is scarce. For example, to keep the blood glucose level constant in the body overnight, when one is not eating (**fasting**), the liver slowly releases glucose from its glycogen stores. After a meal when there is plenty of glucose, the liver stores it again. Similarly when you exercise and need fuel the liver can slowly release glucose to provide energy (see Figure 2.4).

It is also useful to know that insulin (which we shall discuss later) tends to stimulate the liver to take up glucose.

2.3.4 Muscle

There are different sorts of muscle in the body and they have different functions. **Skeletal muscles** are the muscles that, for example, are used for movement in your arms and legs.

Skeletal muscles store glucose as glycogen (Figure 2.4) and are able to use glucose as a fuel. Insulin stimulates muscles to take up glucose, and while exercising, as muscles are used, the glucose is used up. Thus exercise is important for maintaining healthy levels of blood glucose.

- People with diabetes who exercise can find that their blood glucose levels can fall too low. How does this happen?

- Exercise lowers blood glucose levels as muscles use glucose as a fuel. Insulin circulating in the body also lowers blood glucose levels by making the liver take it up. The two factors together can lower blood glucose levels more than expected.

In people without diabetes the body regulates the amount of insulin produced by the pancreas, and production decreases when exercise takes place to stop the blood glucose level from going too low. When tablets are taken for diabetes to stimulate the pancreas to produce insulin, or insulin itself is taken as an injection, then adjustments to therapy may be required when exercise is undertaken. This may not be possible at short notice. If too much insulin is available and insufficient food is eaten when exercise takes place, then the blood glucose level will fall too low and hypoglycaemia results.

Occasionally exercise can result in a high blood glucose level (hyperglycaemia) in people with diabetes. This happens if too little insulin is available when exercise takes place. The various hormones that are released on exercising, such as adrenalin, can act to increase the blood glucose level.

Case Study 2.2 shows how difficult it can be to make appropriate adjustments to insulin and food intake when exercising.

Case Study 2.2

Yusuf Idris is aged 18 years. He was diagnosed with diabetes and started on insulin two months ago. He has been a keen badminton player since the age of 10. His uncle was in the Malaysian national team. Last week he played a match for the first time since his diagnosis. He took his usual insulin at lunch time but ate a large portion of apple pie to try and stop his glucose going too low while playing badminton that afternoon. At the end of the first game he began to feel tired and started to miss shots. He was not sure if it was because he had not played for a while but he checked his blood glucose level and found it to be only 2 mmol/l. For this week's match he has come determined to make sure his blood glucose does not go low again. He has cut his lunchtime insulin dose, eaten extra carbohydrate and brought along a snack to eat at the end of each game. He has also decided to check his glucose level at the start of playing and between games so he can have a better idea about what is happening.

2.3.5 Fat

You may have heard people make comments about their **metabolism**, for example 'I am fat because I have a slow metabolism'. Your metabolism refers to all the things that are going on in your body to keep you alive. Different people do have different metabolic rates. Some people have low metabolic rates and some have high metabolic rates. Metabolic rate may play a part in someone's weight but it is not usually the whole cause of being fat or thin. Glucose metabolism refers to the way in which glucose is processed in the body.

Fatty acids are the breakdown products of fat. **Ketone bodies**, or **ketones**, are some of the products made when fatty acids are metabolised or processed.

Until the mid-1990s it was thought that fat tissue had little function other than as a fuel source. Although fat tissue is indeed a very important fuel source, it is now known that fat tissue also has many hormone-producing functions. Fat tissue is an important store for fat and also for glucose, which can be converted into fatty acids (Figure 2.4).

- What are the other glucose stores?
- Glycogen in the liver and muscles.

Insulin stimulates glucose uptake into fat cells as well as into liver and muscle cells. A lack of insulin results in the release of fatty acids from fat. As already mentioned the body tries to keep the glucose level tightly controlled. Overnight when one is fasting, fatty acids are released and can be used as a fuel. The way fat is broken down from fat stores is complex. Often the body breaks down fat and carbohydrate stores together. Fatty acids are produced which enter the metabolic pathways of the body and are used as fuel. When this occurs ketones are not formed. If fatty acids are broken down when little carbohydrate is available, then they cannot be used as a fuel as carbohydrate is needed for this to happen. Ketones are then produced from the fatty acids, and these *can* be used as a fuel. This may occur overnight when fasting, or in diabetes. If a person does not eat for a long time then the body adapts to use the ketones as a fuel source, but excessive ketone production may be poisonous.

Insulin is very important in determining whether or not ketones are made. After eating, the insulin level is high and this encourages glucose uptake into cells and hence suppresses ketone production. When fasting, the lower level of insulin allows ketones to form, but there is usually enough insulin to stop a build up of ketones. In people with diabetes who do not have insulin, the levels of ketones can build up. When the levels become too high the blood becomes acidic, a condition called **ketoacidosis**, and the person can become seriously ill.

Ketones can be detected in the urine (**ketonuria**) of a person after a prolonged fast, due to fat breakdown in the absence of carbohydrate. In people without diabetes this is not important and just means they have not eaten for a long time. In people with diabetes the presence of ketones in the urine can mean that they do not have enough insulin and that they are becoming unwell (see Section 5.4). Detection of ketones is an important part of helping people to manage their diabetes, especially if they are unwell.

The relationship between glucose, liver, skeletal muscle and fat is illustrated in Figure 2.4.

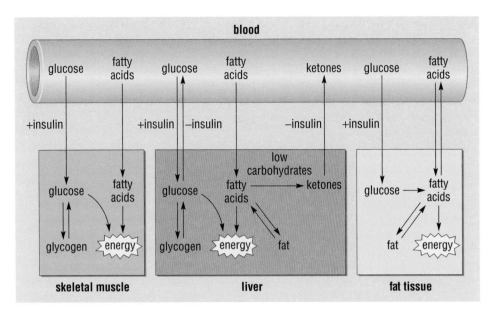

Figure 2.4 The relationship between glucose in the blood and its storage and release from skeletal muscle, liver and fat tissue. Glucose can pass easily between the blood and the liver and back again. This is shown by the two-way arrow. Glucose can also pass easily into the skeletal muscle and fat tissues, but in these cases glucose does not pass back into the blood. In skeletal muscle glucose is converted into glycogen and glucose released from glycogen is used to fuel muscle contraction. Fat tissue converts glucose into fatty acids and thence to fat, and when fat is broken down in normal metabolism fatty acids are produced again, and may be released back to the blood, and taken up by the liver. Here they are metabolised for energy and if insufficient carbohydrate is present ketones may be produced.

Case Study 2.3 illustrates what can happen when someone with diabetes becomes unwell with an infection.

Case Study 2.3

Miss Williams has had diabetes, that has been treated with insulin, for 50 years. She is now aged 80 and lives in a nursing home. Last winter she had a bad chest infection that stopped her from eating. Although she knew the important rule about never stopping her insulin she was too unwell to notice that her carers had not injected her insulin for her. Her carers thought that as she was not eating much, she would not need it. Very quickly Miss Williams became seriously ill. Although she had not eaten for 24 hours, by the time she was admitted to hospital her glucose level was 64 mmol/l (dangerously high), there were large quantities of ketones in her urine, and her blood, when tested at the hospital, contained more acid than it should. She had developed ketoacidosis because she had missed her insulin and glucose could not enter the cells and be used as a fuel.

With intravenous fluids and insulin Miss Williams made a good recovery.

2.3.6 Insulin

Insulin is a hormone produced by the pancreas. It has many actions, but is particularly important in keeping the blood glucose level normal.

● How does insulin help to keep the blood glucose level within the normal range?

○ Insulin allows glucose to enter cells and the tissues of the body (see Offprint 1.1 in Activity 1.1). If there is no insulin then glucose cannot leave the blood and enter the tissues. This means that the blood glucose level just becomes higher and higher. If there is too much insulin, more glucose enters the tissues than it should and the blood glucose level can fall too low. This is what happens when someone takes more insulin than they need.

As insulin helps glucose to enter cells it makes sense that we produce insulin when we eat and the blood glucose level is going up. The insulin prevents the glucose level in the blood from going too high. Between meals and overnight the insulin level drops down. This allows the glucose level to stay within the tight range that the body needs to function normally. If the insulin level did not drop then the blood glucose level would become too low. You have already learnt that the liver, muscle and fat all store glucose when there is plenty about. Insulin allows these tissues to take up glucose and store it. Insulin also stops glucose from being released from the liver.

The brain is the only organ in which glucose uptake is not controlled by insulin. This is important, because otherwise the amount of glucose available for the brain to use would vary as insulin levels went up and down. Instead the brain relies on mechanisms in other parts of the body to keep the blood glucose levels within a narrow range. The brain does not function properly if glucose levels in the blood drop below normal.

It is clear that insulin is needed to stop blood glucose levels from going too high. Diabetes occurs when there is no insulin or not enough insulin (insulin deficiency). Figure 2.5 summarises the actions of insulin and the consequences of a lack of, or insufficient, insulin. Diabetes can also occur when the insulin present does not function properly because the body cannot respond to ('is resisting') its actions (**insulin resistance**). **Obesity** is a common cause of insulin resistance and can lead to diabetes. Obesity is defined as greatly elevated body weight in relation to height (see body mass index in Activity 2.6), to an extent which is associated with a serious increased risk to health.

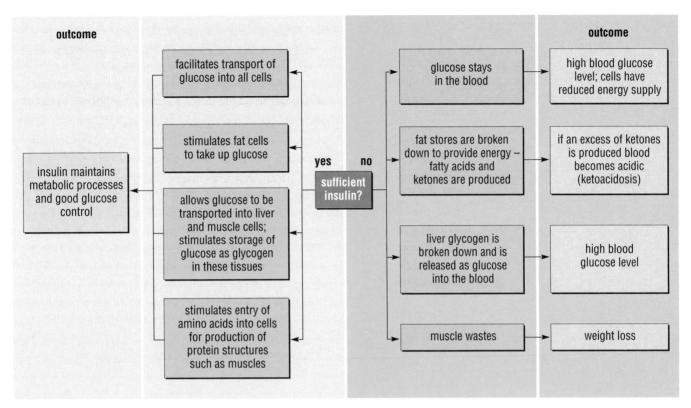

Figure 2.5 Diagram of insulin actions and the consequences of a lack of insulin.

2.3.7 Glucagon

Glucagon is another hormone produced by the pancreas.

● Can you recall which cells make glucagon?

◐ It is produced by the α cells of the islets of Langerhans in the pancreas (see Figure 2.2).

Glucagon causes an *increase* in the blood glucose level. The glucagon level in the blood tends to decrease as the glucose level increases and increases when the level of glucose decreases. It works in the opposite direction to insulin. It stimulates the liver to break down glycogen (its glucose store) and release glucose.

You may wonder why the body needs a hormone to increase glucose levels. Besides having to avoid circumstances where blood glucose is too high, the body also needs to be protected from glucose levels that are too low, as the brain will not function properly in these circumstances, as you saw above. There are lots of hormones that increase glucose levels, and glucagon is one of the most important.

You have been reading about some very complex processes in the body. Try Activity 2.3 to see if your knowledge of the processes involved in diabetes has increased.

Activity 2.3 The effect of drinking a sugary drink – revisited

Suggested study time 10 minutes

Make brief notes on the effect that a drink containing a lot of sugar such as glucose might have on blood glucose level, in: (a) someone with diabetes and (b) someone without diabetes.

Comment

How has your answer differed from that to Activity 2.2? In someone without diabetes, the blood glucose level goes up quickly and then starts to decrease, staying within normal limits. A person with some insulin but not enough, who drinks a sugary drink, will find their blood glucose level goes above the normal limits. (Blood glucose levels can reach 20 mmol/l or more after a sugary drink.) The blood glucose level comes down much more slowly in people with diabetes than in people who have a normal amount of insulin. The level to which it falls after a sugary drink depends on how much insulin is present. If there is no insulin available at all, the blood glucose level remains very high.

2.4 How to diagnose diabetes

Diabetes is a condition that results in an increased concentration of blood glucose and for diagnosis, accurate measurements of blood glucose levels are required. Blood glucose levels can be measured on different samples of blood. Sometimes the whole of the blood sample is used. This occurs when finger prick samples are measured on small personal meters (these are discussed in Section 5.3). For more accurate measurements, the sample of blood is taken to a laboratory and the blood cells are removed. Measurements are then made on the liquid remaining, called **plasma**. (The terms 'plasma glucose' or 'plasma cholesterol' may be familiar to you.) The results using the whole blood sample and the plasma sample will be slightly different because the presence of blood cells affects the test, so it is important to know which is being quoted.

We have already mentioned that the body normally keeps the glucose level controlled. When this control is lost the person has diabetes. It is worth spending a few minutes thinking about how the control of the glucose level might be lost.

- From what you have read so far, describe the possible patterns of insulin production in a person without diabetes.

- Under normal conditions in someone who does not have diabetes, the insulin level usually matches the rises and falls in the level of plasma glucose. The insulin level will therefore be low when the plasma glucose level is low, as illustrated in Figure 2.6.

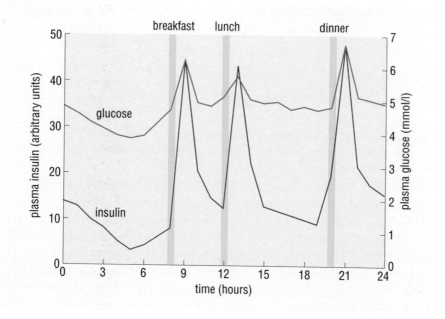

Figure 2.6 Levels of plasma
insulin and glucose over 24 hours
in someone who *does not* have
diabetes. As the glucose level
rises so does the level of insulin.
(The scale for the insulin curve,
in arbitrary units, is shown on
the left-hand vertical axis, the
scale for the glucose curve on
the right-hand axis.)

The level of glucose that is used to diagnose diabetes is defined by the World
Health Organization. The value of the level has been changed over the years and
was most recently updated in 1999 (WHO, 1999).

> **A person with symptoms of diabetes and a venous plasma
> glucose taken at random (i.e. measured at any time) equal to
> or more than 11.1 mmol/l has diabetes.**

If a patient has no symptoms or their random level is not definitely abnormal, then
two abnormal plasma glucose levels are required for a diagnosis. These tests
should be performed on different occasions.

Most commonly, the diagnosis of diabetes is made using fasting plasma glucose
levels. The person having the test should fast for 8–14 hours before the test is
carried out (the test is usually done in the morning after an overnight fast, before
any food is consumed).

> **A fasting plasma glucose greater than or equal to 7.0 mmol/l
> is abnormal.**

When there is uncertainty about the diagnosis an **oral glucose tolerance test
(OGTT)** is used. For example, in someone with fasting plasma glucose between
6 and 7 mmol/l, the doctor may consider performing an OGTT to be sure that the
person does not have diabetes.

The OGTT involves a person (adult) receiving 75 g (grams) of oral glucose, taken in
the form of a drink, i.e. 75 g of anhydrous (dry) glucose in 250–300 ml of water.
'Oral' simply means by mouth. The glucose drink can be taken as a measured
amount of Lucozade®. The manufacturer of Lucozade® provides information about
how much needs to be taken. The drink should be taken over 5 minutes. Plasma
glucose levels are measured prior to the glucose drink and after a period of 2 hours
(the result of this test is commonly termed a '2-hour glucose' by clinicians).

The person having an OGTT should:

- for the three days prior to the test have had an unrestricted carbohydrate diet
- do normal activity on the three days prior to the test
- fast for 8–14 hours before the test is carried out
- not smoke before or during the test.

A '2-hour glucose' after a 75 g oral glucose tolerance test equal to or greater than 11.1 mmol/l is abnormal.

Either the fasting result(s) or the OGTT result(s) can be used in making a diagnosis. However, the doctor needs to be sure of the correct diagnosis and may need to perform further additional tests to confirm it. For example, a person with a fasting glucose of 7.0 mmol/l on two occasions has diabetes even if the OGTT was less than 11.1 mmol/l (for example, fasting 7.0 mmol/l and 2-hour glucose 9 mmol/l). Similarly, if the fasting levels are less than 7.0 mmol/l but the OGTT more than or equal to 11.1 mmol/l on two occasions then the person has diabetes (for example, fasting glucose 6.4 mmol/l and 2-hour glucose 13 mmol/l).

It is not uncommon for one of the tests to be normal and the other to be abnormal and this makes diagnosis more difficult.

People who do not reach the criteria for diabetes may have **impaired fasting glycaemia (IFG)** if their blood glucose levels are 6.1–6.9 mmol/l after fasting (but before the glucose load) or **impaired glucose tolerance (IGT)** if their blood glucose levels are between 7.8 and 11.0 mmol/l two hours after taking 75 g of oral glucose.

These elevated levels are not normal and suggest the person may be at risk of diabetes mellitus in the future. People with these glucose levels are not at an immediate risk of microvascular complications but are at an increased risk of macrovascular complications related to chronic increased glucose levels. **Microvascular** is used to describe the small blood vessels of the body. In patients with diabetes, changes occur within the small blood vessels, particularly those in the eyes and kidneys. Microvascular complications can also affect the blood supply to nerves, leading to nerve damage. **Macrovascular** is a term used to describe the large blood vessels of the body, for example those that go to and from the heart, the arms and the legs. In patients with diabetes, changes occur within these large blood vessels as well as in the small blood vessels. They are described in detail in Chapters 5 and 6. **Chronic** is a term that refers to things that take place over a long period of time.

The threshold levels of blood glucose discussed above have been chosen on the basis of epidemiological data. **Epidemiology** is the study of diseases and risk for diseases in populations. The information has been collected in large populations of people with and without diabetes. One of the reasons that these levels of blood glucose have been chosen is that they are associated with a risk of the complications seen in people with diabetes (see Chapter 6). If people have blood glucose at these levels and above, they are at a much higher risk of developing diabetes complications in the long term compared with someone whose levels are lower.

We shall discuss risk later in this chapter.

2.5 Classification of diabetes

There are several types of diabetes, including two that are common: Type 1 and Type 2. Type 2 is the most common sort of diabetes. Worldwide, about 90% of people with diabetes have Type 2 and about 10% have Type 1. Refer back to Offprint 1.1 *Understanding diabetes* (Activity 1.1) which explains the differences between Type 1 and Type 2 diabetes. The other sorts of diabetes account for very small numbers of people.

2.5.1 Type 1 diabetes

Type 1 diabetes was previously called insulin-dependent diabetes. This is because in people with Type 1 diabetes their pancreas fails to produce insulin and they are dependent on taking insulin for their treatment. It would be useful to look back at Figure 2.5 to remind yourself of the actions of insulin. As we have already discussed, without insulin glucose cannot enter tissues and cells, and so the plasma glucose level increases. When the plasma glucose level is high, glucose is passed out of the body through the kidneys in the urine. At the time of diagnosis, if the urine is tested with a urine testing stick there will be lots of glucose present, whether the patient has eaten or not. Water is required in order to excrete the glucose through the kidneys and patients often pass large amounts of urine and are therefore thirsty. Although there is plenty of glucose in the blood, because it cannot enter the tissues it cannot be used as a fuel source. Instead the body breaks down fat and protein to use as fuel. As a result, the person often loses weight very rapidly for a number of reasons, including loss of fluid, an inability to use glucose as a fuel, loss of muscle as protein is broken down and loss of glucose in the urine. Insulin is required as treatment, and is essential for survival. A person with Type 1 diabetes should never stop their insulin even when they are unwell and not eating.

Type 1 diabetes can develop at any age although it is seen more commonly in children and young adults.

The characteristics that indicate Type 1 diabetes are:

- Rapid development of symptoms of hyperglycaemia (high blood glucose level), that is, frequently passing large amounts of urine, excessive thirst, fatigue and weight loss (see Chapter 7).

- Development of ketones; if left untreated, ketoacidosis develops.

● Can you recall how ketoacidosis develops?

◌ Ketones are produced when the body breaks down fat to use as a fuel. This would normally happen, for example, in a person who did not have diabetes who was fasting. If the level of insulin is not enough to provide sufficient glucose for the tissues to process the ketones, as in diabetes, the level of ketones builds up. This results in increased acid levels in the body – ketoacidosis (Section 2.3.5).

High blood acid levels are harmful to normal body processes, and if left untreated, can cause vomiting and severe loss of fluid. If treatment is not given quickly the person could die. Fortunately death from ketoacidosis is a very rare event in the western world. If ketoacidosis does occur, therapy in hospital is usually successful, correcting the acid level and returning the blood glucose level to normal.

Many conditions are caused by autoimmunity. The body produces substances called antibodies that usually protect the body from disease. If the body is attacked by an organism that it recognises from a previous infection, the antibodies are ready to destroy the organism. If it is a new organism that the body does not recognise, the body produces a new antibody to get rid of it. This may take a few days and, in the meantime, the person may be unwell with the illness. Occasionally the body produces antibodies which, instead of, or as well as attacking organisms, also attack parts of the body – autoimmunity. In the case of Type 1 diabetes the antibodies destroy the β cells in the pancreas. Where Type 1 diabetes is due to destruction in this way, we call it an **autoimmune disease**. Why this happens is unknown, but there is evidence to suggest that **genes** (hereditary factors) may play a part. A person with Type 1 diabetes may also have other autoimmune diseases such as thyroid disease. Environmental factors, for example certain toxins, may also be important in triggering the development of Type 1 diabetes.

Interestingly, worldwide, the **incidence** of Type 1 diabetes varies enormously. Incidence describes how many new cases of a disease have happened over a certain period of time (usually a year). There is a tendency to more diabetes in more Northern countries, with Nordic countries, especially Finland, having a particularly high incidence. The reason for this is not understood.

Activity 2.4, which you should try now, asks you to think about Type 1 diabetes in more detail.

Activity 2.4 Diagnosing Type 1 diabetes

Suggested study time 20 minutes

Read Case Study 2.4, which describes Jennifer's experience. As you read it, think about the features that suggest that Jennifer has diabetes and why it might be Type 1 diabetes.

Comments

Jennifer has marked symptoms of hyperglycaemia. She is thirsty and is passing lots of urine, particularly at night. Jennifer has also had very rapid weight loss.

A random glucose test on a meter in the surgery is high and well above the value needed to diagnose diabetes. If you look back to the WHO classification of diabetes in Section 2.4, only one high glucose level is needed if other symptoms are present. However, the finger-prick blood sample must be confirmed with a laboratory plasma sample. This may be done at the first visit and does not require the patient to return for a fasting test. It is common for people to think that diabetes can only be diagnosed on a blood sample taken first thing in the morning before eating. However, a random blood glucose test result equal to or more than 11.1 mmol/l with symptoms of diabetes is enough to make a diagnosis.

Jennifer did not have ketones in her urine. This does not mean that she does not have Type 1 diabetes, though if they were present it would confirm a diagnosis of Type 1. It depends at what stage the diagnosis is made during the development of Type 1 diabetes as to whether ketones are present. Jennifer's diagnosis has been made early, and ketones have not yet developed. So the speed of the symptoms coming on and the large weight loss would make one think that this patient has Type 1 diabetes. Jennifer will need insulin to control her blood glucose level.

Case Study 2.4

Jennifer is 30 years old. She is married with one child. She works part time as a teacher. Over the last 4 weeks she has lost 6 kg in weight, dropping from 64 kg to 58 kg and is feeling tired. She has noticed that she is thirsty and has to get up frequently at night to go to the toilet. She does not want to go the doctor because she is worried that she may have diabetes. Her mother had diabetes, which was treated with tablets for 10 years, and she was changed to insulin shortly before she died in hospital with a heart attack. Jennifer very strongly associates her mother's death with starting insulin.

Jennifer's husband Gary notices that she is looking unwell and persuades her to see her GP.

The GP immediately considers the symptoms to indicate diabetes. The GP asks Jennifer to provide a sample of urine. He tests it with a test stick, finding lots of glucose but no ketones. He checks a random blood glucose sample on a glucose meter at the surgery. The level is 28 mmol/l. He sends a sample of whole blood to the laboratory to confirm the reading and asks her to return the next day for a fasting glucose test to confirm the diagnosis.

2.5.2 Type 2 diabetes

Type 2 diabetes was previously called non insulin-dependent diabetes. People with Type 2 diabetes produce insulin but it may be in insufficient amounts and/or their cells are resistant to the action of insulin (Figure 2.7). Hyperglycaemic symptoms, such as thirst and passing large amounts of urine, may be absent. Ketoacidosis does not usually develop as there is sufficient insulin to prevent it.

Type 2 diabetes may be present for many years before a diagnosis is made. This is because some people may have few symptoms. Others do not see their thirst or getting up at night to pass urine as a problem. Having diabetes for several years before a diagnosis is made can mean that complications of diabetes, which take years to develop, may already be present at the time of diagnosis. This is one of the reasons why Diabetes UK, the diabetes charity, tries to raise awareness of diabetes and supports screening programmes for this condition.

Figure 2.7 Flow diagram showing the consequences of insulin resistance.

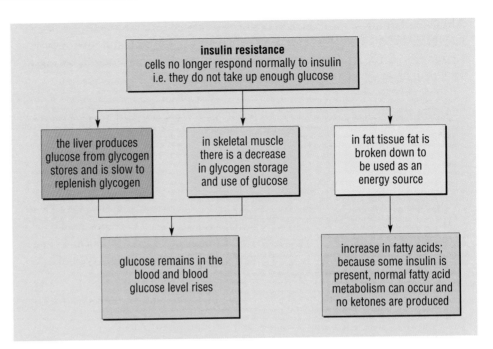

Genes are thought to be important in the development of Type 2 diabetes. In a very rare form of Type 2 diabetes, definite gene defects have been identified. This condition is called **maturity onset diabetes of the young (MODY)**, as it usually occurs before the age of 25 years. Thus in a family with a very strong family history of diabetes occurring before the age of 25 years this diagnosis needs to be considered. Furthermore, certain population groups, for example Asian and African–Caribbean people, are at an increased risk of developing Type 2 diabetes.

Other factors are also important. Obesity and lack of exercise are two particularly important environmental factors thought to be contributing to the rapidly increasing numbers of people worldwide with Type 2 diabetes (Section 2.6.2). Although Type 2 diabetes has usually been considered to be a condition of adults, particularly those over 40 years old, it is occurring with increasing frequency in adolescents.

The amount of insulin that is produced in someone with Type 2 diabetes often decreases over a period of years, although in some people there is a faster decline. In many people the condition is progressive, and eventually, to maintain the correct glucose level with the aim of preventing symptoms and decreasing the risk of complications, insulin is often required. Some people may in fact have slowly developing Type 1 diabetes. Thus treatment of Type 2 diabetes often starts with improvements to diet, i.e. changes in the amounts and types of food, and an increase in physical activity, progressing to tablets and then onto insulin. More tablets are added if required (see Section 4.5).

All diabetes is equally important. A person with Type 2 diabetes who is being treated with modifications to diet alone can develop as many complications as someone with Type 1 diabetes who is being treated with insulin.

Although it may seem quite clear cut, in reality it can be difficult to decide whether a patient has Type 1 or Type 2 diabetes; for example, knowing that someone is on insulin therapy cannot be used to distinguish whether they have Type 1 or Type 2 diabetes. This is illustrated in Activity 2.5.

Activity 2.5 The differences between Type 1 and Type 2 diabetes

Suggested study time 30 minutes

Take a few minutes to quickly re-read the last two sections on Type 1 and Type 2 diabetes and make a list of the differences between the two types. If you have diabetes list the reasons why you fit into one category or another. If you do not have diabetes but know someone who does, try asking them if they would mind if you tried to work out which type of diabetes they had. Are you right?

If your work involves people with diabetes identify two or three of them and try to decide whether they have Type 1 or Type 2 diabetes.

If you kept your notes from Activity 2.1, now would be a good time to reflect on them to see if your understanding has changed.

Case Study 2.5 introduces you to John. As you read it make notes on the clues that indicate that John has Type 2 diabetes.

Comment

Sometimes it can be very easy to tell if someone has Type 1 or Type 2 diabetes. For example, someone on tablets only who has had diabetes for several years has Type 2 diabetes. Someone who comes to hospital or a doctor's surgery with loss of weight and presence of ketones and immediately starts insulin treatment has Type 1 diabetes.

However, it is not always so simple. Someone who has lost only a small amount of weight, and whose plasma glucose level cannot be controlled with tablets and remains high after several weeks of trying to reduce it, may in fact be developing Type 1 diabetes. You would need to have asked the right questions to find out if they had Type 1 or Type 2 diabetes. More and more people with Type 2 diabetes progress to taking insulin injections as well as their tablets as time goes by. They still have Type 2 diabetes but need insulin to control their blood glucose levels.

John fits the bill as the sort of person who would be at risk of developing Type 2 diabetes: he is overweight and takes no exercise. It would be interesting to know his family history, to determine if there is any genetic influence. The high level of glucose in his urine and random blood test is confirmed by his fasting blood glucose level of 9 mmol/l, indicating a diagnosis of diabetes. Without symptoms, two abnormal glucose levels are required. John's lack of symptoms and the absence of ketones make one think that he has Type 2 diabetes rather than Type 1.

Case Study 2.5

John is 30 years old. He is married with two children and is buying his first house. He works as a long-distance lorry driver. He has always been overweight and currently weighs 120 kg. The demands of his job leave little time for exercise. He needs life insurance and his insurers have asked him to have a medical to assess his risk. He sees his GP for the first time in years. He provides a urine sample that shows a large amount of glucose but no ketones. His blood pressure is high, measuring 160/110 mmHg. He does not smoke. A high random glucose test of 13 mmol/l is confirmed by the fasting laboratory blood tests showing a plasma glucose level of 9 mmol/l and a cholesterol level of 8 mmol/l (a high value; ideally it should be about 5 mmol/l).

2.5.3 Gestational diabetes

Gestational diabetes is diabetes that develops during pregnancy. There are no internationally agreed threshold blood glucose levels used to diagnose gestational diabetes. However, there is a trend towards using the IGT (impaired glucose tolerance) test criteria (see Section 2.4). Studies are ongoing to decide what threshold level is important in pregnancy. The increased metabolic demands imposed by pregnancy may just be enough to make a person predisposed to diabetes to 'tip over' into the condition. The diabetes commonly resolves after the baby is delivered, but a few mothers will have had undiagnosed Type 2 diabetes or have developed coincidental Type 1 diabetes. Having had a diagnosis of gestational diabetes, a woman is likely to develop diabetes in future pregnancies and is also more likely subsequently to develop Type 2 diabetes. Lifestyle advice should be given. A change of lifestyle, through increasing exercise and weight reduction, has been clearly shown to delay the development of Type 2 diabetes in those with IGT. During the pregnancy, the woman should be treated for diabetes by changes to her diet and exercise with or without insulin.

Case Study 2.6 describes a person with gestational diabetes. It also introduces the idea of risk, which is discussed in Section 2.6.

Case Study 2.6

Mrs Shah, aged 38 years, is 28 weeks into her fourth pregnancy. During her third pregnancy she developed gestational diabetes. She needed insulin to control her blood glucose level along with a change in diet. After the pregnancy she was very worried about developing diabetes as both her parents had had diabetes. She continued on her new diet. She now weighs 75 kg compared with 110 kg at the same stage during her last pregnancy. She has just had an oral glucose tolerance test for diabetes. The test was normal and she is delighted.

As previously mentioned, a family history of diabetes increases the risk of a person developing diabetes. Asians and some other groups such as African–Caribbeans have an increased risk of developing diabetes compared with Caucasians. Being overweight would increase this risk further. Mrs Shah has done what she can to decrease her chances of developing diabetes. Weight reduction and exercise have been shown in several studies to reduce the risk of developing diabetes and she would have been advised at the end of her third pregnancy to adopt a healthier lifestyle.

2.5.4 Other forms of diabetes

By far the three most common types of diabetes are Type 1, Type 2 and gestational. There are other forms of diabetes but we will not be covering them in any more detail. These are forms due to:

- disease of the pancreas (pancreatitis)
- an excess of hormones that increase blood glucose levels, e.g. excess growth hormone
- drugs, for example, steroid therapy, which tend to oppose the action of insulin
- abnormalities of insulin (rare genetic disorders)
- other associated genetic conditions, for example, cystic fibrosis.

2.6 Genes and risk

Approximately 150 million people worldwide have diabetes, of which 90% have Type 2 diabetes. The incidence of the condition is rapidly increasing. In western countries about 10% of people over the age of 65 years have diabetes. In the UK it is thought that there are between 765 000 and 1 million people with undiagnosed Type 2 diabetes, that is, 29–36% of the total with diabetes (Watkins, 2003). These undiagnosed numbers are based on population samples where everyone is screened using a variety of health tests including those that diagnose diabetes.

2.6.1 Genes

You may have heard of the term 'gene' or 'genetic'. This term refers to the way the body inherits information from each parent. When we are born we receive half our genetic information from one parent and the other half from the other parent. Unless they are identical twins, children from the same parents will have slightly different genetic information giving each of them their own unique character. The important genetic information is packaged in chromosomes. We usually have 46 chromosomes in each cell, and 23 come from each parent. Some conditions are due to a single abnormality in a chromosome. If a child inherits that abnormality from one parent they will also have that condition. This sort of inheritance of a condition (called autosomal dominant) is not common but is important when it occurs: MODY is an example of this sort of inheritance. The mother of person A has the condition and passes it onto to A. In an autosomal dominant condition A has a 50:50 chance of receiving the gene from the parent with the condition (the mother) and therefore a 50:50 chance of having the condition themselves and therefore passing it on to the next generation.

Some conditions need the child to inherit the same abnormal gene from *each* parent before they will develop the disease (autosomal recessive). If they receive the gene from just one parent they do not have the condition but may pass on the abnormal gene if they have a child themselves. This means they are a gene carrier. An example of a condition that is inherited in this way is cystic fibrosis. In this case neither parent shows the condition but they both carry the gene. Each child has a 50:50 chance of receiving the gene from each parent. This will give, on average, one child with two unaffected genes, one child with both affected genes and two children who will each have one affected gene and one unaffected gene. This means that one in four children will have the condition and two will be carriers. This is what happens *on average*, and a family of four children may have no affected children, or more than one affected child, simply by chance.

Many conditions are multifactorial. This means that many factors are important in developing the condition. Diabetes is thought to be a multifactorial condition. Genes may play a part, and it is thought that for most people with either Type 1 or Type 2 diabetes many different genes may be important, although environmental factors are equally or even more important.

2.6.2 Risk

Risk is a difficult concept. Most of what we do in life involves making choices and taking risks. Sometimes the risks are small, and sometimes they are large. It can be difficult sometimes to know what the risk of doing something is. Past experience can also influence the way we think about risk. If one was knocked over by a car crossing the road, then even though the risk of it happening again is small we may remain worried and concerned about crossing the road.

How you explain risk is also important. As mentioned earlier, 10% of people over the age of 65 years have diabetes. That means that 90% do not. Do you think that is a high or a low risk? If it is said that 1 in 10 people has a risk of developing diabetes over the age of 65 years, does the risk sound greater? A 1 in 10 risk is quite high. The risk of developing diabetes is influenced not only by age but by the presence of other risk factors.

For Type 2 diabetes many factors are important.

- Certain ethnic groups, e.g. people of Asian and African–Caribbean backgrounds are at an increased risk (genetic factors).
- A family history of diabetes also increases your chances of developing diabetes (genetic factors).
- Being overweight is a risk factor. The distribution of the fat also appears to be important. A fat abdomen is more of a risk than fat hips (a combination of environmental and genetic factors).

- Lack of exercise. The western lifestyle and progressive decrease in manual jobs have increased the risk of developing diabetes (environmental factors).
- Previous gestational diabetes (a combination of environmental and genetic factors).

For Type 1 diabetes factors that may be important include the following.

- Viruses. There is an increase in cases of diabetes in the months when viruses are more common, although the reasons for this are not fully understood.
- Breast feeding – having been breast fed as a baby may be protective against developing Type 1 diabetes.
- Genetic factors, as previously discussed.

Thus, a 70-year-old Asian Indian man who is overweight and taking no exercise and who has a strong family history of diabetes has a higher risk than a 70-year-old slim Asian Indian man without a family history who takes lots of exercise. The age-adjusted incidence of diagnosed Type 2 diabetes is slightly higher amongst men than women.

Working through Activity 2.6 will help you to think about risk.

Activity 2.6 Risk of developing Type 2 diabetes

Suggested study time 30 minutes

When you are next in your town, take a minute or two to look at people in a shop or restaurant. First, see if you could judge how many of them might be at risk of developing diabetes and why? Then look to see if anyone seems to be at low risk of Type 2 diabetes and why? Finally, measure your own **body mass index (BMI)** (at home, not in the town!) by dividing your weight in kilograms by your height in metres, multiplied by itself, as shown in the equation below. What do you think your body mass index means?

$$BMI = \frac{\text{weight (kg)}}{\text{height} \times \text{height (m}^2)}$$

Comment

A person at higher risk of developing diabetes will tend to be older, overweight and relatively inactive – you might have noticed people not walking very fast, or confined to a wheelchair who were also overweight. Those at low risk will be leaner and more active. A body mass index of 20–25 kg/m² is a healthy one, 25–30 kg/m² is overweight and 30 kg/m² or more indicates obesity. In 1980, 8% of women and 6% of men in the UK were obese – by 1998 that had almost trebled to 21% of women and 17% of men. A further 32% of women and 46% of men were overweight, meaning that most people in the UK are now either overweight or obese (National Audit Office, 2001).

2.7 Summary of Chapter 2

This chapter has introduced the subject of diabetes and how it is diagnosed. It has discussed the structures and processes in the body that are important for controlling blood glucose levels and described what goes wrong when diabetes develops. The differences between Type 1 and Type 2 diabetes and other forms of diabetes have been highlighted. The concepts of genetics, risk and risk management have been introduced.

Questions for Chapter 2

Question 2.1 (Learning Outcome 2.2)

In a few sentences, outline how diabetes is diagnosed.

Question 2.2 (Learning Outcome 2.3)

Complete Table 2.1 to compare and contrast Type 1 and Type 2 diabetes.

Table 2.1 For use with Question 2.2.

Criterion	Type 1 diabetes	Type 2 diabetes
Age at onset		
Treatment		
Presence of ketones		
Cause		

Question 2.3 (Learning Outcome 2.4)

Which hormone is important in the development of diabetes? Briefly describe its role in the development of Type 1 and Type 2 diabetes.

Question 2.4 (Learning Outcome 2.5)

How might you inherit diabetes from your parent(s)?

Question 2.5 (Learning Outcome 2.5)

What factors increase the risk of someone developing Type 2 diabetes?

Question 2.6 (Learning Outcome 2.5)

Explain how obesity is defined and how body mass index is calculated.

References

National Audit Office (2001) *Tackling obesity in England* [online]. Available from: http://www.nao.org.uk/publications/nao_reports/00-01/0001220.pdf (Accessed June 2005).

Watkins, P. J. (2003) *Diabetes and its Management*, Oxford, Blackwell Publishing.

World Health Organization (1999) *Definition, diagnosis and classification of diabetes mellitus and its complications* [online]. Available from: http://whqlibdoc.who.int/hq/1999/WHO_NCD_NCS_99.2.pdf (Accessed June 2005).

CHAPTER 3

AWARENESS OF CARE

Learning Outcomes

When you have completed this chapter you should be able to:

3.1 Define and use, or recognise definitions and applications of, each of the terms printed in **bold** in the text.

3.2 Demonstrate an awareness of the structure of diabetes care, at local and national level.

3.3 Identify the priorities for diabetes care to which the National Service Framework standards refer.

3.4 Suggest methods by which diabetes care may be improved.

3.5 Distinguish between the roles of professionals involved in diabetes care.

3.6 Describe the principles of an empowerment approach to diabetes care.

3.1 Introduction

The previous two chapters have been concerned with introducing diabetes care and providing a brief overview of what is meant by diabetes. In this chapter we consider the structure within which diabetes care occurs, and how the health service is responding to the 'diabetes epidemic', that is the increase in the numbers of people that are being diagnosed with diabetes globally. Professor Sir George Alberti, a leading doctor in diabetes care in the UK, has called this spread 'one of the biggest health catastrophes the world has ever seen' (Boseley, 2003). In the UK, the spread is more rapid in some groups in the population than in others, and in the Asian community in particular. In response to this, new ways of providing diabetes care are being tested.

3.2 Who provides care?

By now you should know that there may be many different people involved in providing care to people with diabetes, as illustrated in Case Study 3.1. Before you try Activity 3.1, refer back to Section 1.3 in Chapter 1 where the roles of various people involved in diabetes care are described.

Case Study 3.1

Jamie's story

Jamie was diagnosed as having diabetes when he was 10 years old. His mother had noticed that he was tired a lot of the time and seemed to be losing weight. He was drinking and passing urine more than usual. She took him to the local health centre where his urine was tested and showed the presence of a large amount of glucose and ketones. A blood test was performed (probably by means of a finger prick) and this showed a blood glucose level of 26 mmol/l. He was referred to the local hospital and was admitted to the children's ward that day as he was vomiting. He stayed overnight before being discharged home the next day. During his stay in hospital he was shown how to inject his insulin and to test his blood glucose levels using a meter. The causes and symptoms of hypoglycaemia (a low blood glucose level – see Section 2.3.2) or 'hypos' were explained to him, and he and his parents were given information about how to treat them if they occurred (this is discussed in Chapter 7). It was thought that he may have needed to have an intravenous insulin infusion (an intravenous drip), but blood results showed that he did not have ketoacidosis (see Chapter 7), so this procedure was not necessary. Advice was given to make sure he had a healthy eating plan. The family were given telephone numbers to use if they had any concerns or questions, and an outpatient appointment at the children's diabetes clinic was arranged for two weeks later.

The following day the family were visited at home and any queries they had were answered. Jamie's blood glucose level was checked, and it had decreased to 11 mmol/l. A series of follow-up visits to monitor his progress and to give further information and advice was arranged. The family were given the contact details for Diabetes UK and also for the local diabetes support group for children and young people. Jamie returned to school the following week.

Marge's story

Marge is in her 60s and has had diabetes for 40 years. She has always taken insulin. Marge used to attend the diabetes clinic at the local hospital, but has recently started to attend her local health centre instead. This was because she felt as though she was 'on a conveyer belt' at the hospital, and rarely saw the same person twice. The result of this was that she felt that she was sometimes given information that was contradictory, and this left her feeling angry and afraid because she was unsure who to believe. The clinic was always very busy and her appointment time was often late, meaning that she was late home for her lunch and sometimes felt hypo when she was driving home. She found visiting the health centre much better, as she knew the staff well, and it was very close to her home. She recently visited for her annual review (see Chapter 6) and met a new member of the diabetes care team who carried out some of the tests that other people had previously undertaken. This meant that they had more time to talk to her about her diabetes and offer further advice and guidance. Her foot examination showed that she had an ingrown toenail which was inflamed, and so she was referred for treatment. She was also invited to join an education group. (These groups are designed to refresh the knowledge of people who have had diabetes for some time and to bring them up to date with recent developments.) As a result of attending the group, Marge made the decision to change to a pen device to take her insulin instead of the needle and syringe that she had used previously.

Abdul's story

Abdul is 48 years old, of south Asian descent, and was diagnosed with diabetes about five years ago. He went for a routine medical examination at work, and his urine was positive for glucose, but no ketones were present. He had a BMI (body mass index) of 32, which meant that he was substantially overweight for his height. He was not unduly concerned about his diabetes, as he believed it to be only 'mild', and only occasionally tested his urine. He had made no significant changes to his eating pattern, and regularly ate food that was high in saturated fat and refined carbohydrate, such as chocolate and sugary cereals. He occasionally attended his local surgery if he was unwell, but not specifically for his diabetes. On a recent visit to the surgery he was feeling tired and generally unwell, and urinalysis showed the presence of glucose and protein. His blood pressure was 170/110 (in units of millimetres of mercury – blood pressure measurements are discussed in Section 5.6). He had a fasting cholesterol level of 7.2 mmol/l. (Cholesterol measurements are discussed in Section 5.5.) He was referred for advice about his eating habits, and for regular visits to review his blood pressure and cholesterol after he had started a course of medication.

Emma's story

Emma is 19 years old and is five months pregnant with her first child. She has had diabetes since she was nine and has always taken insulin. During her earlier teenage years she went through a particularly rebellious phase, and was admitted several times to hospital with ketoacidosis, which occurred because she had stopped taking her insulin and was eating erratically. She is now very worried that this may have affected her unborn baby, as the latest of these episodes was just before she found out that she was pregnant. She was very sick during the first few months of her pregnancy and had been admitted to hospital during this time. She had also had frequent hypos. This stage of the pregnancy means that her insulin requirements will start to increase as the baby grows, and she regularly tests her blood glucose level (i.e. several times a day). She attends the hospital outpatients department every few weeks and is visited at home in between. She will have her baby in hospital and hopes to give birth as naturally as possible.

Activity 3.1 Different roles in diabetes care

Suggested study time 30 minutes

Case Study 3.1 describes four people's experiences of receiving care for their diabetes. Read through these stories, and then make a list of the people who might be involved in providing diabetes care for each person, and what their role would be.

Comment

We hope you found the stories in Case Study 3.1 interesting. They have been provided to demonstrate that there can be not only a wide range of experiences when having diabetes but also that there are a great variety of people involved in diabetes care.

How did you get on with your list? Below is what one course team member wrote after reading these stories. (We do not expect you to have covered so much detail.)

Jamie may have initially seen a practice nurse, a nurse practitioner or a GP when he first went to the clinic with his mother. The practice nurse may have tested his urine and blood, and then referred him on to the GP who would have made the diagnosis. The GP would have contacted the doctor at the hospital and arranged for him to be admitted to the children's ward. On the ward he would have been looked after by nurses and doctors who specialise in the care of children, and they would probably have contacted the nurses and doctors who specialise in the care of people with diabetes – the diabetes specialist nurses (DSN) and the diabetologist. Some hospitals have nurses and doctors who are specifically trained to look after children with diabetes. Laboratory staff would have analysed any blood samples taken. The doctor would have prescribed the type and amount of insulin, and the DSN would have shown Jamie and his family how to inject Jamie's insulin and to test his blood glucose level. A dietitian would have given advice about healthy eating and arranged to see them in the future. Dietitians may work in the hospital and the community so may also visit at home after discharge from hospital. The contact telephone numbers given for use after discharge are likely to have been for these members of the diabetes care team. The DSN and/or the dietitian are likely to have visited Jamie at home. Jamie would see the diabetologist, DSN and dietitian at hospital visits in the future and would also meet the staff who work in the outpatients' department, such as the receptionist, clinic nurses and assistants. He would also have been given an emergency 24-hour telephone number.

Marge would have seen either a diabetologist or more junior doctors when she visited clinics at the hospital. One of the reasons that she may have seen different staff is that the more junior staff rotate among different departments. She would have seen outpatient nurses and clinic receptionists, who may have taken some details and performed tests such as weight and **urinalysis** (analysis of her urine) before she saw the doctor. She may also have seen a DSN and a dietitian at the clinic. When she transferred her diabetes care to her local health centre, she is likely to have seen a practice nurse or a nurse practitioner, and/or the GP who would assess her care and provide further advice and guidance. The new member of the diabetes care team that she met there may well have been a diabetes care technician (DCT) who might have carried out procedures such as measuring her blood pressure, carrying out a foot examination, urinalysis and determining her waist measurement and weight. (Waist measurements are used to determine if somebody is obese – see Section 5.7.) The exact role of the DCT may vary from setting to setting. The education group would probably have been run by either a DSN or the practice nurse, with some input from other members of the diabetes team, who would have taught her how to use the pen device. (Marge's decision to change to a pen device might have been based on evidence that they offer easier, safer, more accurate, and more discrete insulin injections.) Some diabetes specialist nurses run clinics in GP surgeries, rather than the hospital. She would have been referred to a podiatrist (previously called a chiropodist) for treatment of her ingrown toenail and been given advice about how to prevent foot problems in the future.

The care of Abdul's diabetes takes place in a community setting at his local surgery. He is likely to come into contact with any of the professionals mentioned in Marge's story who are based there. The emphasis on his care would be in managing the risk factors for cardiovascular and kidney disease. The potential for the development of complications affecting his eyes would also be of concern, and he may be advised to contact a local optometrist for an initial assessment of the health of his eyes, or be referred to a screening clinic either in a hospital or community setting. He will see a pharmacist when his medication is dispensed who will be able to give him advice about how to take it. Because he has diabetes, he is exempt from paying charges for prescriptions and for eye tests. His wife may come with him to his appointment; this is useful, especially if she does the majority of the shopping and cooking, and an appointment is arranged with a community dietitian. Another worker who may be involved with Abdul's care is the Asian link worker, who has a deeper understanding of dietary and cultural issues. Translators may be employed to work with people for whom English is not the first language.

The care of Emma's diabetes focuses on taking care of both her and her unborn child. The majority of the care is given by nurses and doctors specialising in the care of diabetes and pregnancy. The doctors at the hospital are diabetologists and obstetricians, and she will also see DSNs and midwives – some nurses and doctors have experience in both of these specialisms. (Other areas have clinics where all the relevant professionals are together, meaning that fewer hospital visits are required.) Pregnancy is a time when many women need to pay closer attention to the control of their diabetes, and it may be a chance for Emma to take a long-term view of this. If she continues to have difficulty in managing her diabetes following the birth of her baby, it may be appropriate for her to seek specialist help from a psychologist or a counsellor. She would have been given an emergency contact telephone number.

You will have realised from completing Activity 3.1 that there is a group of 'core' people who are involved to some extent with the diabetes care for all of the examples given above, which nearly always includes a doctor and a nurse. Other people commonly involved are dietitians and podiatrists, and pharmacists as long as the individuals are prescribed medication of some sort. In addition to this 'core' group of professionals, others are involved when there are special circumstances, such as the care of children and during pregnancy. The person with diabetes may also have people other than health care professionals involved with their care, such as family members.

The health care professionals that people with diabetes come into contact with change according to their specific needs at different times. For example, if Abdul needed to start insulin therapy in a few years time, it might take place within a hospital setting, or he might see a DSN, rather than a practice nurse.

● Can you think of any other circumstances which may require specific help?

● You may have thought of times when you, or someone with diabetes, have been admitted to hospital for an operation which was not connected to having diabetes. This is a time when it is very important to make sure that the blood glucose level is controlled, and the diabetes care team and the surgeon and anaesthetist need to work together closely. Another example may be if someone is doing a sporting challenge, such as a long distance run. It would be important then for the diabetes team to link closely with the sports trainer to balance diet and medication with the activity.

3.2.1   New roles in diabetes care

Diabetes care is currently (2005) undergoing a period of change, and this will be reflected in the experience of people with diabetes, both in the way that care is received and by whom it is delivered. New roles are being developed for people who have the necessary skills, but are not registered with a professional body – diabetes care technicians (DCTs) are an example of one such role (see Figure 3.1). As you read in Chapter 1, a DCT carries out some of the functions that previously would have been done by other members of the care team. This means that people such as nurses have more time to concentrate on the more specialist education and treatment of diabetes, and may themselves take on roles that other professionals have previously done, such as prescribing medication. Some of the traditional boundaries between individuals involved in diabetes care are being broken down, as new ways of working evolve.

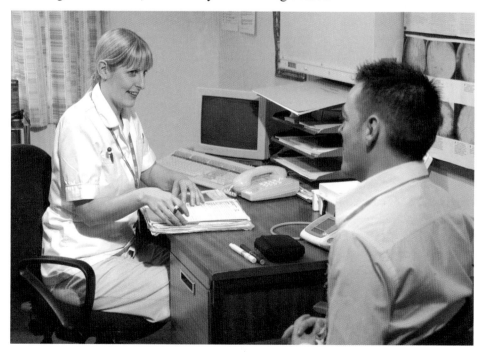

Figure 3.1 Diabetes care technicians often carry out diabetes annual reviews.

The Changing Workforce Programme (NHS Modernisation Agency, 2004) is a national programme that was set up by the Department of Health (in 2001) to help redesign roles (such as the DCT) to improve patient services. As part of this programme, two areas of England have been involved in pilot studies for diabetes care (Department of Health, 2004; NHS Modernisation Agency, 2002).

Another new role being tested is that of the **learning facilitator**, whose role is to deliver a structured education programme to adults with Type 2 diabetes and their carers. There are many groups and agencies involved in the redesign of and support for the new roles in diabetes care work – they include:

*   Diabetes UK – a registered charity providing support and advice to people with diabetes, supporting research and giving advice to health care professionals about good practice in diabetes care
*   the Expert Patients Programme, which enables people with long-term conditions to become experts in their own diabetes management
*   the **National Institute for Health and Clinical Excellence (NICE)**, which provides guidance on best practice and publishes guidelines for health professionals to follow
*   Skills for Health, which is developing competency frameworks that will influence the education, training and qualifications for diabetes care, and
*   the Workforce Development Confederations (WDC), Workforce Development Directorates (WDD) or Strategic Health Authorities (SHA) which develop the delivery of education and training. They influence the ways in which staff are trained and employed.

All these groups and agencies have useful websites where you can gain further information – links are available from the course website should you wish to explore further.

*   What impact do you think the introduction of the new roles may have on people with diabetes?
*   They may not see the person they expect when they attend for clinic appointments, and the new roles will need to be explained. They may find that there is more time to spend with specialist doctors and nurses. Waiting times may also become shorter in clinics.

3.3 A framework for care

The Department of Health has published a Delivery Strategy for putting the National Service Framework for Diabetes (NSF) (Department of Health, 2001) into action (Department of Health, 2002a). The NSF for diabetes was first mentioned in Chapter 1, Table 1.1. Activity 3.2 will help you to find out more about this strategy.

Activity 3.2 A framework for care

Suggested study time 30 minutes

Look at Figure 3.2 to remind yourself of the 12 standards as detailed in the National Service Framework for Diabetes. Now find out about the proposed Delivery Strategy by reading the NSF document, which you will find on the course DVD-ROM.

Make some brief notes on what you think are the main points suggested in the Foreword and Executive Summary in the Delivery Strategy.

Comment

The main points suggested in the Foreword and Executive Summary are as follows.

- The Foreword talks about improving the quality of care for people with diabetes regardless of who they are or where they live. The goals are to increase life expectancy, reduce illness and disability, and to tackle inequalities by helping people with diabetes to manage their care in partnership with others. In order to achieve an improved quality of care,

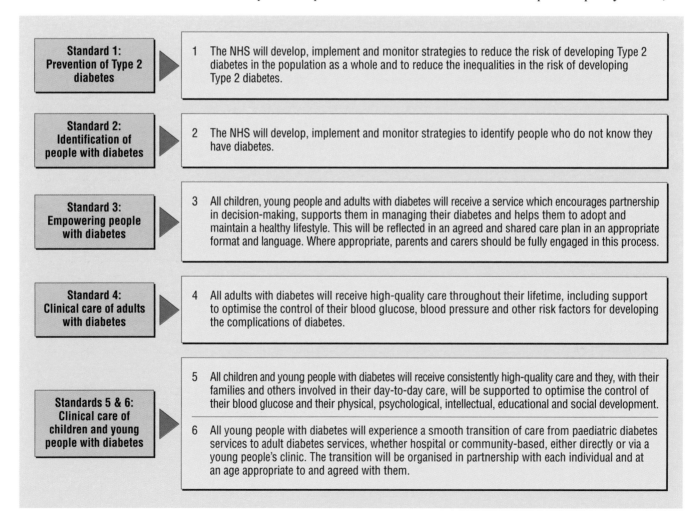

Standard 1:
Prevention of Type 2 diabetes

1 The NHS will develop, implement and monitor strategies to reduce the risk of developing Type 2 diabetes in the population as a whole and to reduce the inequalities in the risk of developing Type 2 diabetes.

Standard 2:
Identification of people with diabetes

2 The NHS will develop, implement and monitor strategies to identify people who do not know they have diabetes.

Standard 3:
Empowering people with diabetes

3 All children, young people and adults with diabetes will receive a service which encourages partnership in decision-making, supports them in managing their diabetes and helps them to adopt and maintain a healthy lifestyle. This will be reflected in an agreed and shared care plan in an appropriate format and language. Where appropriate, parents and carers should be fully engaged in this process.

Standard 4:
Clinical care of adults with diabetes

4 All adults with diabetes will receive high-quality care throughout their lifetime, including support to optimise the control of their blood glucose, blood pressure and other risk factors for developing the complications of diabetes.

Standards 5 & 6:
Clinical care of children and young people with diabetes

5 All children and young people with diabetes will receive consistently high-quality care and they, with their families and others involved in their day-to-day care, will be supported to optimise the control of their blood glucose and their physical, psychological, intellectual, educational and social development.

6 All young people with diabetes will experience a smooth transition of care from paediatric diabetes services to adult diabetes services, whether hospital or community-based, either directly or via a young people's clinic. The transition will be organised in partnership with each individual and at an age appropriate to and agreed with them.

people with diabetes should notice a greater involvement with locally delivered services that are set challenging and measurable targets.

- The Executive Summary sets out a 'vision of diabetes services' where the person with diabetes is at its centre. The care of those with diabetes should be structured and proactive, and staff involved in its delivery should have access to education and training programmes. The summary also mentions targets in Improvement, Expansion and Reform and a Delivery Strategy that enables the NHS to produce the framework and capacity to implement the diabetes NSF.

A National Diabetes Support Team has been formed to enable this framework for care to be implemented, and a National Clinical Director for Diabetes has been appointed to lead this team. The responsibility for planning the provision of care will rest with SHAs, and will be delivered by groups such as Local Implementation Teams or Clinical Action Teams at the local level. These teams will develop protocols and policies for diabetes care in their local area, which will be carried out by people such as those identified in Section 3.1. Primary Care Trusts (PCTs) have the responsibility for delivering diabetes care. They can

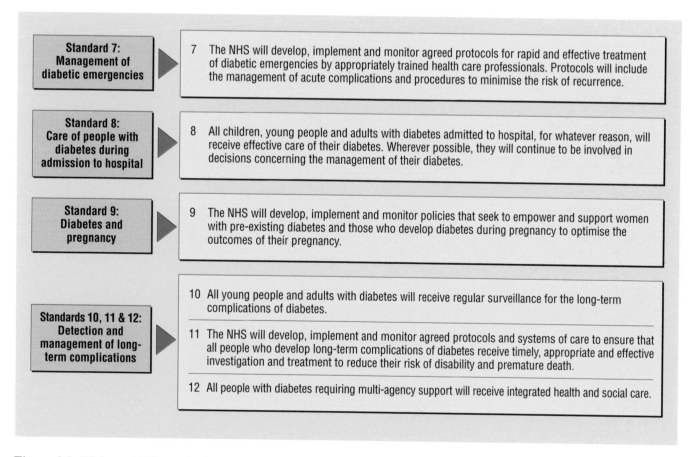

Figure 3.2 Diabetes NSF standards to be reached by 2013.

achieve this either by directly providing a range of services themselves or by commissioning others to do so.

As you now probably realise, there is a bewildering array of organisations (and corresponding websites) promoting strategies for diabetes care. But what does this all mean in practice for you and for people in your locality?

3.3.1 Where is care provided?

Diabetes care is provided in a variety of settings, with the majority being provided in primary care. This includes health centres and GP surgeries. Where more complex care is required, such as for children and young people, or during pregnancy, care is likely to be provided within a hospital setting.

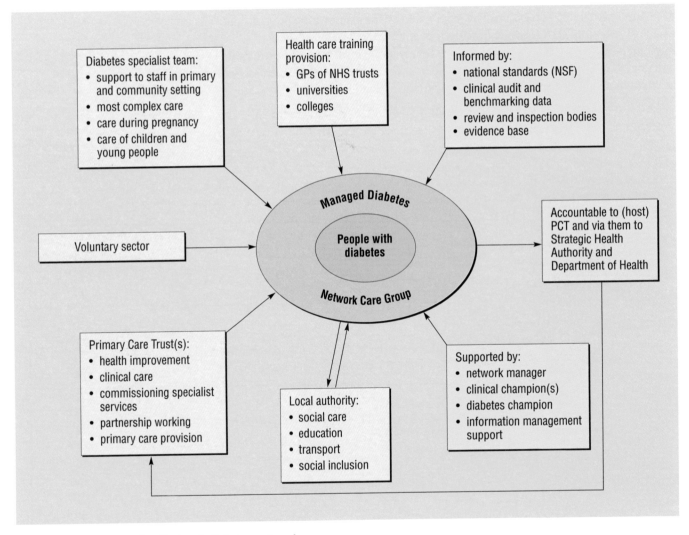

Figure 3.3 An example of a local diabetes network.

● Why do you think that the majority of care is now provided in the community?

○ Because a hospital system would not be able to cope with the increasing number of people with diabetes, especially Type 2. It may be more convenient for people to travel to a local health centre or clinic, rather than go to a hospital that may be some distance away from their home. Quality care can just as easily be provided in the community as in a hospital. Also, people with diabetes may not see themselves as being ill, and would not therefore wish to visit a hospital.

The NSF Delivery Strategy recommends that local 'diabetes networks' should provide care. An example of one such network is illustrated in Figure 3.3, which shows the various people and groups who might be involved in providing diabetes care.

Activity 3.3 Diabetes networks

Suggested study time 1 hour

Look carefully at Figure 3.3. Using this as a guide, draw a diagram that shows an example of a diabetes network in the area within which you work or live. As you are doing this, think about the people involved in providing this care and their roles. Where does the care take place, and are there links with organisations other than those relating to health? You will probably need to look at information available locally, perhaps at your local hospital or health centre. You could try looking at websites produced by your local PCT or SHA. Diabetes UK have a useful website which allows you to look at local care in your area (Dr Foster and Diabetes UK, 2004). Use the link on the course website to access the relevant web page and then follow the instructions given there to find your local information.

Comment

Your diagram will be personal to you. It is likely that you have included a variety of health care professionals such as those mentioned earlier in this chapter, and a variety of locations such as hospitals, health centres and GP surgeries. You may also have included charities such as Diabetes UK, or other aspects such as community education initiatives which may provide sports facilities, etc.

No one would claim that the present level of diabetes care is perfect – there will always be room for improvement. The aim of the NSF is to introduce a high-quality service over a period of 10 years. Figure 3.2 shows what is expected within this time frame.

3.4 Ways of delivering care

Standard 3 of the NSF is about people with diabetes becoming empowered, which means helping people to help themselves by being involved in their own care. The principle of **empowerment** in diabetes care is based on people taking more control of their care, both for themselves as individuals, and also for others by being involved in determining local services and priorities.

Empowerment could be described as the opposite of the experience this woman with diabetes describes:

> 'Doctors don't listen to you as a human being despite the fact that you are the expert because you live with diabetes. They don't give you a chance to ask questions – it is about what they want to do, getting poked and prodded without any explanations. The doctor I saw when I was young was very snooty and had his head in the clouds.'

(Hiscock et al., 2001, p. 25)

An empowerment approach to care takes into account psychological and social factors, as well as medical ones.

Factors that contribute to a good experience include:

A friendly, warm and 'equal' approach to the patient

A willingness to understand the impact of diabetes on other aspects of the individual's life and lifestyle

A 'partnership approach' to treating the condition

A willingness to make time to discuss issues and answer questions

A proactive approach to making referrals to other health care professionals.

(Hiscock et al., 2001, p. 25)

Activity 3.4 Relationships between patients and health care professionals

Suggested study time 15 minutes

Think about the last time you went to see a doctor or nurse. (It can be for any reason.)

Think about the positive and not so positive aspects of the encounter with that health care professional. What contributed to the way you felt about that experience and how might it have been changed?

Try to decide whether you think the encounter was empowering or not, and why.

Comment

It may be that those relationships that you felt were empowering contained elements of sharing information, listening to each others' views and working out a way forward together. Those that were not empowering may have had an unequal balance of power, with one person making decisions and attempting to control the actions of another.

Hiscock and colleagues found that patients felt that services would be improved if health professionals were 'supportive, friendly, accepting, and non-judgemental in their approach' (Hiscock et al., 2001, p. 42). Equality and a partnership approach are essential components of an empowering relationship.

Activity 3.5 takes a closer look at consultations and whether or not they are empowering. You will focus on the communication between health care professionals and people with diabetes in later chapters, but this activity will help you to start thinking about the issues.

Activity 3.5 Some consultations that are not empowering

Suggested study time 30 minutes

Read the two stories in Case Study 3.2, which describe encounters between GPs and two people with Type 1 diabetes. Note down the ways in which you think these two stories differ. Do you think one encounter was more empowering than the other?

Comment

Did you find differences between these two stories? One of the course team wrote:

I could see how Dr Cook, who's obviously got a waiting room full of patients, was anxious to help Jenny quickly. But he didn't give her enough time to talk. In contrast, Dr Kumar attempted to find out more about Sarah and was proactive in referring her to other health care professionals.

Case Study 3.2

Jenny

Jenny is in her early thirties and has had diabetes since she was 11 years old, just as she started senior school. She had always been in fairly good control of her diabetes, until recently when her blood glucose level started to fluctuate. She attended her annual diabetes check-up appointment (her annual review) at her local hospital and was seen by the senior registrar, Dr Cook, after a long wait in the busy outpatients' waiting area.

Dr Cook asked to see her record of blood glucose readings as soon as Jenny went into the room, and noticed immediately that they were high according to the recommended levels for people with diabetes. He asked her what she thought the reasons for this might be, and Jenny admitted she had been eating rather a lot lately, since she and her husband had agreed to separate. Dr Cook reminded Jenny that poor control of her diabetes could lead to all sorts of problems; there had been some important studies showing that high blood glucose levels could lead to blindness, kidney problems and nerve damage.

Jenny started to get upset and blurted out that it was difficult coping with diabetes on top of looking after two kids, with no help from anyone else. She couldn't sleep, and even when she did, she woke up early and couldn't get back off again.

Dr Cook recognised this as a sign of depression and suggested she go on an antidepressant drug for a while, to 'even things out a little for her'. He had read some reports in the *British Medical Journal* that taking certain antidepressants could even improve her diabetes control. Before Jenny could say anything further, Dr Cook wrote out a prescription which Jenny took with relief. Perhaps now she would start feeling better …

Sarah

Sarah is 26 years old, single after recently breaking up with her long-term boyfriend, and working full time as a care assistant in a local residential care centre. Sarah was diagnosed as having diabetes when she was 15, and had found it very difficult to cope with at the time, with her exams coming up and worrying about future employment. She had wanted to train as a nurse but had felt that it might be too difficult now that she had diabetes; being a care assistant was the next best thing in her opinion and she enjoyed her work.

At her check-up with her diabetes consultant, Dr Kumar, she admitted that her blood glucose level was 'terrible', and varied greatly, often on a daily basis. She had never found shift work a problem but just recently it seemed to have had an effect on her diabetes control. She worried constantly about her blood glucose level and often tested her blood four or five times a day – not that she adjusted her insulin as a result, she just wanted to reassure herself that it wasn't too bad. Sarah had never been to see the diabetes nurse and had never received any education about diabetes – all she knew was what she had read in some leaflets she had found at the residential care centre where she worked.

Dr Kumar asked her what other things had been happening in her life recently, and she told him that she had recently split up with her boyfriend. This had been a great strain for her and she had had difficulty sleeping recently, and had resorted to 'comfort eating' in the evenings. The doctor suggested that she see the diabetes nurse, and also the dietitian whilst she was at the hospital, as both of these people could help her to manage her diabetes. As she seemed a bit 'down' he thought she might benefit from an assessment from the nurse to check whether it might be appropriate to refer her for some counselling, to help her sort a few things out. To Sarah's relief, Dr Kumar didn't think that antidepressants were appropriate for her; although they might help her get over her problems, he would rather she talked to the counsellor first and see how things went.

Although Jenny and Sarah had the same type of diabetes and had similar personal problems, a different 'solution' for their care was proposed by their doctors. One of the ways that is suggested for implementing the NSF is that care will be different according to a person's needs at the time. Earlier (in Case Study 3.1) you met Abdul and Emma and you saw how their care had different priorities. The focus in Abdul's care was on the prevention of the development of long-term complications associated with diabetes, whereas in Emma's case it was on the safe delivery of a healthy baby. Other NSF strategies include the following.

- Structured education for people with diabetes.

  This means providing education for people with diabetes that is planned and relevant to their care. They may be linked to research projects such as **DESMOND** (Diabetes Education and Self Management for Ongoing and Newly Diagnosed) or other self-management programmes such as **DAFNE** (Dose Adjustment for Normal Eating). DESMOND is concerned with structured education for people newly diagnosed with Type 2 diabetes, and DAFNE with the principle of people adjusting their insulin dose to fit in with their eating habits, rather than the other way round.

- Development of professional partnerships between people with diabetes and health care professionals.

  For example, for the first time, in 2004, a conference for people with diabetes was linked with the annual professional conference of Diabetes UK.

  The National Electronic Library for Health (NELH) provides examples of care pathways for use by health care professionals when planning and delivering diabetes care. This should mean that a care plan is developed by the person with diabetes and the professionals involved in their care, leading to an integrated approach to their care. There is a Diabetes NSF zone which brings together links relating to NSF implementation. (See the course website for a link to the Diabetes NSF zone.)

Now work through Activity 3.6 to think more about how the NSF standards are being met.

Activity 3.6 Local needs

Suggested study time 1 hour

Read the offprint from the Department of Health (2002b) called *Living with Diabetes – Your future health and wellbeing* in the *Offprint Booklet* (Offprint 3.1).

Make some notes on how far you think the NSF standards are already being met locally, and identify areas where you think there is a need for further improvement. How would you go about making improvements if you were in a position to influence diabetes care?

Comment

Local needs and how they are currently being met vary from place to place. Some areas are already providing very good standards of care, whereas others are still in the early stages of addressing the needs in their area. A good example of how the NSF is being implemented locally is in relation to eye screening, which has been identified as a priority for diabetes care. Someone with diabetes may go to a local optician for screening, or a community venue or a local hospital, depending upon how the NSF standard is implemented in the area where they live.

3.5 Summary of Chapter 3

This chapter has been concerned with the design and delivery of diabetes care, through the NSF. It is a time of change and development, and the need for a changing method of delivery and changes to roles in diabetes care has arisen largely as a response to the increase in the numbers of people with diabetes and the fact that there are limited specialist resources to deal with it.

Traditional boundaries between roles are being challenged and broken down completely in some cases, with the introduction of new roles such as diabetes care technicians and learning facilitators. With these changes it is important that everyone working in diabetes care works to the same guidelines; otherwise people will be given conflicting information, which will make it very difficult for them to make an informed choice about their treatment.

This period of radical change is a challenging time in the history of diabetes care, with the person with diabetes becoming an integral member of the diabetes care team and their expert knowledge of their condition being acknowledged. Any one person in isolation cannot deliver diabetes care; teamwork is an essential feature, at both a local and national level.

Questions for Chapter 3

Question 3.1 (Learning Outcome 3.2)

Name at least three groups or organisations that are involved in planning or providing diabetes care, and describe their role in doing so.

Question 3.2 (Learning Outcome 3.3)

What is the National Service Framework for diabetes?

Question 3.3 (Learning Outcome 3.4)

For any three of the NSF standards suggest ways in which diabetes care relating to them could be improved in your area. You may answer this from personal or professional experience.

Question 3.4 (Learning Outcome 3.5)

Identify four roles that could be involved in diabetes care. Describe the similarities and differences between them.

Question 3.5 (Learning Outcome 3.6)

What does the word 'empowerment' mean to you? What would you expect to find in an empowering relationship?

References

Boseley, S. (2003) 'Diabetes 'catastrophe' warning', *The Guardian*, 25 August 2003 [online] Available from: http://www.guardian.co.uk/uk_news/story/0,3604,1028937,00.html (Accessed April 2005).

Department of Health (2001) *National Service Framework for Diabetes*, London, Department of Health [online] Available from: http://www.dh.gov.uk/assetRoot/04/05/89/38/04058938.pdf (Accessed April 2005).

Department of Health (2002a) *National Service Framework for Diabetes: Delivery Strategy*, London, Department of Health [online] Available from: http://www.dh.gov.uk/assetRoot/04/03/28/23/04032823.pdf (Accessed April 2005).

Department of Health (2002b) *Living with Diabetes – Your future health and wellbeing*, London, Department of Health Publications.

Department of Health (2004) *Delivering the HR in the NHS Plan 2004*, London, Department of Health Publications.

Dr Foster and Diabetes UK (2004) *Your Local Care 2004*, A survey of diabetes services in primary care organisations. A research project by Dr Foster and Diabetes UK [online] Available from: http://www.diabetes.org.uk/yourlocal_care2004/index.html (Accessed April 2005).

Hiscock, J., Legard, R. and Snape, D. (2001) *Listening to Diabetes Service Users: Qualitative findings for the National Service Framework*, London, Department of Health [online] Available from: http://www.dh.gov.uk/PublicationsAndStatistics/Publications/PublicationsPolicyAndGuidance/PublicationsPolicyAndGuidanceArticle/fs/en?CONTENT_ID=4008645&chk=RIZ5wk (Accessed April 2005).

NHS Modernisation Agency (2002) *Workforce Matters – A guide to role redesign in diabetes care* [online] Available from: http://www.modern.nhs.uk/cwp/21135/WM_diabetes_care.pdf (Accessed April 2005).

NHS Modernisation Agency (2004) *Changing Workforce Programme. New ways of working in healthcare* [online] Available from: http://www.modern.nhs.uk/scripts/default.asp?site_id=65 (Accessed April 2005).

CHAPTER 4

MEDICAL MANAGEMENT

Learning Outcomes

When you have completed this chapter you should be able to:

4.1 Define and use, or recognise definitions and applications of, each of the terms printed in **bold** in the text.

4.2 Demonstrate an understanding of the differences in treatment for Type 1 and Type 2 diabetes.

4.3 Describe the role of insulin therapy and outline commonly used insulin regimens.

4.4 Discuss how diet and exercise can help in the management of Type 2 diabetes.

4.5 Describe the range of tablet therapies for diabetes, including their limitations.

4.6 Demonstrate an understanding of the complementary therapies used by some people with diabetes, and their limitations.

4.7 Explain why monitoring blood pressure and cholesterol levels are important in the management of diabetes.

4.1 Introduction

In this chapter you focus more closely on the medical management of diabetes. This is not to say that other aspects of diabetes care are less important; however, the aim of this chapter is to show you some of the broad principles of medical care. This should help you make sense of the confusing array of treatments available and help you negotiate your way around care in both primary and secondary environments. There is no one correct way to manage diabetes and views often differ, both between health care professionals and between the person with diabetes and the health care professionals concerned with their care. However, the aim of the medical management of diabetes is to find the therapy that is most acceptable to the person with diabetes to keep them healthy in the long term.

4.2 Managing diabetes

People's experiences of their diagnosis of diabetes differ and it may depend on the type of diabetes that person has. To illustrate this you return to the stories of some of the people you met in Chapter 2. This chapter introduces what is often called medical management; however, it is not possible to discuss all the different ways that care is given around the UK. Your experience may be different from that described and it is important to remember that there are many different ways to manage diabetes. Let's start with the diagnosis of diabetes before going on to its medical management.

4.3 Diagnosis

Look back to Chapter 2 (Case Studies 2.4 and 2.5) to remind yourself of the experiences of two people with recently diagnosed diabetes, Jennifer and John. Their stories are summarised and extended slightly in Case Study 4.1.

Case Study 4.1

Jennifer is 30 years old, and has been feeling unwell, losing weight, feeling thirsty and going to the toilet frequently. When she went to see her GP, her blood glucose level was found to be 28 mmol/l. A blood sample sent to the laboratory confirmed this result. Jennifer's GP was very concerned and referred her to the hospital's diabetes unit.

John is also in his 30s and, unlike Jennifer, feels well. He is very overweight and goes to see his GP for a medical examination for life insurance, not expecting any problems to be found. A large amount of glucose is found in his urine and he has a fasting glucose level of 9 mmol/l.

As Jennifer has physical symptoms and also a high blood glucose measurement, a diagnosis of diabetes is made. John has no symptoms and as his first fasting blood glucose is only slightly raised he needs to have another blood glucose test before an accurate diagnosis is made.

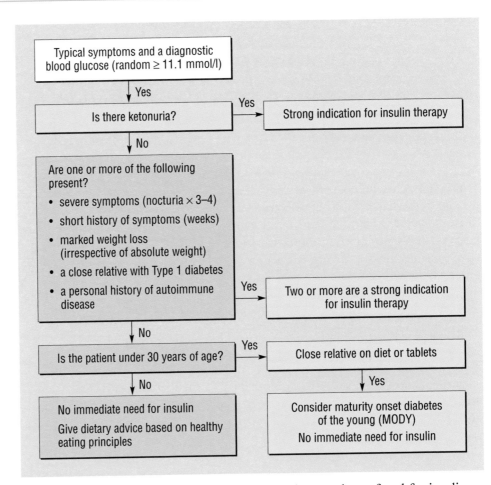

Figure 4.1 Flow chart for deciding whether a patient needs a referral for insulin therapy at the time of diagnosis of diabetes.

Once a diagnosis of diabetes is made, decisions on the management of diabetes need to be reached. To help you see how these processes occur, look at the flow chart in Figure 4.1, which describes how to decide whether a patient needs a referral for insulin therapy.

When deciding on treatment, there are two important decisions to make. First, does the person have diabetes? Second, what sort of diabetes do they have? In Chapter 2 you learned about different types of diabetes. The most common was Type 2 diabetes, followed by Type 1 diabetes. Try the following activity to see how decisions on treatment are made.

Activity 4.1 Diagnosing and treating diabetes

Suggested study time 20–30 minutes

Consider Jennifer and John's stories, referring back to Case Studies 2.4 and 2.5 and 4.1, if necessary. Using the flow chart in Figure 4.1, decide what treatment you would recommend to Jennifer if you were the health care professional involved.

Comment

Jennifer and John went to their GPs for very different reasons: Jennifer because she felt unwell and John for a medical examination for life insurance. This may alter the way they feel when the diagnosis of diabetes is first made. You will consider the social and emotional aspects of diabetes in detail in Chapters 8, 9 and 10.

Jennifer has what are often called 'typical' symptoms and a blood glucose level that confirms the diagnosis. So the answer to the first question on the flow chart is 'yes'. She does not have ketonuria, so we follow the 'no' arrow. In the next box, she has had **nocturia** (passing urine at night), a short history of symptoms and weight loss. We now have a 'yes' to this box, i.e. two or more symptoms that give a strong indication for insulin therapy. The symptoms Jennifer reports suggest that she has Type 1 diabetes.

John has no symptoms. He is very overweight and takes no exercise, both of which are risk factors for Type 2 diabetes. Although he is relatively young (in his 30s) he has nothing else to suggest that he may have Type 1 diabetes. He may initially attend his GP surgery as someone with Type 2 diabetes. We will return to John's diagnosis later in the chapter.

Once a diagnosis of diabetes is confirmed and the type of diabetes is known, treatment or therapeutic options should be considered. The terms treatment and therapy are sometimes used interchangeably as they are considered to mean the same thing.

4.4 Aims of medical management

4.4.1 Blood glucose control

Blood glucose therapy aims to maintain the blood glucose level within approximately normal limits. It involves a range of recommendations. These may include medical therapies such as tablets or insulin but just as important are diet, lifestyle, accurate glucose measurements and other therapies that will help the individual manage their blood glucose level.

Although different therapies will be used for Jennifer and John, the aims of blood glucose management will be similar. Initially therapy will aim to normalise the blood glucose level to make sure that the person feels well. Some symptoms, such as tiredness, may not have been recognised prior to therapy. In the long term near-normal blood glucose control is the aim. This is important to minimise the risk of developing complications, and means aiming for a blood glucose level as close to the normal range as possible, without the side-effects of drug therapy.

Both Jennifer and John will be aiming for a pre-meal blood glucose level of between 4 and 7 mmol/l and a post-meal glucose level of no higher than 11 mmol/l. These aims may not be the same in all patients because age, lifestyle, employment and pregnancy may alter these target levels; the targets will, therefore, need to be discussed and modified to suit each individual (see Chapters 9 and 10).

It is important that people feel well. It is also important that people understand why they are trying to achieve a particular range of blood glucose levels that may seem difficult to attain, especially if they feel well. It is not uncommon for someone to say that they feel well and therefore think their blood glucose level is satisfactory. Achieving tight blood glucose control can take a lot of effort and it is important that people feel able to care for their diabetes and make their own decisions about what they want to achieve. It is also important that support is provided. The level of support that a person may need varies over the years depending on age, life circumstances, particular life events that occur and other medical problems.

- Give an example of a life event that could alter support levels.
- One example is pregnancy (there are others too).

4.4.2 Medical management is more than just blood glucose control

For both Jennifer and John medical management involves not just looking after their blood glucose levels but also making sure that all other factors that influence the development of complications are assessed and treated. At the time of diagnosis, most people with Type 1 diabetes have had high blood glucose levels for a short period of time and complications are unlikely to be found. However, people with Type 2 diabetes may have had raised glucose levels for years and complications of diabetes are commonly found at the time of diagnosis. John may have had diabetes for some time. It is particularly important, therefore, to look for complications early on in his management. You will learn more about this subject in Chapters 5 and 6.

Although the initial care of people diagnosed with diabetes focuses on getting their blood glucose level back to normal, once this is achieved a full assessment of blood pressure, lipids (fats) in the blood and other parameters needs to be made and treatment given appropriately.

4.5 Blood-glucose-lowering therapies

There are a variety of therapies available to lower blood glucose levels. Insulin is an essential therapy for people with Type 1 diabetes.

● Why is insulin therapy essential in Type 1 diabetes?

● Type 1 diabetes is caused by an absence of insulin, therefore insulin must be provided.

● Is insulin therapy essential for Type 2?

● It is not always essential for Type 2.

People with Type 2 diabetes have a larger number of therapies available and may be treated by diet alone, diet with tablets and/or insulin. Many different combinations of therapy can be used depending on the individual's needs.

4.5.1 Insulin therapy

Insulin can only be given by injection. It is broken down by gut enzymes and if taken orally (by mouth) it does not work. This may change as more advanced therapies are developed. Many people, when first told they need to start injecting themselves with insulin, feel very anxious. You consider this issue in the next activity.

Activity 4.2 Anxieties about injecting insulin

Suggested study time 20 minutes

In Chapter 1 you considered how you felt when, or might feel if, you were diagnosed with diabetes. Now consider specifically that you have been told that you need to inject yourself – what questions and concerns would you have?

Are there specific concerns that you think Jennifer might have?

Comment

People have a lot to take in when diagnosed with Type 1 diabetes. There is also often a degree of urgency that adds to the anxiety. People are frequently given a life-changing diagnosis and started on insulin within a few hours. The diagnosis and treatment may take place in a specialist unit but it could take place within a busy Accident and Emergency unit.

What specific concerns would you have? You might be worried about the practicalities of the needle, how to inject and what could go wrong. You might also have questions about how many times a day and where on your body you would need to inject. You may also want to know whether you would always have to inject or if insulin could be given another way. These are all common questions that you would be right to ask and health care professionals should encourage and answer.

You might remember Jennifer associated her mother's death with starting insulin, so it is likely that she is scared that this will happen to her, too. It is most unlikely that there is a connection between the insulin therapy and her mother's death. However, this would need to be carefully explained to Jennifer.

Jennifer's mother had Type 2 diabetes and this is a progressive disorder; for many people it requires a change from tablets to insulin after a number of years. Also, other illnesses often cause an increase in blood glucose levels and tablets may become ineffective.

In the UK it is common to start someone who has been diagnosed with Type 1 diabetes on twice daily medium-acting insulin, e.g. currently (2005) Insulatard® or Humulin I® are used. The description 'medium-acting' refers to the length of time the insulin works for. Human insulin is generally used. Most human insulin is made **biosynthetically**, that is isolated from cells that have been programmed to produce insulin in a laboratory. In small letters after the insulin you may see a term such as emp. This refers to the method used to make the insulin; emp means that the insulin has been produced biosynthetically using bacteria. Some people use porcine (pig) or bovine (beef) insulin. These people were often started on these products before human insulin became available, and have not found changing to human insulin satisfactory. It is important to know how the insulin is manufactured because of religious and other beliefs that may influence their use.

- Insulins can be divided into three groups: short-acting insulins, which have a peak activity approximately 1–4 hours after being injected
- medium-acting insulins, which have a peak activity approximately 4–12 hours after being injected
- long-acting insulins, which last for 24 hours or more.

The short-acting insulins can be divided into two types: (a) quick-acting insulins, which are injected 20–30 minutes before a meal and last for several hours; examples are Actrapid® and Humulin S®; (b) very quick-acting insulins, which have been designed to have a very rapid onset. They can be injected at the time of eating, during a meal or even after eating; examples are Humalog® and NovoRapid®.

Medium-acting insulins such as Insulatard® or Humulin I® are usually taken either once or twice a day depending on the treatment programme (regimen) used. There are many types of insulin available that are a mixture of quick and medium acting. Mixtard® 30 is a mixture containing 30% Actrapid® and 70% Insulatard®.

Long-acting insulins have been available for many years. Insulin glargine and insulin detemir are examples of long-acting insulins.

Unless you are a health professional you will not need to remember the trade names of the different types of drug.

Many different combinations of insulin are used depending on the person's needs. Doses and types of insulin can be altered and adjusted until the best regimen is found. In Case Study 4.2 we return to Mr Idris to see how his changing needs were met.

Case Study 4.2

Mr Idris (see Case Study 2.2) was diagnosed with Type 1 diabetes two months ago. He initially started with two injections a day of medium-acting insulin. He is very active and found that when using this insulin his blood glucose level would be high in the morning, but low in the afternoon. He discussed his glucose level with his health care team and he decided he would prefer four injections a day, so that he could adjust his doses depending on his activity and diet. He now takes very quick-acting insulin with his meals and a long-acting insulin at bed time. This has helped him to control his glucose level better, especially when he plays sport.

Insulin is injected **subcutaneously**. This means that the insulin is injected to a level that is beneath the skin but not so deep that it reaches the muscles. A short, fine needle is used. The usual sites for injection are the thighs, hip area, abdomen, or outer arms (Figure 4.2).

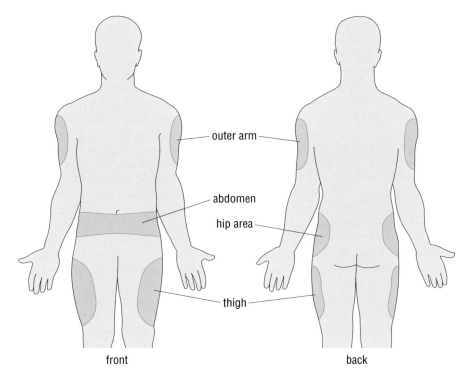

Figure 4.2 Recommended injection sites for insulin.

Insulin can be injected using a syringe with a needle or a pen device (Figure 4.3).

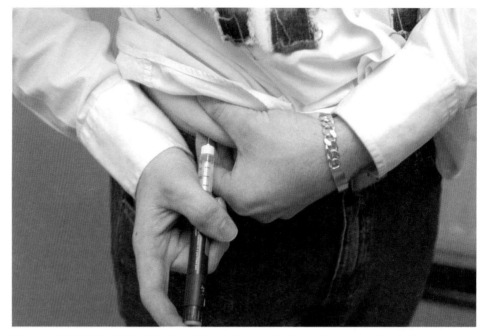

Figure 4.3 Patient injecting into the abdomen to show the correct technique.

There are different sized syringes and needles available. The syringes are designed to be used with a particular strength of insulin known as unit 100 insulin (100 units of insulin per ml)*. This is the usual strength of insulin in the UK. A 1 ml syringe can therefore inject up to 100 units; it is marked in 2 unit marks (Figure 4.4a). The 0.5 ml syringe can inject up to 50 units of insulin and is marked in 1 unit marks (Figure 4.4b). The syringe size is determined by the required dose. The needles attached to the syringes are either 8 or 12.7 mm in length. The 8 mm needle is long enough for most patients to be able to inject subcutaneously.

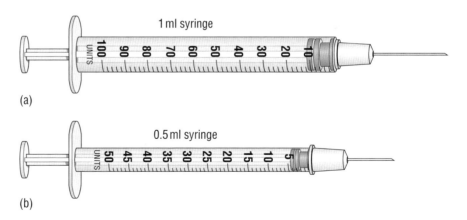

Figure 4.4 Diagrams of syringes showing markings and needle sizes (not to scale). (a) 1 ml syringe; (b) 0.5 ml syringe.

*A unit is an internationally agreed measure of activity (usually of a hormone).

Although people often start their treatment using a syringe with a vial of insulin, many people change to **pen devices** (Figure 4.5), especially when more complex insulin regimens are introduced. Some devices come pre-filled and others require cartridges containing pre-measured units of insulin. Needles for most devices are available separately. They are available in 5 mm, 8 mm and 12.7 mm lengths. Regimens vary across the country and some teams recommend a pen device straight away. There is no evidence to suggest that using a pen is better than a syringe, and practice should depend on the person's needs.

Pumps (Figure 4.6) that continuously deliver short-acting insulin are also available. Pumps have been found to be particularly effective for people who experience difficulty in controlling their blood glucose level as they provide an alternative to multiple injections (Diabetes Control and Complications Trial Research Group, DCCT, 1993). The pump delivers insulin to the body by a thin tube inserted just under the skin, usually on the abdomen, and delivers insulin 24 hours a day according to a programmed plan unique to the wearer. Using a pump can improve diabetes control, which is known to reduce risk of developing long-term complications of diabetes. There is national guidance (National Institute for Health and Clinical Excellence, NICE, 2003) available for deciding on the use of pumps and Diabetes UK also has further information.

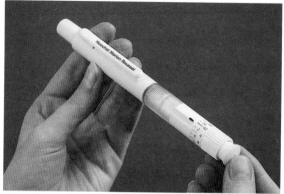

(a)

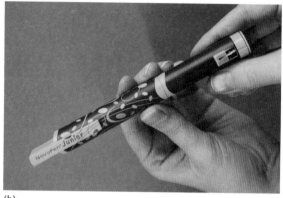

(b)

Figure 4.5 Commonly used pen devices for insulin delivery in (a) an adult, (b) a child. The dose is clicked up and shown on a dial.

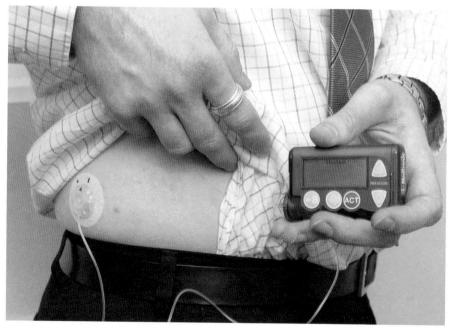

Figure 4.6 Insulin pump in use.

Currently insulin, pen devices, syringes and needles are available on prescription. However, the choice and availability varies from time to time and regionally. It would be sensible to find out what the current arrangements are, for items that you either use yourself or are commonly used locally.

> All people with Type 1 diabetes need to take insulin. They should never stop their insulin even if they are unwell and not eating.

Read Case Study 4.3 to find out how Jennifer manages with her insulin.

Case Study 4.3

Jennifer goes to the hospital to see a diabetologist and a diabetes specialist nurse (DSN). These specialist staff are not always available and some newly diagnosed people see Accident and Emergency and general medical staff. The DSN explains about diabetes and why Jennifer needs to start taking insulin, and shows her how to give herself an injection. This helps to give Jennifer confidence and she draws up her own insulin and injects for the first time. As Jennifer thought that going alone to the hospital would be difficult she brought her husband along with her. Her husband injects himself (with sterile water rather than with insulin) at the same time as Jennifer, which helps him to understand what the injection involves both emotionally and physically. They are both relieved that the first injection has been done and that they were able to do it. Both of them discuss their concerns and anxieties about injections.

Jennifer's doctor suggests that she should start on twice daily medium-acting insulin. The initial dose will be 8 units twice a day. This is a starting dose of insulin and will be adjusted depending on her blood glucose level, which she will need to monitor frequently. She is asked to inject in the morning before breakfast and in the evening before the evening meal. Jennifer has a regular routine and thinks that these injections will fit in. The nurse explains that Jennifer will need to know a lot about diabetes in due course but on the first visit only a limited amount of information is necessary. Jennifer will be seen at the hospital or diabetes clinic and she will not be admitted to the ward unless she is unwell.

The following is a list of useful information given to the patient at the first visit:
- How to inject.
- Where to inject.
- What to do with used needles – some areas provide and collect sharps boxes. Devices that break off and store needles are available. (These are discussed further in Chapter 6.) Needles can be reused by the same individual, although this is not recommended by the manufacturer. If a patient is in hospital the needles should not be reused.

- How to store insulin – in general, the insulin vial or pen being used can be kept at room temperature for up to 28 days. The vials or pens not being used should be stored in a refrigerator (but not frozen).

- Advice on remembering to store insulin safely, especially away from children.

- Information about driving. If Jennifer were a heavy goods vehicle driver, starting insulin would mean the loss of her large goods vehicle (LGV) licence.

- The importance of eating regular balanced meals until further dietary advice is available.

- How to recognise the symptoms of a low blood glucose level and how to treat it. The term 'hypo' is often used to indicate a state of hypoglycaemia.

- A warning that as glucose levels settle vision may become blurred, together with reassurance that the patient is not losing their sight and it will gradually return to normal.

4.5.2 Problems with insulin therapy

There can be an enormous variation in the day-to-day action of insulin due to its rate of absorption from the injection site and activity of the patient. The fastest absorption is from the abdomen and slowest from the thigh. Patients commonly ask why they have 'perfect' glucose levels one day but high or low the next. This is partly due to the action of insulin; for example, its effect can vary depending on the time of day it is injected. Pumps decrease some of this variability and some of the newer insulins available also have less variability.

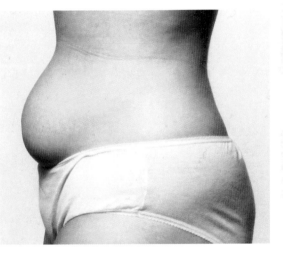

It is important that people who inject insulin vary the injection sites daily. Repeated injection into the same site may result in **lipohypertrophy**. Lipohypertrophy (Figure 4.7) is the term used to describe changes in fat beneath the skin, in which the fat becomes lumpy.

Figure 4.7 The effect of lipohypertrophy on the abdomen.

Lumpy fat can be seen, but it is also useful to feel the injection sites to detect more minor degrees of change. When lipohypertrophy does develop, the site should be avoided and injections at other sites encouraged, because the absorption of insulin becomes variable at lumpy sites.

Concerns about low blood glucose levels are common when starting insulin. People taking tablets can also experience low blood glucose levels. Jennifer may have particular concerns as she is a teacher and she may not want to risk having a hypo in front of her pupils. This worry may affect her ability to control her diabetes tightly.

Read Case Study 4.4 to find out about some other problems that can occur when taking insulin.

Case Study 4.4

Miss Williams, whom you met in Case Study 2.3, is 80 years old and has had diabetes for 50 years. She had no real problems until she moved to the nursing home where she now lives. As she does not do the cooking she is never sure what she is going to eat. When the meals arrive sometimes she just does not like the food and on other occasions she eats a lot. This has caused problems with both low and high blood glucose levels. She has also had problems receiving the injections at the right time because she has not been allowed to keep her own insulin and the drug-dispensing rounds are not at the times that she needs her injections.

Doses of insulin may vary enormously from one person to another. Some people may take 20 units per day; others may be taking more than 200 units per day. The dose taken is the dose that is right for that individual. The individual's dose may also vary from day to day depending on activity, diet and other factors. Unfortunately, even with lots of effort and attempts at fine-tuning the dose, the insulins available are not yet effective enough to stop people sometimes having high or low blood glucose levels.

4.5.3 Non-insulin therapies

You now move on to look at therapies other than insulin for lowering blood glucose level, starting with Activity 4.3.

Activity 4.3 Concerns about the diagnosis of diabetes

Suggested study time 30 minutes

Case Study 4.5 reintroduces John, who has Type 2 diabetes. In this activity you will be asked to compare the experiences of John with those of Jennifer.

As you read the Case Study think about both Jennifer and John and their different experiences of having diabetes diagnosed. Make brief notes on why they each may have problems coming to terms with the diagnosis. What concerns do you think you would have (do have) about having diabetes? How do you think this would affect the management of your diabetes?

Comment

Both Jennifer and John may have difficulty accepting the diagnosis, but this may be for different reasons, linked to the type of diabetes they have and their symptoms. In the last three chapters of this course you focus on the psychosocial impact of diabetes in detail; suffice it to say here, that there are many different factors that might impact on how each person with diabetes adjusts to their diagnosis and manages their condition.

John has no symptoms and so he may have problems accepting that there is anything wrong. On the other hand, there are all sorts of anxieties that he could have, for example concerns about his job, family, other people knowing and the occurrence of complications. It is important to discuss his concerns with him and explore what changes to his lifestyle he thinks he is able to make.

Jennifer does have symptoms of diabetes, and they will improve as her blood glucose level settles. However, she also has anxieties and concerns that need to be addressed.

Case Study 4.5

John's repeat fasting plasma glucose test result confirms the diagnosis of diabetes. His first introduction to diabetes is very different from that of Jennifer. Whereas Jennifer has symptoms of an illness, John feels fine. John will be seen at his local doctor's surgery by the practice nurse and his GP.

At John's initial visit the practice nurse tells him what Type 2 diabetes is and why it occurs. John is obese with a body mass index (BMI) of more than 30 kg/m^2. He is also hypertensive (has high blood pressure) with a raised cholesterol level (level of certain fats in the blood). She gives him advice about a healthy diet and exercise. John is a long-distance lorry driver and is worried about whether he can continue to drive (see Chapter 10). He is also not sure how he can change his diet and take exercise when so much of his time is spent driving a lorry.

It is important to recognise that people who have had symptoms before being diagnosed are often relieved that they know what is wrong with them, rather than living with uncertainty.

Both Jennifer and John, regardless of the specific type of diabetes they have, should aim to follow a healthy diet. In the next section we turn to this thorny subject to discover the dietary recommendations for people with diabetes.

4.5.4 Diet

Our diet is simply what we eat and drink. It does not mean that we are trying to lose weight. Some people say 'I am on a diet' meaning that they are on a weight-reducing diet or some other special diet to suit their needs. What we eat is very important and particularly important in people with diabetes, but actually we are all 'on a diet' of one sort or another. Our well-being is influenced by whether or not we eat a **balanced diet**. A balanced diet is one in which all the food groups are eaten in the quantities and proportions required by an individual to maintain health and normal body weight given their level of activity.

It is recommended that all people with diabetes should meet a dietitian to discuss their dietary needs. The recommended diet is based on the principles of a healthy diet that anyone could eat, and these recommendations are set out overleaf.

Recommendations

Dietitians often recommend frequent small meals. Some people go all day without eating and then eat a lot in the evening. Everyone is different and there may be reasons why people prefer to eat in a particular way. There are also times of the year, for example Ramadan, when people need to change the way they eat. Shift working, travel, etc. also means that eating habits need to be flexible.

Figure 4.8 is a representation known as the Balance of Good Health, which shows the main food groups and proportions needed for a balanced and healthy diet.

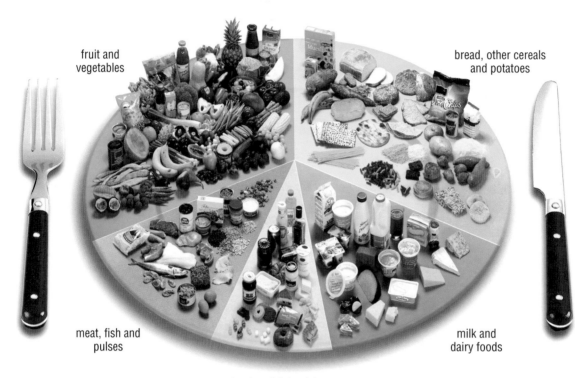

fruit and vegetables

bread, other cereals and potatoes

meat, fish and pulses

milk and dairy foods

food containing fat
food containing sugar

Figure 4.8 The Balance of Good Health, showing the recommended balance of foods in the diet.

- *Complex (starchy) carbohydrates* should be the main part of any meal. This food group includes bread, other cereals and potatoes, etc. Starchy carbohydrates are broken down slowly into sugars. Simple carbohydrates like glucose or fructose are usually absorbed more quickly as they do not need much breaking down.

- Foods containing sugar can be eaten by someone with diabetes although they are not encouraged if the person needs to lose weight. This is because sugar is often found in high fat foods such as chocolate and cakes which are very energy-rich and 'fattening'. Sugary drinks can put up blood glucose levels very quickly – think of the glucose tolerance test – and are not encouraged, but they are very useful for treating low blood glucose levels.

- *Fat* should be limited to help control weight. There are different types of fat. You may well have heard of saturated fat and unsaturated fat. Monounsaturated fats are a particular type of unsaturated fat and are found in olive oil and rapeseed oil. This type of fat is best for maintaining healthy cholesterol levels. (Monounsaturated fats may tend to increase the amount of 'good' (HDL) cholesterol; see Chapter 5.) Grilling, baking, and steaming are better options for cooking than frying. If fat is used for frying or other cooking, the use of monounsaturated fats is recommended.

- *Protein* should be eaten in moderation. Protein is found in meat, fish, eggs, nuts, pulses and dairy products. It is important to eat protein as it is a building block for cells, tissues and organs in the body. Occasionally people with kidney problems may be asked to limit how much protein they eat.

- *Fruit and vegetables* are an excellent source of dietary fibre, vitamins and minerals and at least five portions of fruit and vegetables each day are recommended. It should, however, be remembered that fruit contains sugars (fructose is a fruit sugar) and tends to increase blood glucose levels. People are often surprised at this because fruit is a healthy-eating option.

- *Alcohol* – this should be drunk in moderation. Suggested limits are 14 units per week for women and 21 units per week for men (a unit is equivalent to, for example, half a pint of beer or one glass (125 ml) of wine).

- *Salt* – the general population eats more salt than required as it is present in many processed foods. It is recommended that food should be tasted before salt is added, if necessary, at the table. Limiting salt intake can help decrease blood pressure.

Foods labelled as 'diabetic foods' are often very expensive. They are not recommended because people with diabetes can eat most ordinary food products.

All people, whether they have diabetes or not, should aim to have a body weight that is within the normal range for their height. In Activity 2.6 we looked at body mass index and how to calculate it. There are body mass index charts (Figure 4.9) that show the ideal weight range for an individual of any height.

People who are overweight need to reduce their calorie intake in a balanced way and to increase the amount of exercise that they take in order to burn up calories.

The term **glycaemic index (GI)** may not be familiar to you but it is being used more frequently. It is a way of allocating a score to different foods and drinks according to how much of an effect they will have on your blood glucose when eaten. For example, Lucozade®, which is absorbed quickly and will put your glucose level up quickly, has a high glycaemic index. For people with diabetes choosing slowly absorbed carbohydrates (low GI foods) can help even out fluctuations in blood glucose level. Table 4.1 shows the glycaemic index for a range of foods. It can be very difficult to guess whether certain carbohydrate foods have a high, medium or low glycaemic index. The GI of a food only tells you how quickly or slowly it raises the blood glucose when the food is eaten on its own. In practice we usually eat foods in combinations. Specialist advice in this area is available from dietitians and Glycaemic Index (2005) also contains further information.

Directions: Find your weight in kilograms (or pounds) along the top of the table and your height in metres (or ft and inches) along the left-hand side. Your BMI is the value at the point in the table where they intersect. *NB The chart does not apply to athletes, children, pregnant or lactating women.*

Weight	kg	45.5	47.5	50	52.3	54.5	57	59.1	61.4	63.6	65.9	68.2	70.5	72.7	75	77.3	79.5	81.8	84.1	86.4	88.6	90.9	93.2	95.5
	lb	100	105	110	115	120	125	130	135	140	145	150	155	160	165	170	175	180	185	190	195	200	205	210
Height m (ft, in)																								
1.52 (5'0")		19	20	21	22	23	24	25	26	27	28	29	30	31	32	33	34	35	36	37	38	39	40	41
1.55 (5'1")		18	19	20	21	22	23	24	25	26	27	28	29	30	31	32	33	34	35	36	36	37	38	39
1.57 (5'2")		18	19	20	21	22	22	23	24	25	26	27	28	29	30	31	32	33	33	34	35	36	37	38
1.60 (5'3")		17	18	19	20	21	22	23	24	24	25	26	27	28	29	30	31	32	32	33	34	35	36	37
1.63 (5'4")		17	18	18	19	20	21	22	23	24	24	25	26	27	28	29	30	31	31	32	33	34	35	36
1.65 (5'5")		16	17	18	19	20	20	21	22	23	24	25	25	26	27	28	29	30	30	31	32	33	34	35
1.68 (5'6")		16	17	17	18	19	20	21	21	22	23	24	25	25	26	27	28	29	29	30	31	32	33	34
1.70 (5'7")		15	16	17	18	18	19	20	21	22	22	23	24	25	26	27	28	29	29	29	30	31	32	33
1.73 (5'8")		15	16	16	17	18	19	19	20	21	22	22	23	24	25	25	26	27	28	28	29	30	31	32
1.75 (5'9")		14	15	16	17	17	18	19	20	20	21	22	22	23	24	25	25	26	27	28	28	29	30	31
1.78 (5'10")		14	15	15	16	17	18	18	19	20	20	21	22	23	23	24	25	25	26	27	28	28	29	30
1.80 (5'11")		14	14	15	16	16	17	18	18	19	20	21	21	22	23	23	24	25	25	26	27	28	28	29
1.83 (6'0")		13	14	14	15	16	17	17	18	19	19	20	21	21	22	23	23	24	25	25	26	27	27	28
1.85 (6'1")		13	13	14	15	15	16	17	17	18	19	19	20	21	21	22	23	23	24	25	25	26	27	27
1.88 (6'2")		12	13	14	14	15	16	16	17	18	18	19	19	20	21	21	22	23	23	24	25	25	26	27
1.91 (6'3")		12	13	13	14	15	15	16	16	17	18	18	19	20	20	21	21	22	23	23	24	25	25	26
1.93 (6'4")		12	12	13	14	14	15	15	16	17	17	18	18	19	20	20	21	22	22	23	23	24	25	25

underweight (BMI < 20.0) healthy weight (BMI 20.0–24.9)

overweight (BMI 25.0–29.9) obese (BMI 30.0–39.9) extremely obese (BMI 40 or above)

Figure 4.9 Body mass index chart for adults. Values are in kg/m^2.

Table 4.1 The glycaemic index for some common foods (adapted from Diabetes UK, 2000a).

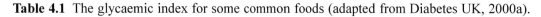

Low GI	Medium GI	High GI
apples, oranges, pears, peaches	honey	glucose
beans and lentils	jam	white and wholemeal bread
pasta (all types made from durum wheat)	Shredded Wheat®	brown rice, cooked
sweet potato, peeled and boiled	Weetabix®	white rice, cooked
sweetcorn	ice cream	cornflakes
porridge	new potatoes, peeled and boiled	baked potato
custard	white basmati rice, cooked	mashed potato
noodles	pitta bread	
All Bran®, Special K®, Sultana Bran®	couscous	

4.5.5 Exercise

In the UK, regular exercise is encouraged for everyone. Current recommendations (in 2005) are half an hour of moderate exercise at least five times per week. Exercise can include mowing the grass or doing the housework. Walking is exercise, of course, and is often preferred to going to the gym or participating in sports such as football or tennis. The easiest way to maintain regular exercise is to make it part of your everyday life.

● Can you suggest ways of increasing daily exercise as part of the normal routine?

◐ Examples are walking or cycling to work, or using the stairs rather than the lift.

Health care professionals can support people with diabetes in their efforts to exercise by helping to work out how they might incorporate exercise into their regular activities.

The benefits of exercise are enormous. It makes people feel good, helps with weight loss, decreases blood pressure, improves insulin sensitivity and can lower glucose levels. Exercise has also been shown to help prevent the development of Type 2 diabetes. Many of the research studies looking at exercise recommend regular exercise on several days a week for it to be beneficial. You gain benefits from exercise even if you start later in life.

When people with diabetes exercise, their glucose levels may fall too low (Case Studies 2.2 and 4.2) and, therefore, adjustments to diet and therapy may be required before exercising. Anxieties about unexpected changes in blood glucose levels are sometimes cited as a reason for not starting to exercise. Try the following activity to help you think about other barriers to changing lifestyle.

Activity 4.4 Barriers to changing lifestyle

Suggested study time 20 minutes

Think about the times that you, or someone you know, have tried to adopt a healthy lifestyle and stopped after a period of time. What have been the barriers to continuing?

Comment

A New Year is often a time when people say they are going to get fit and lose weight. However, many people find this difficult. People are busy, and find it easier to eat 'fast' foods such as pizza and pies, which are often high in calories. It is usually quicker and often easier to take the car rather than to walk or take a bus. Surveys have been done asking people why they do not exercise. Common reasons are:

I'm too fat.	I have an injury.
I'm not sporty.	I need to rest and relax in my spare time.
I haven't got the energy.	I haven't got the time.
There is no one to do it with.	I can't afford it.

Case Study 4.6 looks at how Jennifer and John are given advice about their diet and exercise.

Case Study 4.6

Both Jennifer and John discuss how changes in diet and exercise could help control their diabetes. The advice differs slightly as Jennifer is taking insulin and is not overweight. The advice and information will be personalised, but she will be encouraged to eat a healthy diet and take regular exercise. She will be reminded about the benefits of planning her exercise and making any necessary adjustments in her diet or insulin therapy, so that her blood glucose level doesn't fall too low.

It is very important for John to understand the benefits of losing weight and taking exercise. He needs to be supported with ideas of ways to eat healthily while working as a lorry driver so that he can decide what changes, if any, he would like to make. Should he take food with him or will he be able to buy food on the road? How can he exercise more when he needs to spend all day driving? These are all aspects for him and the health care professionals involved in his care to think through and work out together. John can then consider what changes he can and is prepared to make.

4.5.6 Tablet therapy

Tablets for lowering blood glucose levels are used by people with Type 2 diabetes. One of the main groups of tablet works by making you more sensitive to your own insulin. They therefore lower glucose levels by making your own insulin work better. They tend not to produce excessively low blood glucose levels. This group includes the drugs *biguanides* and *thiazolidinediones* (see below). A second group works by making your pancreas produce more insulin and can potentially produce low blood glucose levels if too much is taken. This group includes the *sulphonylureas* and *post-prandial regulators.* A third, smaller, group, the *alpha-glucosidase inhibitors*, work by delaying absorption of carbohydrate from the gut.

For all of these groups of drug to work, the pancreas needs to be able to produce insulin. With time many people with Type 2 diabetes find that their pancreas does not work very well and that the glucose-lowering drugs work less well. They then need to start taking insulin. Some people will be prescribed tablets and insulin together to lower their blood glucose levels. The doctor and person with diabetes discuss possible therapies and decide together which is most suitable. The various drug groups are described in more detail below.

Biguanides

Metformin is the only available drug in this class. It acts by decreasing liver glucose production and increasing the way glucose is used around the body. It increases insulin sensitivity. It is the drug of choice for patients with Type 2 diabetes who are overweight as it does not promote weight gain. Metformin has been shown to be effective in delaying the development of diabetes in people with impaired glucose tolerance (Section 2.4). It can be used early in diabetes therapy. It is less likely to cause hypoglycaemia if used alone.

Metformin can be used alone or in combination with other drug therapies that lower blood glucose levels, including insulin. It works very well with insulin therapy and often decreases the amount of insulin that someone with Type 2 diabetes needs.

Most tablets with medical benefits have some side-effects, e.g. rashes and headaches. These will usually only be apparent in some people. There are also reasons (**contraindications**) why tablets should not be used by certain people. It is helpful to tell people starting new therapies what side-effects they might experience, and whether they are likely to be important. Patient information leaflets are now regularly given out with tablets and are a useful information source.

Metformin is contraindicated (must not be used) if any of the following are present:

* renal (kidney) impairment
* significant liver impairment or damage, as measured by liver-function tests
* heart disease – the heart is not pumping well and the person is short of breath
* breast-feeding
* if undergoing any X-ray procedures that involve X-ray dyes
* significant illness such as pneumonia.

Side-effects may include:

* nausea
* diarrhoea
* rarely, a condition called lactic acidosis (a type of acid build-up in the blood)
* decreased vitamin B_{12} absorption.

Case Study 4.7 describes John's diabetes therapy.

Case Study 4.7

John has decided that he would like to try and change his lifestyle but is uncertain of how to do it and whether it is really worthwhile. He is given support and helped to make changes when he next sees his doctor. His GP suggests to him that he would also benefit from taking metformin. He agrees and begins by taking one tablet with breakfast as he is told this is the best way to minimise side-effects. Over several weeks he gradually increases his dose until he is taking one tablet with breakfast, lunch and dinner. Although he had some problems with wind he found that over the weeks this improved and then disappeared.

John is now managing to keep his blood glucose level within his target range (see Section 4.4).

Thiazolidinediones (often called 'glitazones')

These drugs work by reducing insulin resistance. They can be used on their own or in combination with either sulphonylureas or metformin. An example is rosiglitazone. The drug needs to be taken for several weeks before an effect on blood glucose is seen.

Cautions and contraindications are as follows:

- liver problems – liver blood tests should be done before therapy, then every 2 months for 12 months and then occasionally while the person stays on the drug
- heart failure
- combination with insulin is currently not allowed in the UK, but this may change
- pregnancy
- breast-feeding

Side-effects may include:

- weight gain
- gut disturbances
- leg swelling
- low numbers of blood cells (reduced blood count)
- low blood glucose levels in combination with sulphonylureas – these sometimes go unnoticed but can be indicated by headaches (see Section 7.3 on hypoglycaemia).

Sulphonylureas

Several sulphonylureas are available and the one recommended depends on local preference, age of patient, kidney function, etc. An example is gliclazide.

These drugs act by increasing the production of insulin from the pancreas. The patient, therefore, needs some pancreatic function for them to be effective. Sulphonylureas can be used in conjunction with most other therapies.

Cautions and contraindications include:

- severe liver failure
- kidney failure – sulphonylureas differ in the way they are broken down. Those broken down by the liver may be used with caution in kidney failure, e.g. tolbutamide and gliclazide
- breast-feeding.

Side-effects may include:

- low blood glucose levels
- weight gain, which can be very discouraging for people who are trying hard to lose weight
- rashes
- nausea
- liver abnormalities
- rarely, blood disorders.

Post-prandial regulators

'Post-prandial' means 'after a meal'. These drugs are so-called as their aim is to decrease the level of blood glucose that occurs in people with diabetes after eating a meal. The drugs stimulate insulin release from the pancreas. An example is repaglinide. They have a faster onset of action and shorter length of action than the sulphonylureas.

Cautions and contraindications include:

- Type 1 diabetes
- pregnancy
- breast-feeding
- kidney problems
- severe liver problems.

Post-prandial drugs have the disadvantage that they need to be taken with meals. As they need to be taken three or four times a day people often forget. However, this is seen as an advantage for people who eat only occasionally. If a meal is missed the dose is not taken which reduces the risk of low blood glucose levels that would tend to occur with sulphonylureas.

Side-effects include:

- abdominal pain
- diarrhoea
- constipation
- nausea
- vomiting.

Alpha-glucosidase inhibitors

Acarbose is the only drug available. It acts by delaying the absorption of carbohydrate across the gut wall.

Cautions and contraindications are:

- pregnancy
- breast-feeding
- gut disease
- kidney and liver disease.

Side-effects include:

- wind
- diarrhoea.

Acarbose should be prescribed at low doses and increased slowly to minimise side-effects. It should be taken with food. Side-effects often limit its usage.

The use of drugs in diabetes is a complex area and it is common for confusion and uncertainty to be experienced by people taking drugs for their diabetes. NICE have produced detailed guidance on the use of these drugs (a link to the guidelines is available from the course website).

An overriding principle should be that if you have concerns then try to find out more about the medication you are prescribed. Always ask the doctor or nurse who is involved with your care, and read the information that you get with the drugs. Keep an eye out for any changes in how you are feeling and go back to your GP or other health care provider as soon as you are unhappy about anything. You can also obtain more information about any drug on the internet. Activity 4.5 looks at some of these issues.

Activity 4.5   Finding out about drugs

Suggested study time 30 minutes

The purpose of this activity is to familiarise yourself with information on drugs in general, using one particular drug as an example. Look inside any packet of tablets that you might have: this might be paracetamol from your medicine cabinet at home, or a diabetes drug or something quite different. Read through the information leaflet and try to answer the following questions. What are the particular reasons for taking this drug? What is the recommended dose for the particular drug you are investigating? What are the contraindications?

A useful place to start finding out more extensively about drugs is the British National Formulary (BNF). This is regularly updated and is available online (a link is provided on the course website). Look up the details of your chosen drug on the BNF database. (You will probably need to register your details beforehand.)

Comment

Were you able to find the information on the use and contraindications of the drug you chose?

Although health care professionals get to know the medications they recommend very well, this is not always the case for people taking the medication. Many people never read the information leaflet that comes with all drugs. Hospital doctors and GPs often use one or two drugs regularly although there may be many available. This allows them and their staff to become familiar with any side-effects. For the person taking the tablets it can be useful to know the types of problem that can occur. They can then bring any concerns to the attention of their health care professional.

4.5.7 Problems with tablet therapy for diabetes

It is common for people to forget to take their drugs. The more complicated the regimen and the more drugs people take, the more likely this is to occur. It is important for people to review their drug-taking regularly. People may not be able to tell that they have not taken their drugs as they simply do not remember. Before adding further tablets and making drug regimens more complex it is important for health care professionals to ensure that drugs are being taken appropriately.

It is important that no blame is attached if problems occur. We all forget things and it is important for health care professionals to encourage and support the patient by giving practical advice about how to remember to take their tablets, for example:

- having them in a place where you will see them at the time you need them

- using special boxes where you put your week's tablets in advance – you can then see if you have taken them at the end of the day

- writing on a calendar in advance when you are going to need another prescription.

Pick up tips by asking people (friends, family and colleagues) how they give themselves cues to remember to take their drugs. Do you have tips you could share with friends and health care professionals? We can all learn from each other. How would you help John to remember to take his tablets? He is frequently away from home. If Jennifer took insulin at lunch time, how could you help her make sure that she had insulin available at school?

4.6 Complementary therapies and diabetes

Most of the complementary therapies available are herbal remedies or nutritional supplements including vitamins, minerals, and related compounds such as antioxidants. Some of those commonly used in complementary treatments include:

- cinnamon
- chromium
- magnesium
- vanadium
- fenugreek
- ginseng
- bitter melon/karela.

None of them have proven efficacy on their own and should be used with caution under appropriate medical advice as they may interact both with each other and with conventional medicines, to give unexpected results. Although there is no scientific or clinical evidence to show that acupuncture or acupressure can cure diabetes (Diabetes UK, 2000b), some people have found acupuncture useful for helping relieve pain in their feet due to changes in the nerves caused by diabetes. Therapies such as aromatherapy and reflexology often make people feel better in themselves, though have not been shown to have any specific effects on lowering blood glucose.

It is important for all those in the diabetes care team to know whether someone is taking complementary medicine as the therapies may interact with prescribed drugs, in particular increasing the risk of hypoglycaemia. Support and help from health care professionals remains important as illustrated in Case Study 4.8.

Case Study 4.8

Mrs Princess Rodgers (see Case Study 2.1) has never liked taking conventional medicines and has decided to make changes to her diet and lifestyle to see if she can treat her diabetes herself. She has read in a magazine that chromium can help and has just started taking it. Over the years she has developed a good relationship with the practice nurse at the health centre. As a result, when Mrs Rodgers goes in for her next appointment she feels able to tell the nurse about what she is taking.

The nurse is glad that Mrs Rodgers has told her about this and puts the information in her notes so that the whole team is made aware of it.

4.7 Medical management of pregnancy and diabetes

Having children is a big decision for anyone. If you are a woman with diabetes (Type 1 or Type 2) and are planning a family, make sure that you ask for pregnancy planning advice from your diabetes care team. Before conception and throughout your pregnancy it is essential that you keep your blood glucose under good control so that the chances are high of conceiving and delivering a healthy baby. As with all pregnancies the first few weeks are important for the baby's physical development and so you need to be particularly careful during this period. Avoid medications that are contraindicated in pregnancy, i.e. are not advisable to take because they have known effects on the baby's natural development inside the womb (as you saw above, these medications include tablets taken by those with Type 2 diabetes). Look after yourself by:

- eating a healthy diet
- if you smoke, trying to stop
- decreasing your intake of alcohol (or even better stopping it altogether)
- having your eyes checked regularly
- checking with your doctor about taking folic acid as sometimes a higher dose than normal is recommended.

Diabetes UK (2005) gives more information about pregnancy and diabetes (see also Chapter 10, Section 10.9).

- Are tablet therapies contraindicated in pregnancy? (See Section 4.5.6.)
- Insulin usually replaces tablets during pregnancy. Medical advice should be taken to check that any tablet therapies are appropriate during pregnancy. If in doubt about your own medication, seek medical advice immediately.

Read the stories of Jennifer and Mrs Shah in Case Study 4.9 which focus on some of the preparations for pregnancy in women with diabetes.

Case Study 4.9

Jennifer, whom you met earlier, has one child. She and her husband want to try for another baby. The diabetes nurse talks things through with Jennifer so that she can decide if it is something that she is ready for and wants to do. The nurse explains that before becoming pregnant Jennifer should try to achieve good blood glucose control. One way in which this can be assessed is by measuring the glycated haemoglobin (HbA_{1c}) level (this is explained in Section 5.3.4). An HbA_{1c} of 7% or less will reduce the increased risk that mothers with diabetes have of their baby having problems.

The nurse also explains that she will have to do many finger-prick blood tests during the pregnancy to provide information to allow her to keep tight control of her blood glucose level. Jennifer will attend the clinic at the hospital many times during the pregnancy to ensure that she will have a healthy baby.

Jennifer knows that there will be a lot of people helping and supporting her through the pregnancy. She is delighted to hear that she will be able to breast-feed if she wants to.

Mrs Shah, whom you met in Case Study 2.6, developed gestational diabetes during her third pregnancy when she weighed 110 kg and took no exercise. At the end of the pregnancy she was very relieved to find that her glucose tolerance test was not in the diabetic range as both her parents had diabetes. However, she knew that if she did not change her lifestyle that it would not be long before she had diabetes. She decided that before any future pregnancies she would lose weight and take more exercise. Over two years she lost 20 kg. She was able to stop her blood pressure tablets. At the start of her fourth pregnancy she had a glucose tolerance test which was normal, and a repeat test at 28 weeks was also normal. Mrs Shah was delighted.

4.8 Other therapies for people with diabetes

The medical management of people with diabetes involves more than just lowering their blood glucose level. The aim is to prevent or at least delay the development of the complications of diabetes. These complications are discussed in detail in Chapters 5 and 6. There are risks of two types.

- Recall from Chapter 2 the two types of complication.

- First, there are the risks that people with diabetes may have of developing problems with their kidneys, eyes and nerves (microvascular complications). Secondly there are the risks that all people have, but which are higher in people with diabetes. This second group includes problems of heart attacks, strokes and other problems with circulation (macrovascular complications) (Section 2.4).

The risks of developing all these complications are decreased if good blood glucose levels are maintained over the years. The risk is not really affected if glucose is high for short periods of time, for example when you are unwell, or the odd day here and there.

The risks are also decreased if the blood pressure and level of fats (lipids) in the blood are kept as normal as possible. In the following sections you read about how blood pressure and lipid levels in the blood can be improved.

4.8.1 Controlling blood pressure

Read Case Study 4.10 to see what was recommended for John's blood pressure.

Case Study 4.10

At John's next clinic he and his doctor discuss his blood pressure. John had a high blood pressure of 160/110 mmHg when he first visited his doctor; however, today his blood pressure is 156/94 mmHg. The doctor wonders if John had been anxious at his first visit. The doctor explains that although his blood pressure is lower today it is still higher than it should be. John has **hypertension**, i.e. repeatedly elevated blood pressure that exceeds 140/90 mmHg. John should aim to decrease his blood pressure to a target of 140/90 mmHg. There are several things that he can do; for example, losing weight, taking regular exercise and decreasing the amount of salt in his diet will all help. John has already discussed ways he can change his lifestyle, with his doctor and practice nurse. He knows that if his blood pressure remains high over several weeks his doctor will recommend drug therapy.

Drugs are commonly used to lower blood pressure. Many different types of drug are used and, like all drugs, they have pros and cons. Except in certain circumstances, it is best to find drugs that suit the patient and that they are happy to take. It is common for people to need three or even four different types of drug to lower their blood pressure. There are many guidelines available for the management of hypertension, and they are frequently updated as new drugs and study results become available.

4.8.2 Reducing blood lipids

Blood lipids are fats found in the blood. **Cholesterol** is a type of lipid that can be found in two different forms (Section 5.5). Cholesterol levels normally range from 3.5 to 6.5 mmol/l; ideally the level should be about 5 mmol/l. Guidelines for treating high cholesterol in people with diabetes are available from NICE. Lifestyle changes in diet and exercise can help to lower the level of fats in the blood and are the first option for many people. Tablets are also often used. The most common groups of drugs used are statins and fibrates. Like all drugs, they can have side-effects such as muscle cramps, and patients are usually warned when starting the tablets to report any problems. To find a full list of contraindications and side-effects if you are interested, go to the British National Formulary website (a link is provided from the course website).

Read Case Study 4.11 to find out what was recommended for John.

Case Study 4.11

John has a cholesterol level of 8 mmol/l. Although he is only 30 years old, treatment may be recommended. It is important to know his family history, because a family history of heart problems at a young age would suggest that he might also be at high risk of heart problems and in this case treatment would be recommended.

If a person already has heart disease or problems with their circulation then they will benefit from treatment, whatever their cholesterol level. John has no evidence of problems with his circulation, and he does not smoke. His risk of having a heart attack over the next 10 years is low and John and his doctor decide that they will continue with lifestyle changes at the moment.

You might be wondering how many different types of tablet John needs to take, or why all this treatment is needed. If John starts metformin he will be taking three tablets a day. Add to this, perhaps three or four different types of tablet for his blood pressure and he could be taking up to seven tablets a day. This could be very hard to remember. John might forget to take his tablets when he was out at work or even when he was at home. Lowering blood glucose level is important to help prevent the complications of diabetes, but lowering blood pressure and cholesterol level are just as important. However, it is also essential that health care professionals recognise that taking medication isn't always top of the list of priorities, as people try to live their lives in the ways most appropriate for them. In addition to the drug therapy, John must also remember to test his blood glucose, and attend clinics to monitor other aspects of health such as blood pressure and cholesterol level, all of which require time and attention that may not be easy to find. Section 4.9 takes a brief look at monitoring.

4.8.3 Aspirin

People with heart or other circulation problems are usually offered aspirin at a dose of 75 mg per day. This is a smaller dose than taken for headaches, etc. This small dose of aspirin has been shown to decrease the risk of having another heart attack or stroke, as it reduces the risk of blood clots forming.

Aspirin is also offered to people who have not had heart problems but who are at high risk. Many people with diabetes fall into this group. Before taking aspirin, as with any drug, the risks and benefits need to be assessed. Blood pressure should be well controlled and it should not be prescribed to people with stomach ulcers, bleeding disorders or allergy to aspirin.

4.9 How do you know if things are well controlled?

This question will be discussed in more detail in some of the other chapters, but it is useful to think about it now. There are several ways to get information about what is happening to blood glucose levels (Section 2.4). First, finger-prick tests can let you know what your blood glucose is at any time. Second, urine tests can be used. Urine tests do not tell you what your glucose level is at the time of testing but are an indication of whether glucose levels are reasonable. Third, the glycated haemoglobin HbA_{1c} blood test can be done at a laboratory. This test can give a measure of glucose levels over the last 2–3 months. Any of these tests and any combination can be used, depending on the individual and their needs.

Blood pressure is monitored either at the hospital or GP surgery. Some people now have their own monitors at home. Lipid levels are measured by blood tests at the surgery or hospital.

Case Study 4.12 shows how different people might monitor their blood glucose levels.

Case Study 4.12

It is important that the health care professionals working with Jennifer and John discuss with them how they want to monitor their diabetes. There is no point in asking them to do things they do not want to do. It is also important to make sure that if they do finger-prick tests they know what to do with the results. It is likely that Jennifer will monitor her glucose level with finger-prick tests as this will allow her to change her insulin from day to day. John, who is taking metformin, may also want to check his blood glucose level. He will not be altering his treatment from day to day, but he might find that knowledge of his blood glucose level is useful to help him learn the effects of eating different foods and increasing his activity levels.

4.10 Risk reduction

Risk was discussed in Section 2.6.2. Much of the management of diabetes and its complications relates to risk reduction. The person with diabetes needs to be part of the decision-making process. This is very important or they will not understand why they need to take so many tablets. The tablets often have side-effects and may make them feel worse rather than better. The reduction in blood glucose levels to targets such as an HbA_{1c} of less than 7% often causes problems associated with low glucose levels. Blood pressure tablets may make people feel tired, cough or feel dizzy. Some of the therapies used may cause impotence. It is important that the person on drug therapy to control blood pressure is aware of the risks and benefits of the various therapies. Suppose they decide that they do not want to lower their cholesterol by taking a tablet? As long as they are fully informed, their decision should be respected – this is an integral aspect of working as part of a diabetes team, with the person with diabetes at the centre.

4.11 Summary of Chapter 4

You have now reached the end of Chapter 4, which has discussed the medical management of diabetes. There are many ways to manage diabetes and experiences differ around the UK. The chapter has covered commonly used therapies and how decisions are made about using them in diabetes care. You've also considered the management of blood pressure and blood lipid levels, and the idea that the medical management of diabetes is much more than just blood glucose control. The next chapter covers more about the medical side of diabetes – this time the annual review. It also looks in more detail at the person's own role in monitoring their diabetes.

Questions for Chapter 4

Question 4.1 (Learning Outcome 4.2)

What are the differences in treatment options for someone with Type 1 compared with someone with Type 2 diabetes?

Question 4.2 (Learning Outcome 4.3)

How do the two types of short-acting insulin differ?

Question 4.3 (Learning Outcome 4.4)

Briefly discuss how diet and exercise can be used to help manage Type 2 diabetes.

Question 4.4 (Learning Outcome 4.5)

What is the drug of choice for people with Type 2 diabetes who are overweight?

Question 4.5 (Learning Outcome 4.6)

What is the benefit of using aromatherapy for someone with diabetes?

Question 4.6 (Learning Outcome 4.7)

Why do people with diabetes often receive treatment for their blood pressure and cholesterol levels?

References

Diabetes Control and Complications Trial Research Group (DCCT) (1993) 'The effects of intensive treatment of diabetes on the development and progression of long-term complications in insulin-dependent diabetes mellitus', *New England Journal of Medicine*, **329** (14), pp. 977–986.

Diabetes UK (2000a) *Glycaemic index* [online] Available from: http://www.diabetes.org.uk/faq/GI.htm (Accessed June 2005).

Diabetes UK (2000b) *Alternative remedies – no miracle cure* [online] Available from: http://www.diabetes.org.uk/news/sept00/herbal.htm (Accessed June 2005).

Diabetes UK (2005) *During your pregnancy* [online] Available from: http://www.diabetes.org.uk/pregnancy/during.htm (Accessed June 2005).

Glycaemic Index (2005) [online] Available from: http://www.glycaemicindex.com/ (Accessed June 2005).

National Institute for Health and Clinical Excellence (2003) *Full guidance on the use of continuous subcutaneous insulin infusion for diabetes* [online] Available from: http://www.nice.org.uk/page.aspx?o=58214 (Accessed June 2005).

CHAPTER 5

MONITORING RISK FACTORS FOR DIABETES COMPLICATIONS

Learning Outcomes

When you have completed this chapter you should be able to:

5.1 Define and use, or recognise definitions and applications of, each of the terms printed in **bold** in the text.

5.2 List the investigations that should form part of a diabetes annual review.

5.3 Discuss the role of different diabetes team members in performing the investigations for an annual review.

5.4 Appreciate the range of results for the various tests carried out at the annual review.

5.5 Explain which risk factors are associated with particular diabetes complications.

5.6 Outline how the person with diabetes can use the annual review to improve their diabetes control.

5.1 Introduction

After reading Chapters 1 and 4 you should have a good understanding about the processes that cause diabetes and how Type 1 and Type 2 diabetes are treated. You have read about the signs and symptoms of the condition, and should appreciate how they would affect the day-to-day life of that person.

The aim of managing diabetes, therefore, is to enable affected people, as far as possible, to feel well enough to live the sort of life they would have lived if they did not have the condition. However, apart from improving the quality of life of the person with diabetes, the correct management of both types of diabetes reduces the risks of the long-term complications that can develop if the condition is poorly controlled. This chapter examines the factors that increase these risks, how they are monitored, and who performs the tests associated with these risks.

5.2 Assessing diabetes complication risk factors

The following story (Case Study 5.1) illustrates that diabetes care is about more than checking your blood glucose level regularly. However, it can be difficult for people to understand why certain tests need to be taken and what the results mean. This can lead to them not following treatment, or indeed not even having the tests done.

Case Study 5.1

Mrs Begum attends a hospital diabetes clinic (such as that signposted in Figure 5.1) for her diabetes annual review. She does not speak English, so she has brought her 14-year-old daughter with her to interpret. She cannot understand why she has been asked to attend the clinic because she only has 'mild' diabetes, treated with tablets. The clinic is so crowded, with people who look much sicker than she is. She does not feel she has anything wrong with her, because she does not feel ill. When she eventually gets to see the doctor, he tells her she must take some more tablets to control her blood cholesterol, because the results of a previous blood test showed it was high.

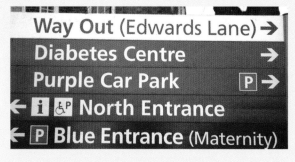

Figure 5.1 Most hospital directions are in English. Finding your way around a hospital is sometimes difficult even if you are able to read English.

Try to imagine what it is like for someone like Mrs Begum (Case Study 5.1) attending a busy diabetes clinic, and not understanding what is being said or done. For example, what difficulties do you think can arise when a family member is used to interpret in this situation? Why does Mrs Begum think she has 'mild' diabetes? Do you think she will take the cholesterol-lowering tablets?

The diabetes annual review consists of numerous tests, which can be confusing or disconcerting for anyone with diabetes who does not understand what they are for. This chapter, along with Chapter 6, describes what these tests are, why they are important, and the purpose of them. Mrs Begum may not get a clear explanation from her daughter who is interpreting for her. This may be because the daughter does not understand the explanation given to her by the doctor, or it may be because her daughter wants to protect her mother from worrying about the results of the tests. This may be the reason why Mrs Begum believes she has 'mild' diabetes. Alternatively, her doctor or nurse may have told her that she has 'mild' diabetes. This can unfortunately happen sometimes in the mistaken belief that Type 2 diabetes is somehow not as serious as Type 1 diabetes, because usually it can be managed, at least in the early stages, by diet or diet and tablets rather than requiring insulin injections.

As you will see in the following chapters, all people with diabetes are at risk of diabetes complications if their diabetes is not controlled. The good news is that the risk factors and early signs of this damage can be picked up at the diabetes annual review, and then the person with diabetes can work with their diabetes team to prevent or limit the damage. You can see, therefore, that without an understanding of what cholesterol is, and what damage it can do, Mrs Begum may not take her cholesterol-lowering tablets.

5.2.1 Discovering the risks

We have already seen that the incidence of diabetes is dramatically increasing both nationally and worldwide. This is of great concern because of the debilitating day-to-day effects of the condition if it is not controlled, but in particular, because of the long-term damage that diabetes causes to blood vessels and nerves in the body.

In the short term, people with poorly controlled diabetes can suffer any or all (or, in fact, none) of the following complications:

- tiredness and lethargy
- depression and change of mood
- thirst
- passing large amounts of urine frequently (a condition known as **polyuria**)
- loss of weight
- genital itching.

Sometimes, as with Mrs Begum, there are no obvious signs or symptoms of the condition. This can make it difficult to see the diabetes as serious and so taking tablets regularly or attending clinics for diabetes checks may not be seen as important.

However, the possible long-term complications (irrespective of any short-term complications) include:

- coronary heart disease (CHD), which includes angina and heart attacks
- cerebrovascular disease (strokes)
- nephropathy (damage to the kidney which can lead to kidney failure)
- peripheral vascular disease (which can lead to gangrene of the feet)
- retinopathy (damage to the blood vessels in the retina at the back of the eye)
- autonomic neuropathy (damage to nerves which can lead to erectile dysfunction (i.e. impotence), chronic diarrhoea, and other problems)
- peripheral neuropathy (damage to nerves to the extremities, causing painful or numb feet).

The investigations for these complications are explored in more detail in Chapter 6. Much of the focus of diabetes management is based on the early detection of these complications and their prompt treatment. However, just as important is the detection of factors in the person with diabetes that increase their risk of developing such damage. By correcting these risk factors, the chance of developing diabetes complications can be avoided, delayed, or the complications reduced in severity. The checks for these risk factors are included in the diabetes annual review.

What are the risk factors? High blood glucose (hyperglycaemia, which you met in Chapter 2) does cause the short-term complications described above, and contributes to some of the long-term damage, particularly to nerves and small blood vessels. As the blood vessels involved are small, these are called microvascular complications. Retinopathy is an example of a microvascular complication. However, high blood glucose is not the only cause of diabetes damage. High blood pressure (hypertension; see Section 5.6) and abnormal blood fat levels (dyslipidaemia; see Section 5.5) are also major contributing factors particularly in the development of complications such as CHD and cerebrovascular disease. These are known as large blood vessel diseases or macrovascular complications because of the blood vessels affected. (Microvascular and macrovascular complications were introduced in Section 2.4.)

● What other factors increase the risk of heart attacks and strokes in the general population?

● You probably thought of smoking, lack of physical activity, being overweight, excessive alcohol intake, an unhealthy diet consisting of high fat, high sugar, high salt, and a lack of fibre.

These factors are all important when considering the risk someone with diabetes has of developing diabetes complications. Other risks may be less obvious and include a difficult social situation, low income level, poor learning ability, a lack of knowledge in self-management of diabetes, old age, mental health problems and stress.

However, that is not to say that every person with diabetes will develop complications if they have high blood pressure, poor long-term blood glucose control and high cholesterol levels. People often cite the person they know who has had long-term high blood glucose but has never developed eye disease (retinopathy), for example. However, many medical studies over the years tell us that there is a greater likelihood of developing diabetes complications if the condition is not well controlled. A complete picture of these factors is therefore crucial to assess the person: to guide medication choice, to identify education needs, to offer other interventions such as advice on giving up smoking, but most importantly, to give the person with diabetes a clear and honest view of their risk so they can make choices about how they manage the condition.

5.2.2 The diabetes annual review

The function of the diabetes annual review is to identify risk factors. The GP or a doctor in the hospital diabetes team may perform this review, while other members of the team, for example the practice nurse in the GP surgery, or the diabetes care technician in the diabetes clinic, carry out many of the tests.

Although some of the risk factors can be identified by physical tests (examples include blood tests to check cholesterol level, or measuring blood pressure), much of the information required to judge risk factors (such as dietary and smoking history, or home blood glucose monitoring results) is obtained by careful discussion between the health care professionals and the person with diabetes. (See Case Study 5.2.)

Case Study 5.2

Janet has had Type 2 diabetes for four years. She takes her diabetes tablets regularly each day, tries to eat a healthy diet, and usually has a brisk walk on most days. She checks her blood glucose level with a meter several times a week, and feels satisfied that her diabetes control is within the target range she agreed with the doctor. She has arrived for her annual review with a urine test, her medications, and her blood glucose record book. She had some blood tests taken two weeks ago so the results would be available to discuss with her doctor. Although she feels well, she is keen to find out if her diabetes is as well controlled as she thinks it is.

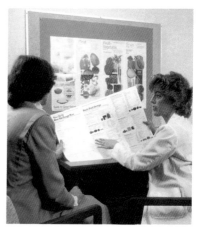

Figure 5.2 As part of an annual review, the person with diabetes sees a number of health care professionals, including a dietitian.

You can see then, that an annual review is a team effort, with the person with diabetes as the focus (Figure 5.2).

Activity 5.1 Sharing personal information

Suggested study time 10 minutes

It is important that people with diabetes feel able to share information with their health care team, about their lifestyles and the difficulties they may be facing as they try to make changes.

Describe to someone the food you ate yesterday. Make a note of their reactions to what you had eaten and any responses they give. Did the person react in a non-judgemental way or did you feel they disapproved of any of the foods you ate? How did you know? Did they use words like 'naughty' or did you notice a change in their facial expression?

Comment

We've suggested discussing food for this activity because diet can be an emotive subject, with many people having a reasonable knowledge about what they should be eating, and feeling guilty if they are not using this knowledge. Hopefully, every health care professional, when asking the patient to share honest information, will ensure privacy and confidentiality and receive information in a non-judgemental way (we discussed communication skills in Section 1.5). Comments like 'what?!' and 'really?' express disbelief and incredulity, and therefore are judgemental. If you have diabetes this may discourage you from sharing information, which may create barriers to having useful conversations with health professionals.

Apart from diet, information on many of the risk factors mentioned above needs to be obtained through discussion with the person with diabetes and/or their partner or carer. This process is described as taking the patient's history. It includes collecting information on smoking history and units of alcohol consumed, family history of diabetes and related diseases like heart problems, and the amount of exercise taken weekly. It is often done formally and noted in the medical records by a doctor, but is also done informally, for example by the nurse or diabetes care technician asking how someone is managing with dietary changes when weighing them at the clinic. Some information can be more difficult to obtain, particularly if it relates to stressful situations at home that may impact on other risk factors like adherence to a healthy diet or number of cigarettes smoked. This information may be offered later when a trusting relationship has developed between the health care professional and the person with diabetes.

- What could prevent you giving information to a doctor or nurse at the clinic?

- You may have thought of several factors, but probably a lack of privacy and trust will be among them. You may not want to discuss the number of cigarettes you smoke for example, if you think the doctor will reprimand you.

5.2.3 What monitoring is carried out at the annual review?

The diabetes annual review consists of a series of tests to monitor risk factors as well as the presence of any signs of diabetes complications. It also involves an assessment of the self-management skills of the person with diabetes, and their understanding and control of blood glucose. It therefore gives the opportunity for the early detection of diabetes complications and identification of risk factors for developing them – these risk factors are outlined in the following sections.

5.3 Monitoring blood glucose levels

Most people with diabetes are encouraged to keep their day-to-day blood glucose level between 4 and 7 mmol/l before meals. This is very similar to the blood glucose range of someone who does not have diabetes. However, this can be very difficult to achieve, and if you have diabetes, you should agree the ideal range for you with your diabetes team.

Two large diabetes research trials have shown that by maintaining a blood glucose range as near to the normal range as possible, the chances of developing long-term complications can be prevented, reduced or delayed. These trials were conducted in the **Diabetes Control and Complications Trial** (**DCCT**, 1993; see Box 5.1) and the **UK Prospective Diabetes Study** (**UKPDS**, 1998; see Box 5.2).

Box 5.1 The Diabetes Control and Complications Trial (DCCT)

This trial compared people with Type 1 diabetes who had intensive treatment to keep very good control of their blood glucose level, with people with Type 1 diabetes who had conventional treatment, and did not manage to achieve such good control. Intensive treatment involved four injections of insulin daily, frequent home blood glucose testing, regular visits to clinics, and telephone calls from diabetes nurses. The trial, which reported in 1993, was conducted in the USA over a period of nine years, with over 1000 people involved. It demonstrated very clearly that keeping good control of blood glucose dramatically reduced the risk of developing diabetes complications involving small blood vessels (i.e. microvascular complications), and slowed the progress of damage in people who already had complications like diabetic retinopathy (eye disease) and nephropathy (kidney disease).

Box 5.2 The UK Prospective Diabetes Study (UKPDS)

This study looked at the effect of blood glucose (and blood pressure) control in people with Type 2 diabetes. It was carried out over 20 years in the UK, reported in 1998, and involved over 3000 people. Like the results from the DCCT, it also showed that keeping good control of blood glucose reduced damage to small blood vessels and nerves. However, it concluded that even with a lot of support from the diabetes team, it can actually be very difficult to achieve good control.

The evidence from these two studies has been used to encourage people with diabetes to make and maintain lifestyle changes, take medication regularly, and to adjust insulin doses or seek advice if their blood glucose is not staying within their agreed limits. Assessing whether this is being achieved can be done in two ways:

- self-monitoring of blood glucose (Section 5.3.1) or for the presence of glucose in the urine (Section 5.3.2)

- regular monitoring of HbA_{1c} (glycated haemoglobin, Section 5.3.4).

5.3.1 Self-monitoring of blood glucose

Many people with diabetes are encouraged to monitor their blood glucose as it gives them immediate feedback to help them in the day-to-day management of the condition. It can help them to make decisions about lifestyle changes and choices, and to adjust their medication as required (Figure 5.3). It can therefore be a powerful education and empowerment tool if the person using it has been trained properly in how to do the test correctly and to know what to do with the test results. (Empowerment is an important concept in diabetes management and involves people managing their condition themselves, and making informed choices about their treatment.) However, at the time of writing (2005), there is considerable controversy about whether only people on particular diabetes treatments should be encouraged to do the tests. This is because the cost of the blood testing equipment is relatively high, and in some areas, more money is being spent on the equipment than on the tablets used to treat diabetes. Unfortunately, many people test their blood glucose regularly but do not use the results constructively (often because they have not been shown how to adjust their medication or where to access advice), and therefore the expense of the tests is not justified by an improvement in blood glucose control and a reduction in diabetes complications.

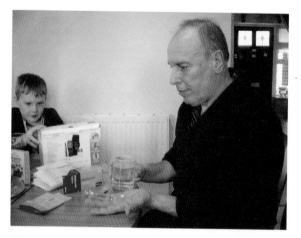

Figure 5.3 People with diabetes adjust their medication as required depending on their blood glucose level.

Activity 5.2 What does Diabetes UK, which represents people with diabetes, say about self-management?

Suggested study time 20 minutes

Look at the Diabetes UK website (accessible from the course website) and read the position statement on 'Glucose Self-monitoring in Diabetes' (Diabetes UK, 2003). This paper is available on the course DVD-ROM.

Comment

You will see that Diabetes UK takes the stance that all people with diabetes should be able to test their blood glucose as often as they feel is necessary. However, the National Health Service has a limited budget, and money spent in one area of care means less money for another area. **Primary Care Trusts (PCTs)**, which control budgets for prescribing, may try to limit the number of blood glucose strips being prescribed by the GPs in their locality. Primary Care Trusts are made up of GPs and other health care professionals and are responsible for planning health care services for a local population.

To monitor their blood glucose, people may be given, or may purchase from a pharmacy, a **blood glucose meter**. This is a device for analysing the glucose content of a small sample of capillary blood, usually obtained from a finger, which is placed on a disposable testing strip and then inserted into the meter. There is a variety of meters available (Figure 5.4), each using a particular blood glucose-testing strip. The strips are available in containers of 50, and are supplied on prescription from the patient's GP via their local pharmacist.

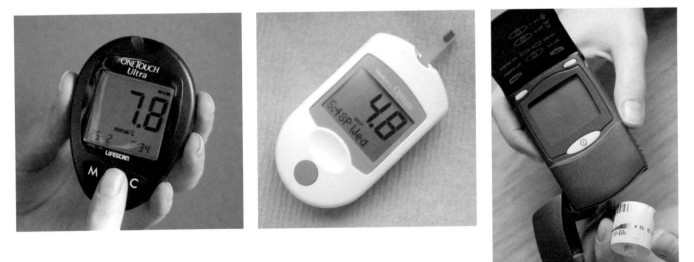

Figure 5.4 Three of the many blood glucose meters available.

Activity 5.3 Finding out about choosing a blood glucose meter

Suggested study time 30 minutes

The next time you are out shopping, visit a local pharmacy and look at the range of blood glucose meters available, or if you have access to your local diabetes centre, ask to see their selection of meters. Compare their size, weight, price, the technique for using them, and the blood glucose strips recommended for use with them. Look at the Diabetes UK website again to see the full range of meters available in this country.

Comment

You may find several meters on display in your local pharmacy. They vary in price depending on additional functions. Some are very small and can be carried discreetly in your pocket. However, for people with poor eyesight a meter with a large display may be more suitable.

A person using a blood glucose meter must learn how to use the device correctly (Box 5.3), especially if they are then using the results to adjust medication. As you saw from Activity 5.3, there are several types of blood glucose meter available, all with different methods of use, and all requiring a particular brand of blood glucose-testing strip. If you have diabetes, it is important to find a meter that you find easy to use, and has the functions you require to manage your diabetes. For example, some meters have a large memory, which means the results can be downloaded onto a computer. This is useful if you want to look at trends in your blood glucose level over a period of time.

Box 5.3 Accurate blood glucose monitoring

Some procedures are common to all blood glucose meters, whether you or your carer is doing the test.

- Make sure you have the correct strips for the meter you are using. They are all brand-specific, and a meter will not work accurately with the wrong strips.

- You must always wash your hands before testing your blood glucose. Any substance on your fingers will contaminate the strip and can give an inaccurate reading.

- The meter must be correctly calibrated for the strips in use. This may involve inserting the chip included in the strip packet into the meter each time a new box is opened, or typing in a code number stamped on the package.

- Check that the strips have not expired, and that they have been stored at room temperature.

- Make sure you have an appropriate device for pricking your fingertip. Needles should not be used. Lancets are available on prescription and should be used once only.

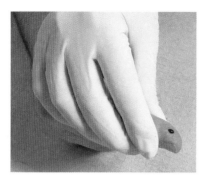

Figure 5.5 Blood samples are taken by pricking the side of the finger.

- You should prick the side of your finger (Figure 5.5), avoiding the thumb and forefinger as the skin on these digits is tougher from greater use. Using the side is also less painful than the centre of finger pads. Allow a few seconds for bleeding to start, to allow a sufficient drop of blood to form.

- Read and follow the meter instructions carefully!

The sharp lancets that have been used to obtain the blood sample from the finger, or alternative site, must be disposed of carefully. As discussed in Chapter 1, safe disposal of sharp devices that can transport viruses and infection from one person to another is extremely important. In the diabetes clinic or surgery, sharp devices (lancets and needles) can be safely disposed of in designated sharps boxes or bins (Figure 5.6a). Unfortunately, you may find that the procedure for disposing of lancets, blood-contaminated strips and tissues, and used needles from insulin devices, is not straightforward outside the hospital or clinic environment. Some local councils provide a sharps disposal service by supplying individuals with sharps boxes and collecting them when they are full. Other areas recommend the use of a 'safe-clip', a small device for clipping off the needle and lancet point, which is then retained within the clip (Figure 5.6b). The remainder of the lancet, needle base, and blood contaminated tissue and strips should be stored in a screw-top container such as an empty bleach bottle (Figure 5.6c). When the clip and bottle are full, they are placed in the household rubbish.

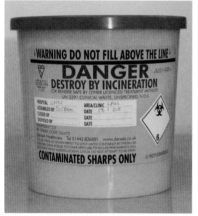

(a)

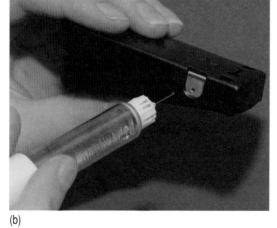

(b)

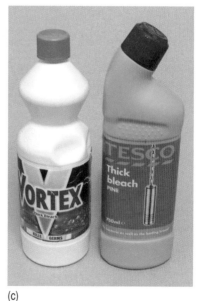

(c)

Figure 5.6 Devices for safe disposal of used lancets and needles: (a) a sharps box; (b) a 'safe-clip'; (c) bleach bottles.

- Can you think of any disadvantages of having a sharps box delivered and collected from an individual's house by the local council refuse department?

- The person may be concerned about their privacy. They may not want their neighbours to know they have diabetes. What happens if the person was out when the box is to be collected? Would it be safe to leave the full box on the doorstep?

If a blood glucose meter is used competently, home blood glucose results provide valuable information about the user's daily management of their blood glucose level and this often helps to increase their understanding about the condition. The results are usually recorded in a blood glucose monitoring book or can be downloaded from a computer and printed out as a graph. The record contributes to the assessment carried out during the annual review. As seen in the DCCT and UKPDS studies, long-term complications from a persistently high blood glucose level can occur particularly in small blood vessels.

5.3.2 Self-monitoring of urine glucose

Some people may choose not to test their blood glucose. They may instead test for the presence of glucose in their urine as a measure of blood glucose control. In someone without diabetes, the amount of glucose in the blood does not reach such a high level that the kidneys start to transport it into the urine. This level is called the **renal threshold** and in most people, is about 10 mmol/l. If the level of glucose rises to above this amount in the blood of someone with diabetes, then glucose starts to appear in the urine. By testing their urine at regular intervals, someone with diabetes can see if the amount of glucose in their blood has risen above the normal range (i.e. 10 mmol/l) since they last passed urine. If their diabetes is well controlled, they would find most of their urine tests would be negative (i.e. no glucose in the urine). Of course, to be effective, this test assumes that the person has a normal renal threshold. If their kidneys do not start to remove glucose into the urine until the level of glucose in the blood reaches, say, 15 mmol/l, they may have negative urine tests (i.e. a 'normal' result) despite having poorly controlled blood glucose. This can occur commonly as people get older, and is described as having a high renal threshold. Sometimes, people have a low renal threshold, where glucose appears in the urine when the blood glucose level is normal. Both high and low renal thresholds can occur in healthy kidneys, and does not necessarily mean there is kidney damage, but it does mean that urine testing is not a suitable method for blood glucose monitoring.

● Why would someone choose not to test their blood to check his or her diabetes control?

● Blood testing can be painful. Some people with poor vision or manual dexterity problems (severe arthritis, for example) may not be able to use a glucose meter. Some people feel anxious about the results they get, especially if they do not know what to do about them. In addition, some GPs restrict the prescriptions of blood testing strips to people using certain types of diabetes treatments because of the costs of testing strips (as mentioned above).

5.3.3 Venous blood sampling

The most accurate method for measuring blood glucose is to take a sample of blood from a vein (a venous sample) that is then tested in a laboratory. (This will result in a plasma glucose level, as discussed in Chapter 2.) This is always done when diagnosing diabetes – a capillary sample used with a blood glucose meter or a urine test is not accurate enough for a diagnosis. Venous samples are also used for many other blood tests which are important in identifying changes which may lead to long-term complications in people with diabetes.

Veins are large, thin-walled blood vessels which carry blood back to the heart. The most commonly used vein for venous blood sampling is found in the antecubital fossa, that is the area inside the bend of the elbow (Figure 5.7a). As you can see in this diagram, there are many veins in this area that are close to the surface of the skin. If there is difficulty in getting blood from these veins, other sites such as the back of the hand may be used.

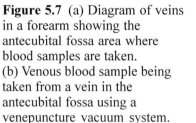

Figure 5.7 (a) Diagram of veins in a forearm showing the antecubital fossa area where blood samples are taken. (b) Venous blood sample being taken from a vein in the antecubital fossa using a venepuncture vacuum system.

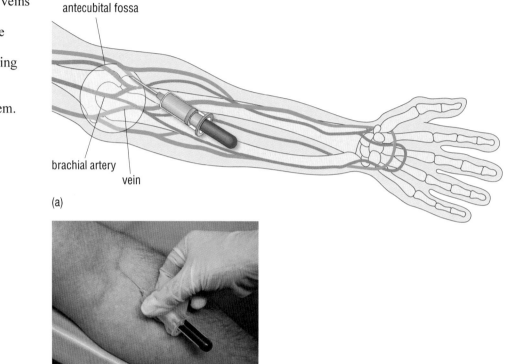

antecubital fossa

brachial artery

vein

(a)

(b)

The equipment needed to take a venous blood sample is of two sorts. Either a syringe and needle is used, or a closed vacuum system and needle. The closed vacuum system (also known as a **venepuncture** vacuum system) has the advantage of enabling several samples to be taken safely at any one time by reducing the risk of blood spillage and needle-stick injury to the person taking the sample (Figure 5.7b). Venepuncture literally means 'puncturing the vein' and is used to describe a needle entering a vein through the skin.

Before blood is taken, it is important that the person with diabetes understands what is going to be done and why, and has given their consent. (Informed consent was discussed in Section 1.6.) The person taking the blood should always wash their hands before they start the procedure and wear a fresh pair of gloves.

The equipment used in taking a blood sample includes:

- disposable gloves
- alcohol swab
- tourniquet
- needle and syringe, or venepuncture vacuum system
- specimen tubes

- sharps box
- cotton wool balls and adhesive tape
- forms
- plastic bag.

● Can you think what all these items are required for?

● You probably thought of at least some of the following:

Disposable gloves: these are used to protect the person taking blood from any accidental blood spillage. In Chapter 1 you read about infection risks from blood; gloves offer some protection should a spillage happen. They also help to protect the patient from any bacteria on the health professional's hands, though this person should always wash their hands even when using gloves.

Alcohol swab: this is used to clean the patient's skin before it is punctured to take the blood sample. The alcohol should be left to dry for at least five seconds before the sample is taken; this kills most of the bacteria on the skin so that they cannot enter the blood when the needle enters the vein through the skin.

Tourniquet: this is an elasticated strap used to compress the vein above the proposed site of the injection, allowing the vein to be seen more easily and felt more readily. The tourniquet should be put on tightly enough to raise the vein but not so tightly that arterial blood flow is stopped. Tourniquets should not be left in place for any longer than two minutes, in order to avoid injury. Tourniquets that are left on too long can make the arm quite painful.

Venepuncture vacuum systems: these are closed systems used for collecting blood samples. The vacuum in the specimen tube causes the blood to be drawn directly into it (see Figure 5.7b). Risk of blood spillage is reduced as each specimen tube can be attached in turn to the system.

Needles and syringes: these are used to obtain the sample of blood when a venepuncture vacuum system is unavailable or not suitable, such as when the patient's veins appear fragile. Needles and syringes come in various sizes and a suitable size should be chosen. The needle should remain sheathed when being applied to the syringe and until the sample is about to be taken. It should not be resheathed after use as this increases the risk of a needle-stick injury. Used needles should be placed in a sharps box.

Specimen tubes: blood samples are placed in these after collection by the needle and syringe method. There are different types of sample tube depending on the laboratory test to be done. Labels on the specimen tubes must be accurately completed, including the patient's name and identification number. (See, for example, Figure 5.8.)

Sharps box: this is needed for the safe disposal of needles and other used equipment. (See, for example, Figure 5.6a.)

Cotton wool balls and adhesive tape: these are needed to apply pressure to the vein following the procedure, to avoid haematoma formation (the leakage of blood forming a large bruise) at the site. A small adhesive dressing may be used after bleeding has stopped.

Forms and plastic bags: the forms accompany the specimens to the laboratory in plastic bags to give the patient's details and request the required tests. An appropriate form, accurately completed, accompanies each specimen. In the laboratory, the details on the specimen tube are checked with the details on the form, to make sure the correct tests are performed for the correct patient.

Figure 5.8 Specimen tubes colour-coded for different blood tests.

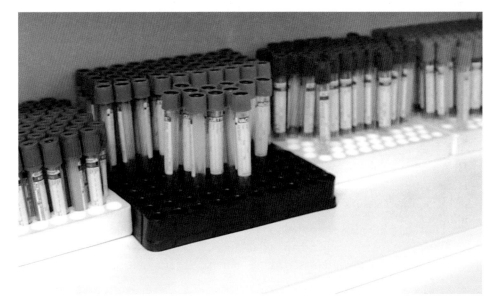

5.3.4 HbA$_{1c}$ levels

Another way of assessing blood glucose control is by measuring the **glycated haemoglobin**. This test is abbreviated to **HbA$_{1c}$** (first mentioned in Section 4.7). Haemoglobin is a protein that is found in red blood cells and its function is to transport oxygen around the body. Red blood cells are functional for about 90 days, after which they are broken down in the spleen, along with the haemoglobin contained within them. Glucose reacts with protein over time, changing it (or 'glycating' it). By taking a sample of red cells and measuring how much of the haemoglobin within them has been changed by this process, the result gives an idea of what the blood glucose level has been like in the last two to three months for that person. If the blood glucose level has been high, a greater proportion of the haemoglobin will have been in contact with glucose and will have become glycated than if the blood glucose level has been normal or low. This is a process that occurs even in someone without diabetes, so there is a 'normal' range of glycated haemoglobin. The aim of diabetes treatment is to enable someone to control their blood glucose as well as possible so that their HbA$_{1c}$ result is similar to that of someone without diabetes. The result is measured as a percentage of total haemoglobin changed, and depending on the techniques used in your local laboratory, the normal result is usually less than 6.5%. Guidance from NICE (the National Institute for Health and Clinical Excellence) recommends that most people with diabetes should aim for results of between 6.5 and 7.5% or less (NICE, 2002). The GMS2 (General Medical Services) contract also encourages GPs to help at least 50% of their patients to get this result. However, it is very difficult for most people to achieve, particularly if the risk of hypoglycaemia is too high. If you have diabetes, and are not able to achieve this target, you should be reassured that *any* reduction in HbA$_{1c}$ will reduce your risk of developing microvascular complications.

Activity 5.4 Finding out about HbA$_{1c}$ testing

Suggested study time 10 minutes

Find out what is considered to be the normal range for HbA$_{1c}$ at your local diabetes clinic. If you have diabetes yourself, do you know what your last result was, and is it within the target range? Also, check how HbA$_{1c}$ is measured at the clinic.

Comment

HbA$_{1c}$ can be checked using a venous blood sample which is sent to the laboratory, or your diabetes clinic may use a machine that analyses a finger-prick capillary sample of blood, where the result is available within a few minutes.

5.4 Monitoring ketone levels

In Chapter 2 (Section 2.3.5), you read about the formation of ketones when fats in the body are broken down. Ketones are an alternative energy source, and are usually only present when there is insufficient glucose to meet the body's energy requirements. They can occur in small quantities in someone without diabetes, after prolonged fasting. The presence of insulin, however, normally suppresses the production of significant amounts of ketones. In people with Type 1 diabetes who are deficient in insulin (perhaps because they have forgotten to take their insulin injections, for example), ketones can be produced in large amounts because, although there is plenty of glucose available in the blood, the body is unable to use it for energy without insulin. Ketones accumulate in the blood, altering the acidity (the pH level). They are removed from the body in the urine and via the lungs in the breath. They have a distinctive 'pear-drop' smell or nail varnish type odour, which you may notice on someone's breath when you are close to them.

In people with diabetes, ketones are a sign of very poor diabetes control. If ketones build up in sufficient quantities in the blood, the condition of diabetic ketoacidosis (DKA) develops (as discussed in Section 2.3.5), which is a medical emergency. Testing for ketones when the blood glucose is high, especially if the person with diabetes is unwell, is essential to identify DKA, or to prevent it developing further, by treatment with fluids and insulin.

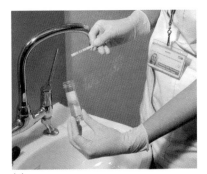

(a)

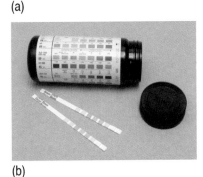

(b)

Figure 5.9 (a) Reagent strips are used to test urine samples.
(b) The pads on the strip test for the presence of different substances (including ketones) in urine – the intensity of the colour change is judged against the scale given on the side of the bottle.

Ketones can be detected in the urine by using a reagent strip (Figure 5.9). Usually the testing strip consists of a white plastic strip with a coloured pad stuck to it. The pad for ketones may be one of several pads for various tests if the urine is being tested at the GP surgery or hospital clinic. The pad is dipped briefly into a specimen of urine, and then examined after the recommended time (usually about 30 seconds) for a change in colour. The intensity of the colour change depends on the amount of ketones in the urine. No colour change means there are no ketones in the urine, and is said to be a negative result. A very strong colour change means that ketones are present in high quantities, and treatment to prevent DKA is required urgently.

People with Type 1 diabetes can obtain ketone testing strips on prescription from their GPs. It is useful to have a supply available to test for ketones during periods of illness, when people may be more likely to develop DKA. By frequently testing the blood glucose and ketones, the person may be able to make decisions about adjustments to their insulin dose to avoid hospitalisation with DKA, or at least recognise that they need to contact a health care professional for advice.

The presence of ketones in the blood is usually tested in a hospital laboratory. However, at the time of writing (2005), one blood glucose meter on the market has the facility for home testing of blood ketones using specific strips. However, most people use urine testing to detect ketones.

5.5 Monitoring lipid levels

Another common blood test that is often taken at the same time as the venous blood sample for HbA_{1c} is for the lipid profile. Lipids are fats, and they can be found in the blood. The target for ideal blood lipid level has changed recently, as new evidence is gathered from research. This test measures the total level of cholesterol in the blood, what proportion of that cholesterol is made up of LDL (low-density, harmful, lipoprotein) cholesterol and HDL (high-density, protective, lipoprotein) cholesterol, and the level of another type of fat called **triglycerides**. Abnormally high levels of lipids, in particular triglycerides and LDL cholesterol, and low levels of the protective HDL cholesterol, are common in people with Type 2 diabetes. This abnormal profile is termed **diabetic dyslipidaemia** and increases the risk of CHD, and so these factors are checked at least annually to ensure the results are well within the normal range. Drug treatment is recommended, in conjunction with a healthy lifestyle, to reduce the person's risk of CHD by trying to achieve as near normal a level of blood lipids as possible. The treatment includes drugs called statins and fibrates. The proportions of the different lipids in the blood determine the GP's choice of medication.

Activity 5.5 Finding out about cholesterol levels

Suggested study time 5 minutes

Do you know what your cholesterol level is? Ask some of your friends and colleagues if they know their levels.

Comment

You may be surprised at how many people know their cholesterol level. People without diabetes can have abnormal cholesterol levels too, and there is an increased public awareness nowadays of the risk of a raised cholesterol level. (Ideally, the level of LDL-cholesterol should be about 5 mmol/l. See Section 4.8.2.) Some pharmacists offer on-the-spot cholesterol tests, which anyone can use. If someone has high blood pressure, for example, his or her practice nurse may also have checked their cholesterol as part of their CHD risk profile.

5.6 Blood pressure monitoring

High blood pressure (hypertension) is another common problem in people with diabetes, particularly Type 2 diabetes. Along with dyslipidaemia, it is strongly associated with a high risk of developing CHD. As a consequence, blood pressure should be checked at least annually, but is usually checked at every diabetes clinic visit, especially if it is above normal. Blood pressure in people with diabetes should be 140/80 or less, and they may need to take several different tablets to get to this level. (**Blood pressure** is measured in units of millimetres of mercury (mmHg) but normally the units are not quoted.) If you have diabetes, you may have been advised to try and attain an even lower level, particularly if you know you have diabetes complications. Like blood glucose control, it can be very difficult to achieve the desired target, but again, any reduction in blood pressure is beneficial. The UKPDS (see Box 5.2) showed that reducing blood pressure was more effective than control of blood glucose in reducing macrovascular disease (such as heart attacks and stroke).

Blood pressure simply means the force with which the blood pushes onto the walls of the blood vessels as it flows through them. This force is produced by the pumping action of the heart pushing the blood around the body, and the elastic nature of the blood vessels which allows them to stretch as the blood is pumped into them, and spring back afterwards when the heart is relaxing to push the blood onwards. If you had no blood pressure you would be dead; this would occur if the heart stopped pumping. However, if the blood vessels become less elastic, the heart has to work harder to pump the blood through them and this can lead to many problems, such as heart failure. People with diabetes are very prone to developing inelastic blood vessels as a result of the build up of **atheroma**, a fatty substance which causes narrowing of the arteries and also makes them much less elastic. This can then result in problems such as heart attacks and strokes. High blood pressure is an indication that the arteries are becoming less elastic (although there may be other reasons for high blood pressure). This is why it is so important that the blood pressure is checked regularly and accurately, and treatment started if the blood pressure is higher than normal. It is also very important that the equipment is properly maintained so that accurate readings are obtained.

Blood pressure is measured by using a manual or electronic measuring device (a sphygmomanometer), which measures the pressure of blood in the arteries (Figure 5.10).

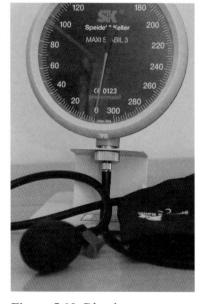

Figure 5.10 Blood pressure measuring device (sphygmomanometer) with pressure cuff.

The two numbers given when quoting blood pressure refer to the pressure of blood in the artery when the heart is contracting (systolic pressure) and the pressure of blood in the artery when the heart is relaxing (diastolic pressure).

● Which do you think is the higher measurement?

● The systolic is the higher reading because this is when there is a surge of blood into the arteries.

Many people are used to having their blood pressure measured. However, for some people, the annual review may be the first time their blood pressure has been measured and they may be quite worried about it. Other people who have had their blood pressure measured before may also be worried in case they have high blood pressure. It is important therefore that the person taking the blood pressure explains what is going to happen, and why it is being done, and that the person being checked consents to the procedure. The blood pressure may also be raised if the person tested is very anxious or has been rushing to get to the appointment, so the person should be given time to relax before having their blood pressure measured.

● Mrs Ferguson's blood pressure was always higher when Dr Jones took it than when the nurse checked it. Why do you think this could happen?

● You may have heard of 'white coat syndrome', where a patient's blood pressure is higher when the measurement is taken by a health care professional than when the patient is relaxed in a familiar environment. Perhaps Mrs Ferguson feels more relaxed with the nurse or the nurse talks to her for a few minutes before checking the blood pressure.

Blood pressure is measured by wrapping a cuff round the arm and inflating it, to compress the artery so that there is no blood going through the artery (Figure 5.11). This means that if the cuff is left inflated, it will be painful as the blood supply to the arm and hand is interrupted. As the cuff is slowly deflated and the pressure in the cuff gradually reduces, blood can start to pass back down the artery. By listening through a stethoscope held over the brachial artery in the antecubital fossa, the person doing the procedure can hear sounds from the time the blood re-enters the artery (systolic pressure) until the blood is flowing freely through the artery (diastolic pressure). This is the manual system and for this, a mercury or aneroid (air-filled) sphygmomanometer is used. Mercury, or more specifically its vapour, is highly toxic and therefore mercury sphygmomanometers are being phased out. If an electronic device is used, a cuff is still applied but the reading is taken automatically following automatic inflation and deflation of the cuff.

Once the reading has been taken, it should be documented clearly in the record of the person with diabetes. If it is either too high or too low, the doctor may start treatment or adjust the current medication.

Whenever your blood pressure is taken, it is important you know what the result is. This information will help you to make choices about your diet and exercise, and may give you some incentive to lose weight or try to give up smoking if these are problems for you. If you are concerned about the result, you should be able to discuss your worries with your doctor or nurse.

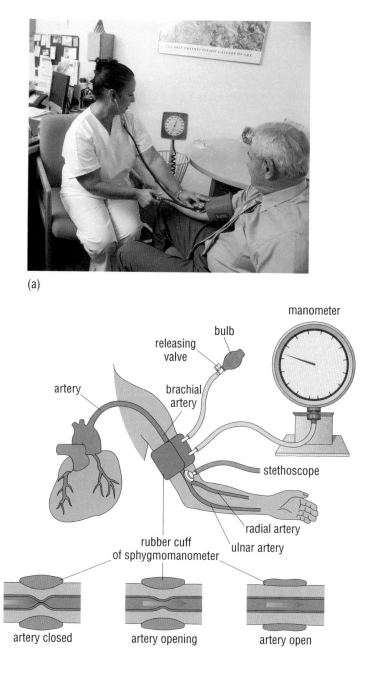

(a)

(b)

Figure 5.11 (a) Measurement of blood pressure using a sphygmomanometer. (b) The pressure in the cuff is increased until the blood flow stops, and then the flow gradually returns as the cuff is slowly deflated.

There are devices available for people to check their blood pressure at home. They can take the blood pressure at the arm or wrist. The normal range of measurements varies according to the site where the blood pressure is taken and the age of the person. As with the use of blood glucose meters, it is essential that the user knows how to use the device properly, and knows what to do with abnormal results. If you are using one of these devices, you may find it helpful to take it with you when you attend your diabetes clinic appointment. You can then compare the result you obtain with your device with the result obtained at the clinic.

The increased risk of CHD in people with Type 2 diabetes cannot be over-emphasised. Any of the factors that cause CHD must be identified and treated if possible, because people with diabetes have such a high risk of developing the condition. Along with identifying hypertension, hyperglycaemia, and dyslipidaemia, lifestyle risk factors need to be assessed, and the person advised on behaviours that increase CHD risk. It may be very difficult to change behaviour, but people need to be aware of the risk involved and empowered to make changes if they choose, through education and initiatives such as support to give up smoking.

5.7 Calculating body mass index

Being overweight is another risk factor for CHD, as well as a risk factor for developing Type 2 diabetes. Assessing whether somebody is overweight can be done in two ways. Simply weighing someone may not accurately determine if they are overweight. For example, two people may weigh 70 kg but one may be of an average weight whereas the other person is obese. Height is an important factor in determining if the person's weight is healthy for them. To take this into account, the relationship between weight and height is determined by calculating the body mass index (BMI) – introduced in Activity 2.6.

A BMI of between 20 and 24.9 kg/m^2 is desirable. A BMI of 25 kg/m^2 or higher is overweight, and over 30 kg/m^2 is classed as obese. (See Figure 4.9.)

The distribution of fat on the body is also significant; carrying fat around the abdomen is associated with highest risk. This is termed 'central obesity' and people with this distribution are described as 'apple-shaped'. A simple assessment for central obesity is to measure waist (or girth) circumference in centimetres using a tape measure (Figure 5.12c). Ideally, waist circumference in men should be less than 94 centimetres (cm), and less than 80 cm in women. (You may see other values quoted in other sources as the exact value is open to debate.) If these values are exceeded it is an indication of excessive body fat around the abdomen. A further calculation that can be made is the waist to hip ratio. The waist should be measured at the level of the umbilicus (belly button) and the hips at the widest point. The waist measurement is divided by the hip measurement. Ideally the ratio should be 1.0 or less in men or 0.8 or less in women.

● Mrs Soames has a BMI of 29 kg/m^2 with a waist measurement of 92 cm. Her husband has also has a BMI of 29 kg/m^2 with a waist measurement of 92 cm. Who has the higher risk of coronary heart disease?

● Mrs Soames has the higher risk. Although both of them are overweight, Mrs Soames has central obesity, with a waist measurement higher than is ideal for a woman.

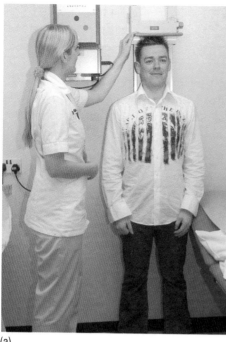

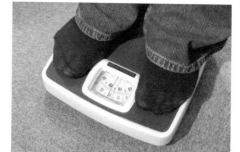

(b)

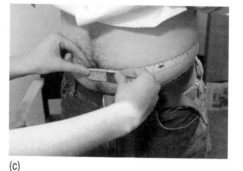

(c)

Figure 5.12 Determining risk by calculating BMI and measuring the waist circumference.

(a)

5.8 Making sense of the measurements

It is clear that there are several risk factors that contribute to diabetes complications, and that must be assessed at least annually, and treated if possible to reduce the risk of damage. The risk factors for CHD are particularly important because of the very high risk that people with Type 2 diabetes have of developing this complication. To make sense of all the factors we have discussed above, a calculation can be made from measurements of blood pressure and lipids, and from taking into account factors like smoking, which can give a prediction of relative risk of having a coronary event in the next 10 years. This is called the Framingham CHD risk score. People having a high risk on this score need to have their risk factors treated aggressively. Unfortunately, most people with Type 2 diabetes fall into this category.

We discussed in Chapter 1 that the person with diabetes is the central and most important member of the diabetes team. It is important that they are aware of their targets for blood pressure, HbA$_{1c}$, and lipids, what their values actually are, and the presence of other risk factors for diabetes complications. With this information, they may decide to make changes in their behaviour and lifestyle, to reduce their risk of other health problems. It is their choice, but without all the information they cannot make that choice. It is therefore important that they are informed of the result of any test performed on them. If they do not understand the significance of this information, an appropriate health care professional like a GP or nurse should explain it to them. All test results should also be clearly marked on their patient-held record card so they can compare their progress over time.

5.9 Summary of Chapter 5

This chapter covered the annual review for people with diabetes. You have seen that even if someone feels they are in good health, they may still have risk factors that could increase the chances of getting diabetes-related complications. It is important to create a plan, which is agreed between the person with diabetes and the health professional, to show what actions need to be taken to reduce risk factors or maintain low risk.

The diabetes annual review is an opportunity to check for factors that will increase a person's risk of developing diabetes complications, so they can address them before damage occurs. The idea is very much that 'prevention is better than cure'. It is also an opportunity for the person with diabetes to get feedback on how well they are doing (and recognition if they are struggling with aspects of their condition).

Every person with diabetes must have an annual diabetes review. It can be delivered at the hospital diabetes clinic, or for most people, by their local GP and practice nurse. The person with diabetes should not be a passive element in the process: they are supplying much of the information from their own monitoring and experience of living with the condition. They should have the results of the tests performed on them, and be given explanations about their meaning. They then have the information about how well they are managing their diabetes, and are able to make choices about any changes they may wish to make about their management.

Studying this chapter will have built on your knowledge of diabetes and diabetes care systems, and the personal impact of having diabetes, as well as helped you to think about underlying risk factors for complications. The next chapter covers in more detail the tests done to detect the presence of the complications themselves.

Questions for Chapter 5

Question 5.1 (Learning Outcomes 5.1, 5.2 and 5.3)

List the investigations that are likely to take place during a diabetes annual review and the various team members involved.

Question 5.2 (Learning Outcome 5.2)

Which tests in the diabetes annual review check for coronary heart disease risk?

Question 5.3 (Learning Outcomes 5.4 and 5.6)

Mrs Smith feels her diabetes is well controlled because her home blood glucose test results are all in single figures. When she attends the diabetes clinic with her GP for her annual review, she is shocked to find her HbA_{1c} is well above target. Can you suggest possible reasons for this?

Question 5.4 (Learning Outcome 5.4)

Explain how the HbA$_{1c}$ result can give a picture of diabetes glycaemic (i.e. the level of glucose in the blood) control.

Question 5.5 (Learning Outcomes 5.1 and 5.4)

When would you expect to find ketones in urine?

Question 5.6 (Learning Outcome 5.5)

Jane weighs 70 kg and is 1.75 m tall. Nina weighs 70 kg and is 1.52 m tall. Who is at greater risk of CHD, based on their BMI?

References

Diabetes Control and Complications Trial Research Group (DCCT) (1993) 'The effects of intensive treatment of diabetes on the development and progression of long-term complications in insulin-dependent diabetes mellitus', *New England Journal of Medicine*, **329** (14), pp. 977–986.

Diabetes UK (2003) *Glucose Self-monitoring in Diabetes* [online] Available from: http://www.diabetes.org.uk/infocentre/external/ndst1.pdf (Accessed April 2005).

National Institute for Health and Clinical Excellence (2002) *Inherited Clinical Guideline H. Management of type 2 diabetes: Management of blood glucose*, London, National Institute for Health and Clinical Excellence.

UK Prospective Diabetes Study (UKPDS) (1998) 'Group Intensive blood glucose control with sulphonylureas or insulin compared with conventional treatment and risk of complications in patients with type 2 diabetes (UKPDS 33)', *Lancet*, **352**, pp. 837–853.

CHAPTER 6

SCREENING FOR COMPLICATIONS OF DIABETES

Learning Outcomes

When you have completed this chapter you should be able to:

6.1 Define and use, or recognise definitions and applications of, each of the terms printed in **bold** in the text.

6.2 Describe how risk factors are related to the long-term complications of diabetes.

6.3 Briefly describe the different types of eye and kidney disease associated with diabetes.

6.4 State the types of cardiovascular disease which are more likely to occur if a person has diabetes.

6.5 Describe how diabetic neuropathy can affect the feet.

6.6 List the basic principles of good foot care.

6.7 List the screening measures carried out at the annual review to identify long-term complications.

6.1 Introduction

In previous chapters you have explored the nature of diabetes, and have considered the risk factors which can increase the likelihood of developing long-term complications of diabetes. In this chapter you examine further these long-term complications, their effect on the person with diabetes, and the screening which is carried out to detect them. You will also explore the relationship between the risk factors described in the previous chapter and the complications of diabetes.

6.2 Becoming aware of the complications of diabetes

Case Study 6.1 describes an active professional man who has already adapted his lifestyle very effectively to cope with the onset of diabetes complications. Also, in common with many people with diabetes, he is now developing other complications, which he has not yet noticed. Read his story to help you explore the onset and management of these complications.

Case Study 6.1

Mr Sam Evans is 65 and has had Type 1 diabetes since he was 30. He has never allowed diabetes to stop him playing an active role in the life of his family, or in his job in the finance department of a university, though over the last few years his deteriorating eyesight has forced him to travel by public transport rather than cycle or drive as before. Mr Evans is now due to retire from his job. While dressing for work one morning he was somewhat dismayed when his wife noticed an ulcerated area (open sore) on his foot, of which Mr Evans had been previously quite unaware.

As you see, Mr Evans is experiencing some health changes which are likely to be related to his diabetes. Carry out Activity 6.1 to explore the impact of the onset of these complications.

Activity 6.1 Facing up to complications

Suggested study time 15 minutes

Read through Mr Evans' story again.

Mr Evans has continued to lead a very productive life since the diagnosis of diabetes 35 years ago. Which long-term complications may he now be exhibiting and how may these affect his lifestyle?

Comment

It is likely that after 35 years of having Type 1 diabetes Mr Evans has eye disease. He has enough sight to manage his everyday life and his job but not enough to be able to drive or cycle safely. It is possible that Mr Evans may experience progressive deterioration in his sight over the coming years, which he may find restrictive.

The fact that Mr Evans has a wound on his foot, which he has not felt, suggests that he has some loss of sensation in his feet, which is another common long-term complication of diabetes. His visual difficulties may have meant that he did not see the ulcer either, and but for his wife it might have continued to be unnoticed and untreated. There may also be another factor contributing to the foot ulcer, that of poor circulation to the feet, which is often seen in diabetes, especially when it has been present for a long time as in Mr Evans' case. He used to cycle and this would have benefited his overall health including his circulation, but his eyesight is now not adequate for safe cycling. Prompt, effective treatment of the foot ulcer should result in its healing, and continued good foot care will be needed for Mr Evans to keep his feet healthy. He may need his wife's help with this.

It is very common for people like Mr Evans to develop complications, especially if they have had diabetes for many years. It is not always possible to prevent them, though it is important to try, but it is essential that complications are detected and treated as quickly as possible. In Mr Evans' case, for example, this would prevent further deterioration of his condition and promote his continued active lifestyle. Screening for complications is an important part of helping people with diabetes to remain as healthy as possible.

As you know there is no such thing as 'mild' diabetes. Some people talk about having 'mild' diabetes, or even 'a touch of diabetes'. However, as you have discovered in a previous chapter, all forms of diabetes are potentially life threatening and complications can be devastating, affecting a person's health and ability to cope with all aspects of their everyday life. Anyone with diabetes can develop complications, particularly if the condition is not well controlled. Unfortunately, some people do not realise that damage to blood vessels and nerves can be happening over a period of time even when there are no obvious symptoms. By the time symptoms occur (e.g. loss of sight or a heart attack), serious damage has already taken place. Therefore, anyone with diabetes, whether they are managing their condition by diet and lifestyle changes, or by taking tablets or insulin, should have an annual review. As you read earlier, the purpose of the annual review is to screen and start treatment for risk factors predisposing to the development of complications (e.g. high blood pressure and abnormal blood lipid levels). It is also used to check ongoing blood glucose control and adjust treatment as appropriate. This is particularly important in Type 2 diabetes, which has a natural tendency to worsen over the years; a person who at first is able to manage their diabetes by changes to diet and lifestyle is likely to need the additional help of medication at a later stage. Early complications can also be identified so they can be treated before becoming a major problem (e.g. laser treatment can prevent blindness when used at the appropriate time) and these aspects will be discussed in this chapter.

As you read in Chapter 5, the annual review may be led by the GP and practice nurse, the community diabetes specialist nurse, or by the hospital diabetes consultant (see Figure 6.1). Different members of the multidisciplinary diabetes team are involved in the review, with the person with diabetes being central to the team. For example, a technician in the diabetes centre may carry out eye screening using a digital camera, or in the community a trained optometrist may do this. It is therefore important that there is good communication between the different team members to ensure that the annual review is fully completed and any abnormalities noted and treated where possible. In order for you to understand further the importance of annual reviews, we now move on to consider the possible complications of diabetes in more detail.

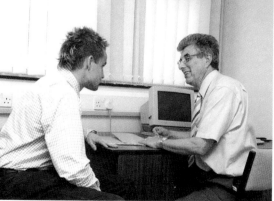

Figure 6.1 Different members of the diabetes team (such as the diabetologist) are involved with the annual review.

6.3 The types of complication associated with diabetes

The long-term effect of a high level of glucose and abnormal levels of lipids in the blood, and high blood pressure, is to cause damage to the blood vessels throughout the body. This in turn brings about deterioration in the functioning of organs and tissues such as the kidneys and nerves. This damage can be compounded by factors such as cigarette smoking and physical inactivity.

As you read in Section 5.2, the complications of diabetes can be divided into two broad groups called microvascular complications (involving small blood vessels) and macrovascular complications (involving large blood vessels).

Microvascular complications mainly affect the eyes, kidneys and nerves as these structures all rely on small blood vessels in order to work properly. For example if there is damage to the small blood vessels in the back of the eyes, **diabetic retinopathy** can result and may lead to deterioration of sight and eventually blindness.

It is worth noting that the ending -*opathy* occurs quite frequently in medical terms. It literally means 'suffering' and is used to show that there is something wrong with a particular part of the body. In the case of *retinopathy* it indicates that something is wrong with the retina.

Similarly, damage to the blood vessels in the kidney can lead to kidney damage (**diabetic nephropathy**; *nephro-* refers to the kidney), which can result in renal failure. Damage to the small blood vessels supplying the nerves causes **diabetic neuropathy** (*neuro-* refers to the nerves or nervous system) that results in loss of sensation and other nerve changes. All these are called microvascular complications of diabetes because they involve small blood vessels.

The other complications of diabetes associated with blood vessels are known as macrovascular complications as these involve the large blood vessels in the body, particularly those of the heart, brain and legs. Macrovascular complications can lead to heart attacks, strokes, pain in the legs when walking, and gangrene of the feet. Approximately 75% of people with diabetes die as a result of macrovascular complications such as a heart attack or stroke (Warren, 2002).

Some complications are more common than others, and this chapter focuses on those which most frequently occur. We will start by considering diabetic eye disease.

6.4 Diabetes and eye disease

For many people with diabetes the loss of sight is one of the most feared complications, partly because this is often the complication of which people are most aware. For example a person with diabetes may have a friend, acquaintance or relative who already has visual difficulties as a result of diabetes. Diabetes is still the commonest cause of blindness in people under the age of 65 in the UK (MacKinnon, 1998) though in fact very few of those registered blind are completely blind. Many have severely limited useful vision, or may be able to distinguish only light and dark. The development of eye disease is related to the length of time that the person has had diabetes. About 80% of patients show at least some signs of eye disease after having diabetes for 20 years (MacKinnon, 1998). Control of blood glucose during this time has a very important influence on the extent of the damage; poor control being associated with severe sight-threatening damage. The Diabetes Control and Complications Trial and the United Kingdom Prospective Diabetes Study, which were discussed previously (Boxes 5.1 and 5.2), both showed that maintaining good blood glucose control prevented or slowed down the progression of diabetic retinopathy in the long term (DCCT, 1993; UKPDS, 1998).

Before we consider the possible eye diseases associated with diabetes, we need to consider the eye itself.

6.4.1 Structure of the eye

The **cornea** is a clear covering over the front of the eye (Figure 6.2), which allows light through, protects the eye and helps the eye to focus light. The eyelid, eyelashes and eyebrow also protect the eye. Light passes through the **aqueous humour** (a watery fluid) in the front of the eye, through the **pupil** to the **lens**. The pupil is surrounded by the **iris**. The iris is made up of muscle fibres running in two different directions: in a circular direction around the pupil and radiating outwards from the pupil. The pupil is made smaller or larger by the contraction and relaxation of these muscles. This enables the amount of light entering the eye to be controlled. If the light is very bright the pupil is made smaller thus restricting the amount of light entering the eye, whereas if the light is dim then the pupil is made larger thus allowing more light to enter. In this way the retina receives the correct amount of light to enable vision, but not so much that the retina is damaged by the intensity of the light.

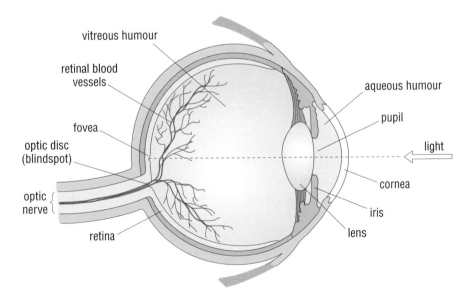

Figure 6.2 Diagrammatic cross-section through the eye showing the internal structure. (*Note*: the blood vessels lie in the wall of the eye, not the vitreous humour.)

The lens has the ability to bend the light rays as they pass through it. It can be varied in thickness by the ligaments and muscles that support it. This enables the image to be focused on a particular area of the **retina** known as the **fovea**. The retina is the area at the back of the eye that absorbs the light entering the eye. It contains many blood vessels, and receptors that respond to the incoming light to produce the sensation of sight. (Figure 6.3 shows an image of a healthy retina.)

Many of the light receptors (photoreceptors) are concentrated in the fovea. This is the area of central vision which gives the clearest image. The rest of the retina contains receptors that are not as concentrated as those in the fovea. The **optic nerve** takes signals from the light receptors to a particular area at the back of the brain known as the **visual cortex**, where the brain interprets what you see. The **vitreous humour** in the eye provides support to the eye structure, and because it is a clear liquid, allows the passage of light across to the retina. The optic disc is the area where the blood vessels and nerves enter the eye, so creating a 'blindspot' in the retina.

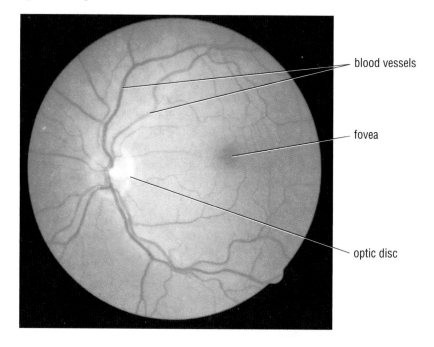

blood vessels

fovea

optic disc

Figure 6.3 Photograph of a healthy retina showing the position of the fovea, optic disc and associated blood vessels.

6.4.2 Diabetic retinopathy

A high blood glucose level, as well as other abnormalities such as high blood pressure, gradually damages the small blood vessels in the retina, eventually causing retinopathy. Retinopathy usually develops slowly and can be classified according to various characteristics seen during an eye examination. Three types of retinopathy are described below.

Background retinopathy is a condition in which small blood vessels in the retina become closed off and other blood vessels nearby dilate to compensate. Examination of the retina reveals small bulges in the blood vessels (these are called microaneurysms), slight leakage of blood from the blood vessels (haemorrhages), and hard exudates (see Figure 6.4). Exudates are similar to tide marks that show where fluid containing lipids (fats) has leaked out of the weakened blood vessels. The person is not aware of this damage and their sight will seem perfectly normal at this point.

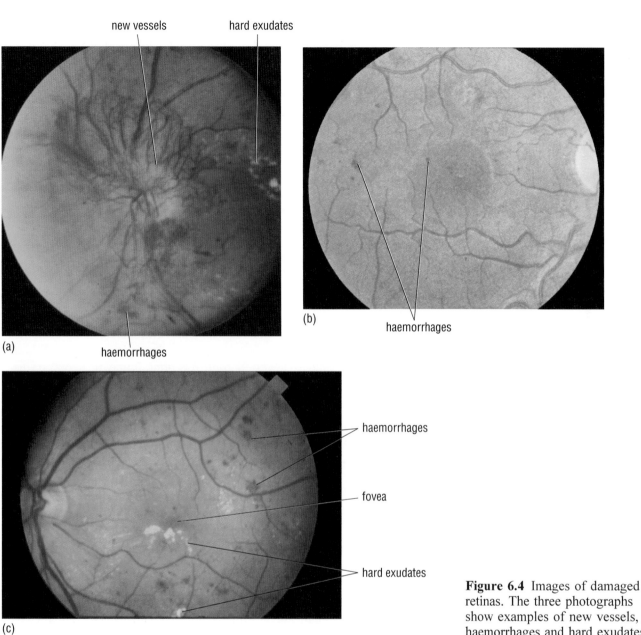

Figure 6.4 Images of damaged retinas. The three photographs show examples of new vessels, haemorrhages and hard exudates.

Pre-proliferative retinopathy includes the development of abnormal, irregularly shaped blood vessels, and 'cotton wool spots'. These are white areas of nerve damage that have occurred due to poor blood supply to areas of the retina. Again, the person usually has no symptoms to indicate the presence of this type of retinopathy.

Proliferative retinopathy is very serious as it can cause loss of vision with little or no warning. There is a proliferation (growth) of new blood vessels in the retina. These vessels are weak and therefore very prone to bleeding, especially if they grow forward into the vitreous humour in the eyeball instead of lying flat over the retina. Bleeding can be severe.

- Suggest what might happen if the eye fills with blood?

- Blood is not clear, therefore light cannot pass through it. This will impair vision.

There may be some improvement in vision after the bleeding has stopped since some of the blood is gradually re-absorbed. However, repeated episodes of bleeding lead to further deterioration in sight and can cause detachment of the retina from the back of the eyeball. If this is not treated quickly it may result in permanent blindness.

Since diabetic retinopathy can be present without symptoms, an annual eye examination is essential to identify the condition at an early stage, when it can be treated. Damaged blood vessels can be closed off by laser treatment, reducing the risk of bleeding in the eye. Laser treatment does not restore lost vision; but it can prevent further deterioration. If background retinopathy is treated quickly vision should be maintained. In addition to laser treatment of the damaged blood vessels, blood glucose and blood pressure control should be reviewed. If control is poor, it may be necessary to make adjustments to diet, exercise and medication regimes.

The annual eye examination involves several different tests, including visual acuity and retinal screening. Visual acuity is tested by asking the patient to read a standard eye chart, such as a Snellen Chart (Figure 6.5) from a fixed distance. This test checks the accuracy of central vision, that is, what you look at when you focus straight ahead. Near vision (needed for reading and close work) can be tested using a reading chart. Visual acuity should be tested before dilating drops (necessary for subsequent eye tests) are put into the eyes. If visual acuity has deteriorated since the last check, it may indicate diabetic retinopathy. However, the patient may just need new spectacles or may be developing cataracts, another common problem in diabetes, in which the lens becomes cloudy so that the person feels as if they are looking through a fog.

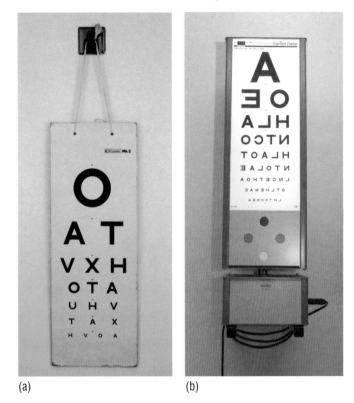

(a) (b)

Figure 6.5 (a) A traditional Snellen Chart. (b) A more modern version of a Snellen Chart. Note that this is viewed in a mirror so the letters are reversed.

Retinal screening involves an examination of the retina of the eye. This can be done by the doctor or eye specialist looking into the eye using an ophthalmoscope. You will have had this done if you have visited the optician to get your eyes tested. However, this test does not provide a permanent record and people with diabetes should have their retinas examined by having a photograph taken using a digital camera (Figure 6.6). The photograph can be studied and comparisons made on subsequent visits so that small changes can easily be spotted. This may be done in the diabetes centre if suitable equipment is available, or at an eye clinic, usually in the hospital.

To ensure a good view of the blood vessels in the retina, tropicamide eye drops are inserted into the eyes about 20 minutes before the examination. These drops dilate the pupil, thus allowing a clear view of the retina. Dilating drops should be used with caution as they can damage the eyes if glaucoma is present or the person has had eye surgery, such as lens implants for the treatment of cataracts. In glaucoma the circulation of the aqueous humour at the front of the eye is affected so that aqueous humour accumulates and the pressure inside the eye increases, eventually damaging the optic nerve. Dilating drops can further restrict the circulation of the aqueous humour leading to an even greater build-up of pressure and the possibility of sudden severe damage to the optic nerve.

Following the addition of the drops, patients find they are intolerant of bright light. This is because the drops dilate the pupil, overriding the ability of the iris muscles to make it smaller again. This allows more light into the eye and onto the light-sensitive retina. Patients must be warned about this before the drops are inserted, and should not drive until the effect has worn off. This may take two hours or longer.

6.4.3 Cataracts, glaucoma and blurred vision

In addition to retinopathy, people with diabetes are also more likely to develop two other common eye conditions, cataracts and glaucoma. A **cataract** occurs when the lens of the eye becomes cloudy or opaque so that the person can no longer see clearly through it. The commonest reason for this is ageing, but having diabetes increases the likelihood of developing cataracts. The treatment is surgical removal of the natural lens and replacement with an artificial one. This can usually be done under a local anaesthetic.

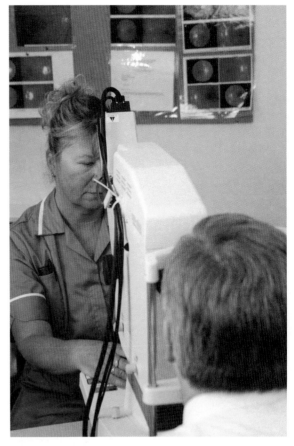

Figure 6.6 A technician using a digital camera to screen someone's eyes. The images in Figures 6.3 and 6.4 were taken with this sort of camera.

Glaucoma is a serious, sight-threatening condition in which the pressure inside the eyeball increases.

- What effect does this have?
- It puts pressure on the optic nerve, which may suffer sudden damage. If it is left untreated, glaucoma will certainly cause optic nerve damage.

Many patients with glaucoma are unaware of its presence until the damage has already been done so it is important that eye screening, including pressure testing, is done regularly. Checking for glaucoma is also carried out as part of any routine eye test, whether or not the person being tested has diabetes.

Some people notice that when they are first diagnosed with diabetes or during periods of poor control, their eyesight is blurred. This can be very frightening because they may think they are losing their eyesight. However, blurred vision is a temporary symptom caused by glucose accumulating in the lens of the eye, and, as a result, the eyeball becoming a little dehydrated. Blurred vision does resolve but it may take several weeks to do so. It is therefore important that the affected person does not spend money on new glasses at this time, because their vision will change as the blood glucose level stabilises. Any concerns about vision can be discussed with the GP or nurse at the diabetes clinic.

6.4.4 Coping with blindness

The author Sue Townsend has diabetic retinopathy and is registered blind. She has talked about this to journalist Martin Cullen (Cullen, 2002). Activity 6.2 asks you to think about how Sue has had to adapt to her blindness.

Activity 6.2 Adapting to life with little sight

Suggested study time 30 minutes

Read Offprint 6.1 'Vision and Values' from the May/June 2002 issue of *Balance* and note how Sue realised she had problems. How has loss of sight affected Sue's life?

Comment

Sue is registered blind but she still has some vision left; she is able to see light and shapes but very little else. Most people who are registered blind still have some residual vision; this varies in amount and usefulness between different people. Sue is still very positive and is able to continue her work though she is much slower now, as she has to write in very large letters and use a magnifying machine to read. She manages well at home where she is in familiar surroundings, but finds it difficult to go out alone. Sue is very sensitive to the reactions of other people to her blindness. You may have noticed that Sue admits her blood glucose control has been poor and that she is a smoker. As you may recall from Chapter 5, these are two important risk factors for the development of various complications associated with diabetes.

Sue Townsend uses aids such as a white stick and a magnifying machine. If a person is registered blind there are numerous aids available to help them cope with everyday situations. Organisations such as Sight Concern and the Royal National Institute for the Blind provide support and advice for people with visual difficulties. Sue appears to have coped very well with her loss of sight; however some people need a great deal of support to help them come to terms with losing their sight, and clearly it is much better if the problem can be prevented in the first place.

6.4.5 Screening for eye disease in people with diabetes

Some people may be able to get their eyes screened in the community, either by a local optometrist who has been trained to do diabetes eye screening, or in a mobile eye-screening unit. Whether the annual eye screening is carried out in a hospital or in the community is unimportant; the important issue is that the screening is done in order that maximum useful sight is preserved. Activity 6.3 will help you to be aware of your local facilities for this service.

Activity 6.3 Eye screening in your locality

Suggested study time 30 minutes

Find out what eye screening facilities are available in your area for people with diabetes, and where they are located.

Comment

The answer will obviously depend on your locality. However, you have probably discovered that eye screening is offered annually in the diabetes clinic or eye clinic at the hospital, at community diabetes clinics or by local optometrists.

Not everyone with diabetes attends their annual screening. As this is such a beneficial test in terms of helping to prevent deterioration in eyesight it is important to find out why this is so. There may be many reasons, such as difficulties with transport or care of a child or dependent elderly relative; or there may be fear of what will be found at the screening appointment, especially if for some reason the diabetes control is not as good as the person might wish. Fear of blindness may even result in avoiding eye appointments; this may be a way of denying that there is any special need to take care of the eyes and thus pretending that there is no risk to the eyesight.

We now go on to look at the kidney condition known as diabetic nephropathy. Nephropathy is often found in people with diabetes who have retinopathy, as both conditions reflect the fact that microvascular disease is present in the body. Thus if a person with diabetes is found to have retinopathy they should be checked for nephropathy, and vice versa.

6.5 Diabetes and renal disease

6.5.1 The structure of the kidney

Kidneys are reddish-brown bean-shaped organs, about 10 cm long. They are found at the back of the abdominal cavity, one each side of the spine (Figure 6.7). They have a very rich blood supply which is important to the functioning of these organs. Each kidney is made up of about a million small structures called **nephrons**, which filter the blood, remove waste products and unwanted substances, control the amount of water in the body and make urine. The urine is carried from the kidney to the **bladder** along a tube called a **ureter**. The bladder stores the urine until it can be passed. By testing the urine, it is possible to find out some things about the body as a whole and about how well the kidneys are working.

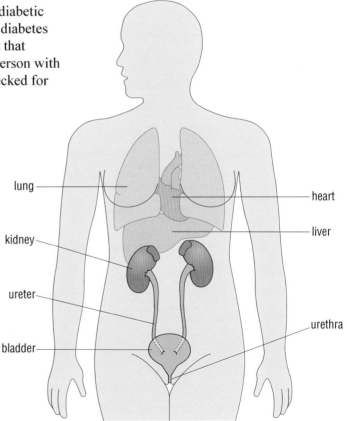

Figure 6.7 Diagram showing the position in the body of the kidneys, ureters and bladder in relation to other organs.

The kidneys have a crucial function in maintaining health by filtering waste matter (produced by all the cells that make up the body) from the blood. They also maintain the correct level of salts (**electrolytes** such as sodium, potassium and chloride ions), water and acidity so that the cells and other organs in the body can function efficiently. Waste matter (including urea), excess water and salts, and other substances (e.g. drugs) are removed from the body as urine. This process is called **excretion**.

6.5.2 Diabetic nephropathy

Nephropathy (renal disease) occurs when the small blood vessels forming the filtering part of each nephron become damaged. This means that the kidneys gradually become less and less efficient at removing waste from the body. The blood pressure also increases because the kidneys have a role in regulating blood pressure; failing kidneys try to improve their own blood supply by bringing about a general increase in blood pressure in the body. However, hypertension (high blood pressure, discussed in Chapter 4) itself damages the kidneys because of the increased pressure in the renal blood vessels. Anaemia also develops in the late stages of diabetic nephropathy because the kidneys play a role in the formation of red blood cells and the ability to do this deteriorates as the renal function declines. Eventually, the patient goes into complete renal failure (**end-stage renal failure**, sometimes called stage 5 renal failure, in which the kidneys are carrying out virtually none of their normal functions) and requires dialysis and/or a kidney transplant if the condition of the patient favours this and a donor organ becomes available. Patients in end-stage renal failure, even if they are on dialysis, are in a poor state of health and have to manage their diet and fluid intake with extreme care to reduce the work their kidneys have to do.

As with all complications of diabetes, early detection of diabetic nephropathy and treatment to control risk factors will slow down the progression of the damage.

- Why is good control of blood glucose and blood pressure aggressively targeted when signs of diabetic nephropathy are detected?

- Both high blood glucose and high blood pressure damage the small blood vessels of the kidney so strenuous efforts to correct these are beneficial in reducing the rate of progression of nephropathic changes.

6.5.3 Screening for nephropathy in people with diabetes

There are two main ways of screening for nephropathy – checking for protein in the urine, and checking the blood for abnormalities caused by renal deterioration.

Urine testing

In the healthy kidneys, protein molecules (including albumin, a protein which is formed in the liver and is one of the plasma proteins) are too large to be filtered from the blood into the urine via the kidney filtering system. However, if diabetic nephropathy develops and the blood vessels begin to be damaged, the filtering system develops larger 'holes' so that the smallest protein molecules begin to be filtered from the blood into the urine. They can be detected by very sensitive urine testing strips or tests (see Figure 5.9). This is called **microalbuminuria** testing, as it detects minute amounts of protein in the urine. Urine samples can be tested in the clinic using microalbumin strips or can be sent to the clinical biochemistry department to be tested. The presence of microalbuminuria is an early indication that the person is starting to develop diabetic nephropathy. Improved control of blood pressure and blood glucose at this stage slows the progression of the disease.

When more severe diabetic nephropathy is present, larger amounts of protein are present in the urine and can be detected using the routine urine testing strips found in a diabetes clinic. The person with diabetes may be completely unaware of the damage and have no symptoms. However, the presence of protein in the urine indicates potentially serious kidney damage and the need to review the management of diabetes generally. The person may value the opportunity to discuss this with a doctor or diabetes specialist nurse and receive support in making positive decisions to adjust their lifestyle, diet and medication as appropriate. Such changes will have a beneficial effect on health and will slow down the progression of renal damage, though at this stage it may not be possible to reverse the damage which has already occurred.

Sometimes patients may have a urine infection, and this also gives a positive result on testing the urine for protein. To check this, a further fresh sample called a mid-stream specimen of urine (MSU) may be obtained from the patient. This is sent to the laboratory to be tested for infection.

If it is confirmed that there is no infection, the patient may be asked to collect all the urine they pass over a 24-hour period, to see exactly how much protein they are losing. (Special containers are available in which to collect 24-hour urine production.)

Blood tests to detect renal damage

Normally, the kidneys precisely regulate the level of electrolytes (salts) in the blood by filtering out excessive amounts and passing them from the body in the urine. As the kidneys become less efficient, the levels of certain electrolytes begin to become abnormal. Blood tests are usually taken at least once a year, as part of the annual review, to detect any changes in these levels. You may see this test written as U + Es on the clinical biochemistry request form. It stands for urea and electrolytes. (Urea is a major constituent of urine.)

Creatinine is another substance present in the blood as a result of muscular activity in the body. The blood creatinine level is normally lower than 130 mmol/l because the kidneys constantly clear creatinine from the blood, as fast as it is produced. If the creatinine level is rising, it suggests that the kidneys are working less efficiently.

It is usually a combination of urine and blood test results, rather than just one test that enables a diagnosis of diabetic nephropathy to be made.

6.6 Diabetic neuropathy

Neuropathy is another very common complication of diabetes and it can be extremely difficult to treat. (This was defined in Section 6.3.) **Peripheral neuropathy** refers to damage to the nerves supplying the extremities, or periphery, of the body. The nerves picking up sensations can be affected and this can then lead to pain or numbness.

- Why are these seemingly opposite effects both caused by the same thing?

- The symptoms depend on the type of nerve damage.

The nerves that convey pain and touch sensations from the extremities to the brain are called **sensory nerves**. Nerves which send instructions from the brain to the rest of the body, known as **motor nerves**, can also be affected. Damage to these nerves is known as motor neuropathy. In severe cases this can result in joint wasting and joint changes leading to an abnormally shaped foot. There are other nerves, which supply the internal organs such as the heart and the digestive system. These nerves are known as **autonomic nerves** and they control all the 'automatic' functions in the body, for example the movements in the digestive system which aid the digestion of food and enable it to progress through the length of the gut from mouth to anus.

6.6.1 Autonomic neuropathy

Autonomic neuropathy affects the autonomic nervous system. This system is essential to life as it maintains all the automatic systems in the body which happen without you thinking about them.

- What functions does your body carry out without you thinking about them?

- We already noted above that digestion and the passage of food through the gut is controlled by the autonomic nervous system. In addition, breathing (although you can hold your breath for a while, when you are asleep breathing is automatic), heart beat, temperature control, sweating, blood pressure control and size of pupils in the eye are the main functions you might have thought about. Elimination of urine and faeces is partly under voluntary control but there is an important element of this controlled by the autonomic nervous system. Likewise sexual function and erections are partly controlled by the autonomic system.

Autonomic neuropathy can therefore cause a variety of distressing conditions such as an erratic heart beat, chronic diarrhoea, delayed stomach emptying, bladder problems, impotence, difficulty controlling body temperature and sudden unpredictable drops in blood pressure (this can cause fainting attacks).

6.6.2 Erectile dysfunction

Also known as impotence, **erectile dysfunction** is a form of neuropathy suffered by many men with diabetes. The ability to obtain and maintain an erection to enable sexual intercourse is impaired, often resulting in difficulties in relationships between the affected sexual partners. The person who has the erectile dysfunction may feel worried and frustrated, while the partner may suffer from feelings of rejection. If the couple is not able to talk about the problem this may result in each becoming isolated from the other. In many cases there is effective treatment for the condition, but it depends upon the affected person being able to discuss the problem with a health care professional. This can only happen if there is an open and relaxed atmosphere at the clinic appointment, with open questions being used and time given to allow the problems to be discussed. Another essential requirement is privacy, so it is vital that consultations are not interrupted by other people entering the room. In Chapter 1 the difficulty of talking about personal problems was discussed. There are many types of treatment for impotence available, including tablets such as Viagra®, injections, counselling and mechanical devices.

In an article published in the magazine *Balance*, reporter Alyson Jones talks to Keith and his wife Florence (Jones, 2004). Keith has had Type 1 diabetes for 13 years and is aware of increasing difficulties in keeping an erection. Activity 6.4 helps you to think about the emotional and physical help that is needed by people who are experiencing problems like these.

Activity 6.4 Losing (and regaining) that loving feeling

Suggested study time 20 minutes

Read Offprint 6.2 'You've lost that loving feeling' from the March/April 2004 edition of *Balance* and notice how Keith and Florence felt about their problem. What help did they eventually receive?

Comment

It is of note that the reporter spoke to both Keith and his wife, as both partners are affected when one has erectile dysfunction. You probably noticed that the erectile dysfunction was making both Keith and Florence feel very isolated, as they were not able to discuss the problem together. Keith felt embarrassed and angry and was keeping Florence away in case she wanted to make love. Both partners were suffering greatly, as is often the case with such a problem.

Keith did eventually pluck up the courage to visit his doctor, and for most people a great deal of courage is needed to enable them to talk about their problem. Keith also received some helpful advice from the Sexual Dysfunction Association. They were able to explain the reason for Keith's difficulties and also encouraged him to talk to Florence, which was clearly a turning point in their relationship. Keith is aware that because his erectile dysfunction is caused by neuropathy his condition is not curable. However, he has tried a number of treatments and has now found some tablets which suit him well and enable him and his wife to enjoy a sex life. Florence did not know where to find help, and it is important to be aware that when erectile dysfunction is present, the partner may also be in need of help such as counselling or some advice.

Some of the treatments which Keith tried did not help him, and some even caused him pain. However different treatments suit different people, even when the underlying cause of the erectile dysfunction appears to be the

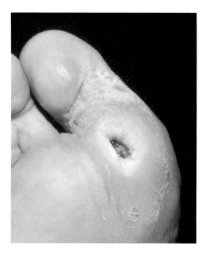

Figure 6.8 People with diabetes are at risk of developing foot ulcers such as this, which can take a long time to heal.

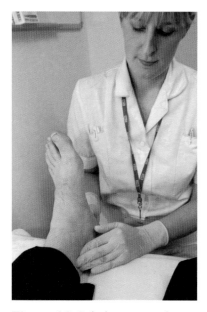

Figure 6.9 It is important that feet of people with diabetes are checked regularly.

same. Like Keith, people should not become discouraged if the first attempts at treatment do not appear to be successful, as it is very likely that with persistence a helpful solution to the problem can be found. Other factors such as stress, anxiety and fatigue can worsen the erectile dysfunction, even though the underlying cause may be neuropathy, so it is important that these matters are also discussed.

Erectile dysfunction is a specific type of problem linked to neuropathy. There are other types of neuropathy which put the feet particularly at risk, and these are discussed in the next section.

6.6.3 Peripheral neuropathy and foot problems

Peripheral neuropathy puts the person with diabetes at particular risk of damage to their feet, especially if they also have poor circulation in this area. The nerve damage gradually reduces the sensitivity of the feet, which means the patient may not notice a foreign object such as a drawing pin or a stone in the shoe, or a badly fitting shoe rubbing the foot. This causes damage to the skin, which allows infection to enter the foot leading to gangrene in severe cases. Commonly, ulcers (open sores) form on the foot that take a long time to heal (Figure 6.8). The nerve damage can also lead to muscle weakness (this is known as motor neuropathy) and changes in blood flow which can lead to abnormality in the shape of the foot and subsequent bone damage. This makes ulcer formation highly likely because the abnormal shape of the foot and abnormal walking patterns produce high-pressure points on the weight-bearing areas of the foot.

Another reason that people with diabetes are at high risk of foot problems is that they may have a decreased blood supply to the foot. As you saw in Chapter 5, people with diabetes are prone to atheroma and this can lead to a 'furring up' of the blood vessels supplying the feet. (We will return to this issue in the next section when we discuss CHD.) The effect of this is to reduce the blood supply to the feet, resulting in feet which are pale and cool to touch, with reduced or absent pulses. If an ulcer then develops on the foot, healing is much slower than normal because of the reduced blood supply.

Because of the risks described above, it is extremely important that people with diabetes look after their feet well, and that they have access to appropriate services so that their feet can be checked regularly (as in Figure 6.9) and treated promptly whenever it becomes necessary. Activity 6.5 will help you become aware of what is available in your own area to help people with diabetes keep healthy feet.

Activity 6.5 Caring for feet in your locality

Suggested study time 30 minutes

Find out what facilities are offered by your local podiatry (or chiropody) service and how people can access it. This can be based at your nearest hospital or at your GP surgery or there may be services at both places.

Comment

People with diabetes are entitled to free podiatry services, though in some areas there is a shortage of podiatrists leading to long waiting times for routine treatment. Services are usually based in secondary care, at hospitals, but some PCTs offer their own services. However, if a person with diabetes does have even a minor foot problem they should be able to get an emergency appointment at the hospital. They do not have to get a GP's referral for this.

At least once a year (usually as part of the annual review), the person's feet are examined for changes in shape, colour, warmth, and areas of pressure (as seen by areas of hard or thickened skin). The person is asked about any pain, tingling, or numbness they may have noticed. Some or all of the following tests are used to check sensation.

- The tip of a 10 g plastic thread called a **monofilament** (Figure 6.10a) is pressed into various areas of the foot, until the monofilament bends. The person is asked before the test begins to tell the examiner when he or she can feel the pressure. If they are unable to detect the monofilament, this demonstrates a reduction in sensation.

- A **neurotip** (Figure 6.10b) has a sharp and a blunt end. Each end is pressed on to the person's foot in varying areas, and they are asked to say whether they think the sharp or the blunt end is being used.

- A **tuning fork** (Figure 6.10c) is tapped against a hard object and then as it resonates it is placed against the foot. The person should be able to feel the fork vibrating.

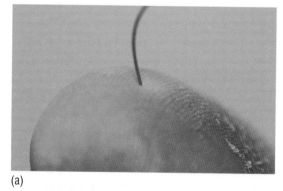
(a)

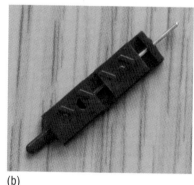
(b)

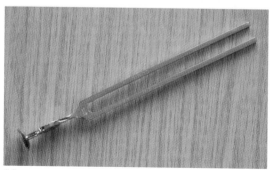
(c)

Figure 6.10 (a) A monofilament being applied to the surface of the skin. (b) A neurotip, about 2 cm in length, showing the sharp and blunt ends. (c) A tuning fork, about 10–15 cm in length. The disc at the end of the fork is held against the skin as the prongs vibrate.

- Why is more than one test sometimes applied to the feet?

- The monofilament, neurotip and tuning fork each test a different sensation, touch, pain and vibration. Sometimes there can be loss of one or more sensations due to the damage of the associated nerve fibres.

Warmth and coolness are also applied to the foot. The person should be able to tell the difference. If they are unable to distinguish between the two, the test is a good education tool as it makes them aware of the dangers of putting their feet against hot water bottles, near fires, or in hot bath water.

All these tests can be used to assess how sensitive the feet are. If nerve damage is present, sensation is reduced, and the person's feet are 'at risk'. Depending on previous history of ulceration, amputation, circulation, and their ability to care for their feet, the person is graded as low, medium or high risk. Education on self-care is crucial, as is care from a registered podiatrist.

6.7 Care of feet in people with diabetes

6.7.1 Footwear examination

Ill-fitting footwear is one of the most common causes of foot ulceration, particularly in older people, and is frequently a contributing factor to callus and blister formation. However, it is probably one of the most difficult areas to address due to fashion, finance, social stigma and peer pressure.

Anyone who has diabetes should check the inside of their shoes each time they are put on. This shoe check may also be carried out as part of the overall foot assessment. The shoes should be checked by feeling inside for rucks, seams and crinkled inner soles, as all these can cause trauma to the foot. If the toes have made an impression in the upper of the shoes they do not fit correctly, being too shallow, too short or too large, allowing the foot to slide back and forth in the shoe. It is not uncommon for people with neuropathy to wear shoes that are a size or two smaller than their feet because then the shoe squashing their feet stimulates the working nerves and lets them know the shoe is on the foot.

People with diabetes, even if they have no obvious foot problems, should avoid walking barefoot and should also avoid slip-on shoes or slippers. Trainers have most of the hallmarks of a well-fitting shoe (as outlined in Box 6.1) and are more suitable than slippers for indoor use.

Financial considerations may prevent some people from changing their footwear even if they wanted to. However cost is not the only consideration, as expensive shoes are not necessarily well-fitting shoes.

6.7.2 Basic foot care advice

The information below is an example of some basic foot care advice, which might prove useful for people with diabetes.

Box 6.1 What makes a good shoe?

The following characteristics make a good shoe:

- uppers made of a breathable material (e.g. leather)
- no more than 2 cm heel height
- long enough so that there is a 1 cm gap between the longest toe and the end of the shoe
- wide enough so as not to press on the widest part of the forefoot
- deep enough so as not to press on any of the toes
- shape of the front of the shoe should be a semicircle or D-shape
- soles should be made of rubber rather than leather or a thin hard material
- there should be no prominent seams or lining joins.

Importantly, there should be some form of fastening such as a lace or strap, as close as possible to where the foot joins the ankle. Ideally, laced shoes should have more than three pairs of eyelets to ensure adequate support.

Nail cutting

- Cut your nails to follow the shape of the end of your toes, not straight across.
- After cutting them, file away any sharp edges.
- There should be about 1 mm of white showing – avoid cutting them too short.

Your skin

- Use a bland moisturising cream on your feet every day, but not between your toes.
- If you have hard skin, try to remove it with either an emery board or pumice, but never with anything sharp.

Hygiene

- Wash your feet daily in warm water and use a mild soap.
- Dry well, especially between the toes.
- While washing and drying your feet, have a good look at them to check for any cuts, abrasions, blisters, splits or oozing.

Caution

- Avoid going barefoot.
- Avoid putting your feet on or near direct sources of heat (such as hot water bottles, fires and radiators) even if your feet feel cold.
- Avoid using medicated products for removal of hard skin or to treat ingrown toenails.

The basic advice on foot care for a person with diabetes is fairly simple, though it is vital that these procedures are carried out carefully every day so that good foot health is maintained. Many products are available over the counter for the treatment of foot conditions, or for general foot comfort and care (such as those shown in Figure 6.11). Activity 6.6 is about checking whether these products are suitable for use by people with diabetes, and can be done when you are out shopping one day.

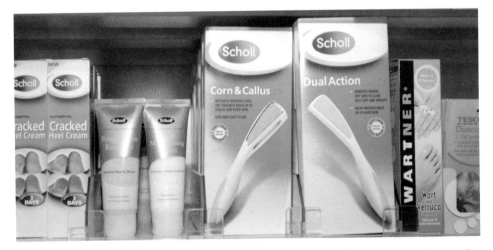

Figure 6.11 There are numerous foot care products available in supermarkets and pharmacies.

Activity 6.6 Choosing foot care products wisely for people with diabetes

Suggested study time 15 minutes

Go to your local pharmacy, or the pharmacy section of your supermarket, and look at the products on sale for foot care and treatment of minor foot conditions. How many state that people with diabetes should use them with caution, or not at all?

Why do you think these products should be used with caution in diabetes?

Comment

Many products sold to treat corns or verrucas on the foot contain caustic substances to treat the problem. However, these substances are damaging to normal skin and if used by someone with diabetes could result in skin breakdown, infection, ulceration and ultimately the possibility of amputation. Some cleansing and moisturising products may also be highly perfumed, or too harsh, and are not suitable for use by people with diabetes.

6.7.3 The impact of foot problems for people with diabetes

Foot problems have been shown to be one of the most serious of all the diabetes-related complications. Foot ulcers (open sores) are common, affecting approximately 15% of people with diabetes, and if not treated quickly they can lead to amputation (Rayman and Rayman, 1999). In fact, in people with diabetes a foot ulcer is the main precipitating cause of over 85% of all lower limb amputations (Apelqvist and Larsson, 2000). The good news is that if foot ulcers can be prevented, so can the majority of lower limb amputations to which they lead. Information gathered from research studies from all around the world has shown that where a structured foot care system is in place, that includes screening, health education, podiatry, multidisciplinary team working, adequate footwear and fast-track referrals to special ulcer clinics, amputation rates can be reduced significantly.

The basic formula for achieving success is team working, with an understanding that everyone within the team is very important no matter what his or her individual role. The list below gives a simplified formula to achieving success. (Who is involved with any of these activities will vary from place to place.)

- Annual foot inspection and examination of all people with diabetes.
- Foot health education for people with diabetes and, where appropriate, their carers.
- Identification of the at-risk foot.
- Regular inspection of all identified at-risk feet.
- Ensuring that those people identified with foot problems are receiving appropriate foot care.
- Footwear examination and provision of appropriate footwear.
- Rapid referral for treatment of all open sores, infections, or blood-stained hard skin.
- Good communication.
- Fast access to emergency treatment for foot problems.

6.8 Cardiovascular disease

Cardiovascular disease is the biggest killer of adults with diabetes, with the risk of a heart attack, and death from a heart attack, being much higher than in people who do not have diabetes (MacKinnon, 1998). Some people who survive a heart attack have such severe damage to the cardiac muscle that they remain very breathless, even at rest, and feel very tired. This may mean that they are unable to work or play an active part in their family life. Other people, even if they have not had a heart attack, may suffer from angina, which is discussed in the next section. The UK Prospective Diabetes Study (UKPDS, 1998) demonstrated that controlling risks for heart attacks (for example, blood pressure and cholesterol) is at least as important as controlling blood glucose. Before we discuss cardiovascular diseases further, we need to look at the structure of the heart.

6.8.1 Structure of the heart

The heart is described as a double pump (Figure 6.12). The left side of the heart collects oxygen-rich blood from the lungs and pumps it around the body to provide all the organs and cells of the body with oxygen. Meanwhile the right side of the heart collects oxygen-poor blood from the organs and cells of the body (where some of the oxygen has been used up) and pumps it to the lungs where it collects more oxygen. This cycle repeats about 70 times each minute (the heart rate) and continues throughout life. Measurements of heart rate are usually taken when you are at rest and when seated. Many things can alter heart rate – exercise, stress or anxiety can all increase heart rate.

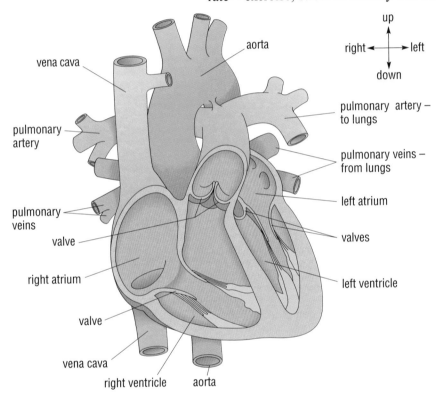

Figure 6.12 A cut-away diagram showing the internal structure and major blood vessels of the heart. (*Note*: The arrows at the top right of the diagram indicate the position in the body if we are looking at the person from the front.)

So that it can carry out this continuous pumping action, the heart is made of a special type of muscle called cardiac muscle or **myocardium**, with a very smooth lining (endocardium) that ensures that blood flows smoothly through the heart. As you can see from Figure 6.12, the heart is divided into four chambers: the left **atrium** and **ventricle**, and the right atrium and ventricle. On each side of the heart, the blood first enters the atrium which contracts to squeeze the blood through a central valve into the ventricle. The ventricle then contracts to deliver the blood into the **pulmonary artery** (on the right side of the heart) and hence to the lungs, and into the **aorta** (on the left side of the heart) and then all around the body. Both atria contract together, followed by both ventricles. The left ventricle has the thickest, most muscular wall as it has the most work to do in pumping the blood right around the body, from the top of the head to the ends of the toes and fingers.

6.8.2 Coronary heart disease

In order to be able to carry out its work, the heart must have a blood supply of its own so that the myocardium (heart muscle) can receive the oxygen and nutrients it needs for energy. This blood supply to the heart muscle is called the coronary circulation. Coronary arteries carry oxygen and nutrient-rich blood to the myocardium. Sometimes the coronary arteries become narrowed with atheroma (see Section 5.6), which stops the coronary arteries from carrying sufficient blood for the heart's needs. If this happens the person will suffer from **angina** (chest pain) or may have a **myocardial infarction** (heart attack). In such cases the person is said to have **coronary heart disease (CHD)**.

Atheroma is caused by abnormal blood lipids, high blood glucose, and high blood pressure (plus poor diet, lack of exercise and smoking) and can occur in all arteries. The presence of atheroma in arteries in other parts of the body can itself cause high blood pressure, contributing to the vicious circle of damaged blood vessels and hypertension.

● What do you understand by the term 'blood pressure'?

○ Everybody has blood pressure. The term blood pressure refers to the force with which the blood pushes against the walls of the blood vessels as it flows through them. This force is produced by the pumping action of the heart. When a person's blood pressure is measured using a sphygmomanometer or electronic measuring device, it is the pressure in the arteries (arterial blood pressure) that is measured. (Blood pressure was discussed in Sections 4.8.1 and 5.6.)

You can see that high blood pressure is both a risk factor for developing damage to blood vessels, and also a sign of existing damage. For these reasons, patients may have to take three or four different anti-hypertensive tablets to control their blood pressure. Adequate blood pressure control is essential in breaking the vicious circle of hypertension and arterial damage and is also very beneficial in preventing or slowing the progress of other complications of diabetes, such as nephropathy.

6.8.3 Strokes

Earlier in this section it was noted that atheroma can affect arteries throughout the body. This includes the arteries that supply the brain. Narrowing of these arteries restricts the flow of blood to the brain, and if an artery is completely blocked the area of the brain it is supplying with blood will die. This is called a **cerebrovascular accident (CVA)**, or stroke, and is due to progressive damage to the major blood vessels supplying the brain. This is called **cerebrovascular disease (CVD)**. The results of a stroke include speech difficulties, limb weakness or paralysis, confusion and difficulty swallowing. Some of these effects may improve over time, but some people are left with a permanent disability. If a large area of the brain is affected the person may die.

As you saw above with CHD, a person may suffer from angina, due to reduced flow of blood through the coronary arteries causing chest pain. In a similar way a person with atheroma affecting the cerebral arteries may experience **transient ischaemic attacks (TIAs)**. These occur when the blood flow to the brain is temporarily reduced, producing symptoms similar to a stroke but which resolve within 24 hours. A person with diabetes is at increased risk of suffering from TIAs and strokes. At the annual review it is important that questions are asked in such a way that any such episodes are identified.

6.8.4 Screening for CHD

Screening for CHD may be included in the annual review, especially if the patient complains of chest pain or fainting attacks. The commonest test is an electrocardiograph or ECG. This detects the electrical pattern of the heart's pumping action to see if there are any weak parts in the muscle, or an abnormal rhythm. The ECG may be checked while the patient walks on a treadmill, to see if the pattern changes with exercise (Figure 6.13). If the ECG suggests there may be a change in the shape of the heart because of damage to the muscle, the patient may have a scan of the heart so that more information can be gained.

Figure 6.13 (a) The ECG is measured while the patient is exercising. (b) An illustration of a typical ECG trace.

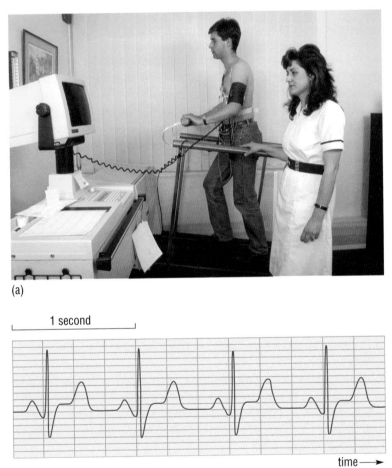

(a)

1 second

time ⟶

(b)

6.9 Summary of Chapter 6

We have explored the various long-term complications of diabetes in this chapter. These include a greater risk of damage associated with microvascular and macrovascular complications. They can have devastating effects and may even be life threatening. However, screening to detect early signs of these complications means that active treatment can be implemented with the aim of slowing the progression of the complications. In some cases early intervention will prevent serious consequences such as blindness, end-stage renal failure or amputation.

Questions for Chapter 6

Question 6.1 (Learning Outcome 6.2)

List the common long-term complications of diabetes.

Question 6.2 (Learning Outcome 6.2)

How are the risk factors (identified in Chapter 5) related to these complications?

Question 6.3 (Learning Outcome 6.3)

Name and briefly describe three main types of eye disease associated with diabetes.

Question 6.4 (Learning Outcomes 6.1 and 6.3)

Define diabetic nephropathy. What blood and urine changes are associated with this complication, and why do they occur?

Question 6.5 (Learning Outcome 6.4)

People with diabetes have a higher incidence of cardiovascular disease. Why is this, and how may this disease be recognised?

Question 6.6 (Learning Outcomes 6.1 and 6.5)

What is meant by diabetic neuropathy, and what effects can it have on the individual?

Question 6.7 (Learning Outcome 6.5)

Explain the main ways in which diabetes can affect the feet.

Question 6.8 (Learning Outcome 6.6)

At the beginning of this chapter you were introduced to Mr Evans, who had developed a foot ulcer. What advice would be given to Mr Evans about foot care?

Question 6.9 (Learning Outcome 6.7)

What screening measures are carried out at the annual review to identify long-term complications?

References

Apelqvist, J. and Larsson, J. (2000) 'What is the most effective way to reduce incidence of amputation in the diabetic foot?', *Diabetes–Metabolism Research and Reviews*, **16**, suppl.1, pp. S75–S83.

Cullen, M. (2002) 'Vision and Values', *Balance*, no. 187, May/June, pp. 25–28 [online] Available from: http://www.diabetes.org.uk/balance/187/187sue.htm (Accessed April 2005).

Diabetes Control and Complications Trial Research Group (DCCT) (1993) 'The effect of intensive treatment of diabetes on the development and progression of long-term complications in insulin-dependent diabetes mellitus', *New England Journal of Medicine*, **329** (14), pp. 977–986.

Jones, A. (2004) 'You've lost that loving feeling', *Balance*, no. 198, March/April, pp. 40–42, London, Diabetes UK.

MacKinnon, M. (1998) *Providing Diabetes Care in General Practice: a practical guide for the primary care team*, 2nd edn, London, Class Publishing.

Rayman, G. and Rayman, A. (1999) 'Avoid the distress caused by foot ulcers', *Practice Nurse*, **18** (9), 19 November, pp. 603–610.

UK Prospective Diabetes Study (UKPDS) (1998) 'Group Intensive blood glucose control with sulphonylureas or insulin compared with conventional treatment and risk of complications in patients with type 2 diabetes (UKPDS 33)', *Lancet*, **352**, pp. 837–853.

Warren, E. (2002) 'Diabetes', *DoctorUpdate*, 17 January, pp. 13–23 [online] Available from: http://www.doctorupdate.net/du_reference/ du_refarticle.asp?ID=5334# (Accessed April 2005).

CHAPTER 7

HYPERGLYCAEMIA AND HYPOGLYCAEMIA: LIVING ON THE EDGE?

Learning Outcomes

When you have completed this chapter you should be able to:

7.1 Define and use, or recognise definitions and applications of, each of the terms printed in **bold** in the text.

7.2 State the possible causes of hyperglycaemia and hypoglycaemia.

7.3 Describe simple physiological mechanisms that occur in hyperglycaemia and hypoglycaemia.

7.4 Identify who is at risk of hyperglycaemia and hypoglycaemia, and when they may be vulnerable.

7.5 Recognise the signs and symptoms of hyperglycaemia and hypoglycaemia.

7.6 State the general principles of treating hyperglycaemia and hypoglycaemia, depending upon the setting.

7.7 Give simple instructions about prevention, awareness and treatment of hyperglycaemia and hypoglycaemia.

7.8 Give simple instructions about self-management of sick days.

7.1 Introduction

Earlier chapters have provided you with an introduction to what diabetes is, how it can be managed medically and how to go about screening for risk factors and for the development of complications. We now move on to examine hyperglycaemia and hypoglycaemia (introduced in Chapter 2) in more detail, and consider some general principles for treating high and low blood glucose levels. We also examine some of the situations that cause variations in blood glucose control and how people with diabetes can manage them.

7.2 Hyperglycaemia

First of all, let us consider the possible causes of hyperglycaemia (you met this in Section 2.3.4) – that is, a high level of glucose in the blood. Start this section by reading, in Case Study 7.1, about the experiences of Mrs James.

Case Study 7.1

Mrs James is aged 72 and lives alone. She has been feeling very tired for the past few months and has put this down to getting older. Everything is a real effort, and she really cannot be bothered to go out with her friends anymore. To try and get some energy, she has been drinking an energy drink because she's seen the advertisements about this product.

Another reason why she hasn't been going out is the problem she has developed with her water works … she needs to keep spending a penny, and sometimes she just doesn't get to the toilet in time, which is so embarrassing. She has been trying not to drink so much to see if that will help, but her mouth has been so dry lately.

- What do you think is wrong with Mrs James?

- She has probably developed Type 2 diabetes which has resulted in hyperglycaemia.

Hyperglycaemia occurs when the blood glucose level is above the normal limit. You will recall from Chapter 2 that the blood glucose level is maintained between about 4 and 7 mmol/l in someone without diabetes, no matter what they have eaten. Hyperglycaemia can occur in people with Type 1 and Type 2 diabetes, either because there is insufficient insulin available in the blood, or the insulin they have is not working effectively. There are several reasons why this may happen.

Mrs James clearly demonstrates the signs and symptoms of high blood glucose. She is tired because the glucose in her blood is not an available energy source. She is passing large amounts of urine (known as polyuria, Section 5.2.1) as her kidneys remove the excessive glucose from her body – a process known as **osmotic diuresis**. This results in her becoming dehydrated, which is why her mouth is dry and she is thirsty. These symptoms have been developing slowly over several months, which is a common feature of newly diagnosed Type 2 diabetes. As she lives by herself, no one has noticed her gradual deterioration. Unfortunately, she has been trying to compensate for the tiredness by taking a sugary energy drink, which has increased the glucose level in her blood and made the symptoms worse!

The signs and symptoms of hyperglycaemia in Mrs James seem quite obvious to an informed observer. She was conscious of changes in her well-being but did not realise what the changes meant. Sometimes, however, someone may have hyperglycaemia but not notice any symptoms, as you will see as you read the story in Case Study 7.2.

Case Study 7.2

John has recently been to the optician, as he hadn't had his eyesight checked for a while. After examining his eyes, the optician advised John to see his GP for some blood tests as he could see changes at the back of John's eyes that suggested he had diabetes. The GP confirmed that John's blood glucose level was high and that he had probably had diabetes for several years as he had already developed diabetic retinopathy.

John has obviously had a high blood glucose level for some time. It has not been high enough to cause him distress. However, the high blood glucose will still have damaged his body. This is why it is recommended that people with diabetes monitor their blood glucose level, both by urine or blood tests and by annual glycated haemoglobin blood tests. You cannot rely on how you feel to tell how well controlled your diabetes is.

●   Can you recall the test for glycated haemoglobin?

●   It is the HbA_{1c} test (see Section 5.3.4).

7.2.1 Causes of hyperglycaemia

Hyperglycaemia is likely to be present at the time of diagnosis of diabetes, but once the condition is treated it can still reoccur.

There are particular times when people are more vulnerable to hyperglycaemia, as you will consider in Activity 7.1.

Activity 7.1 Causes of hyperglycaemia

Suggested study time 10 minutes

Think about a time when you have had hyperglycaemia yourself, or talk to someone you know who has had it. Think about what might have happened to cause the hyperglycaemia.

Comment

Events that might contribute to the development of hyperglycaemia in people with diabetes include:

- undiagnosed diabetes
- being stressed or upset about something, or a traumatic event like an accident
- being unwell, having an infection, or after an event like a heart attack
- surgery
- taking particular medicines, e.g. steroids
- going through the later stages of pregnancy
- stopping insulin injections or diabetes tablets
- taking insufficient insulin, perhaps because the insulin pen device is not functioning properly, using expired or damaged insulin that has lost some of its potency, or injecting into an area of skin that does not absorb the insulin properly
- eating too much carbohydrate-containing food
- decreasing the usual amount of exercise taken
- gaining weight.

- Why does weight gain cause a high blood glucose level in someone with Type 2 diabetes?

- Being overweight causes insulin resistance, which makes any insulin present less effective. This results in a high blood glucose level. (See Section 2.3.6.)

Any of the events listed in Activity 7.1 could result in insulin levels being too low to deal with the amount of glucose circulating in the blood, with the result that glucose cannot pass into the cells to be used as a source of energy. While it stays in the blood, the level of glucose can be estimated by blood glucose monitoring. When insulin levels are inadequate to cope with this level of glucose, the liver, muscle and fat cells are not able to take up sufficient glucose from the blood to maintain a normal blood glucose level. A low insulin level also causes glucose to be released by the liver into the blood – a process that is normally suppressed by insulin. The effect of all this is to keep the blood glucose level high.

Stress, whether physical or emotional, also raises blood glucose because of the actions of the stress hormones **adrenalin** and **cortisol** (one of the steroid hormones). Steroid hormones are chemical messengers that occur naturally in the body, or in the case of cortisol, may be prescribed for the treatment of conditions such as asthma or arthritis; collectively the steroid hormones that raise blood glucose are called **glucocorticoids**.

A person with Type 1 diabetes who is severely deficient in insulin (perhaps because they have forgotten to take their injection) starts to break down fats in the body. This occurs because the body still has a need for energy, and glucose is unavailable because of the lack of insulin. However (as discussed in Section 2.3.5) fats cannot be broken down completely without enough insulin to allow glucose to enter cells, and as a result ketones are produced. Although these ketones are used as an alternative energy source for the body (particularly the brain), they make the blood more acidic than normal. If the level of ketones builds up, a dangerous condition called diabetic ketoacidosis can result. (This was discussed in Section 5.4.) This condition results from the blood becoming so acidic that all the normal processes in the body, which are very sensitive to how acidic the blood is, are not able to work properly. Ketoacidosis usually only occurs in people with Type 1 diabetes who produce no insulin of their own. In Type 2 diabetes some insulin is still produced, and so ketoacidosis is less likely. Ketoacidosis is a potentially life threatening condition in the short term, and requires urgent treatment, usually in a hospital.

Case Study 7.3

Susan

Susan is 26 years old and has had Type 1 diabetes for 12 years. She has had an upset stomach for the last 24 hours and has been sick. As she was not eating, she stopped her insulin because she thought her blood glucose level might drop too low without food. This morning, her blood sugar was 28 mmol/l despite not eating since breakfast time yesterday. She is still being sick and has tested her urine for ketones. The test shows she has large amounts of ketones present.

Joe

It is bedtime and Joe, who has Type 1 diabetes, has had a great Christmas Day. He knows he has eaten too much and really those mint creams on top of the mince pies were a big mistake! He has had to pass urine four times in the last hour so he knows his blood glucose level is high. He checks it and finds his blood glucose is 24.6 mmol/l. He also tests his urine for ketones but this is negative. He knows that he has had his usual insulin dose (which is why he does not have any ketones in his urine) but he has had far more carbohydrate than usual which is why his blood glucose is so high.

Activity 7.2 Who is most at risk?

Suggested study time 20 minutes

Having read the two stories in Case Study 7.3, who is at most risk of becoming seriously ill, Joe or Susan?

Comment

Susan is at most risk because her lack of insulin is not only causing hyperglycaemia but also the production of ketones. This is a medical emergency. Joe does not have ketones in his urine, despite his high blood glucose level. His blood glucose will gradually return to normal over the next 24 hours if he returns to his normal diet and continues with his insulin.

An increased blood glucose level in people with Type 1 diabetes is associated with a greater chance of developing the long-term complications of diabetes. This was demonstrated in an important study called the Diabetes Control and Complications Trial (DCCT, 1993), as was described in Chapter 5 (Box 5.1). Another study, the UK Prospective Diabetes Study (1998; see Box 5.2), showed that having a high blood glucose level over several years also caused damage in people with Type 2 diabetes. The daily experience of having high blood glucose is described in Chapter 1 – hyperglycaemia can affect relationships, the ability to work, and quality of life because it can make the person tired, irritable, lacking in energy, and depressed.

Another consequence of hyperglycaemia is that children born to mothers who have persistently high blood glucose during pregnancy have a greater chance of having a high birth weight, and in some cases an increased risk of stillbirth and birth defects. An increased risk of birth defects is related to pre-existing diabetes in the mother, but all the other problems referred to have the potential to also occur in gestational diabetes, a form of diabetes that is only present during pregnancy.

7.2.2 Prevention of hyperglycaemia

As hyperglycaemia occurs because of a lack of insulin (either complete or relative lack), it follows that it is important that the body has enough insulin to deal with the requirements of the body in certain situations. The amount of insulin may need to be increased during vulnerable periods, or the demand for insulin can be reduced (for example, by eating less carbohydrate or increasing the amount of exercise taken) depending on the cause of the high blood glucose.

If someone with Type 1 diabetes is vomiting, they should continue to have insulin injections. However, because of the effects of being unwell, they will require *more* insulin than usual, even though they may not be eating. This is due to the hyperglycaemic effects of the stress hormones produced during sickness, and is why Susan (Case Study 7.3) had a raised blood glucose level despite not eating. In cases of severe hyperglycaemia, insulin is usually given by intravenous infusion (a 'drip') in hospital. A dextrose (or glucose) infusion is also available should the blood glucose level go too low. The rate of the insulin infusion can be adjusted quickly, as required, when it is given intravenously. Once the person is able to eat and drink normally, and has stopped being sick, the intravenous infusion is stopped and the usual regimen of insulin injections is resumed. Surgery is another occasion when intravenous insulin is commonly used in people with Type 1 diabetes.

People with Type 2 diabetes may need to go to hospital and have intravenous insulin too, particularly if they normally require a large dose of diabetes tablets, are having major surgery, or are vomiting and unable to take their usual tablets. Although people with Type 2 diabetes still produce some insulin, and may keep their blood glucose level within the normal range with a healthy diet and diabetes tablets, they may not be able to continue to do so when they are ill, or if their body is producing large amounts of stress hormones.

Of course, everyone has periods of relatively minor illness, like colds or a urinary tract infection, for example. These ailments can still cause an increase in the blood glucose level, even if the person is taking their usual amount of insulin and eating normally. Again this is the effect of the stress hormones. People with diabetes, particularly those with Type 1 diabetes, need to know how to manage their diabetes during periods of illness, so that they avoid the development of ketoacidosis and admission to hospital for intravenous insulin.

There are a few simple instructions given to help people manage their diabetes during illness. You may hear them described as the 'sick day rules'. The instructions include the following:

- Do not stop your insulin or tablets.
- Try to drink plenty of sugar-free fluids to avoid dehydration.
- If you are unable to eat normally, try easily digested foods, for example, nibble on biscuits, drink soups and milky drinks, sip Lucozade®, or eat ice cream.
- Test your blood glucose at least four times a day while unwell.
- Test your urine or blood for ketones.
- If the blood tests show your blood glucose level is persistently high, especially if you have ketones either in your blood or urine, then be prepared to take extra quick-acting insulin.
- If you are vomiting, or your blood glucose and ketone levels are not improving, you *must* seek emergency medical help.

Activity 7.3 Sick day rules

Suggested study time 1 hour

Discuss the sick day rules with the people you meet (or know) who have diabetes. Some people still believe they should stop their insulin if they are not eating. (These people should be referred to their local diabetes specialist nurse for advice, or, if they are not under the care of a hospital clinic, to the person with responsibility for diabetes care at their GP practice.) Find out if the diabetes department you or someone you know attend or work in has written guidance on coping with illness and diabetes, particularly about how much to increase insulin doses.

Read Offprint 7.1 from *Balance* entitled 'When you are ill' (Diabetes UK, 2003) (Figure 7.1) to see what advice Diabetes UK gives for dealing with diabetes when you are ill.

Comment

Sick day rules apply to all people with diabetes, including those with Type 2 diabetes taking diabetes tablets or managing their diabetes with diet alone. They should continue taking their tablets, but sometimes they may need to change to insulin treatment temporarily during illness if their blood glucose level is very high. As the *Balance* article says, if there is any doubt or concern about what to do when ill, always contact your GP or health care team for advice.

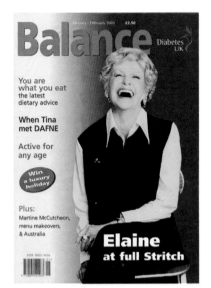

Figure 7.1 The cover of the January/February 2003 issue of *Balance*, where the article 'When you are ill' appears.

7.2.3 Recognising hyperglycaemia

If hyperglycaemia is not too severe, there may be no apparent symptoms. (You read about such a situation in John's story in Case Study 2.5.) Although John had diabetes, he experienced no symptoms. This can be dangerous because if the diabetes remains untreated, long-term complications may be developing without the person being aware. This is the reason why the annual review is so important (as you saw in Chapters 5 and 6), to screen for risk factors and for the development of complications.

In contrast, Jennifer, whom you also met in Chapter 2, was experiencing discomfort as a result of her symptoms. (If you cannot remember what these symptoms were, turn back to her story, in Case Study 2.4, to remind yourself of them.)

If hyperglycaemia in those people with Type 1 diabetes remains untreated, symptoms such as those experienced by Jennifer become more severe. They develop quite slowly, over a period of hours and days rather than minutes. The symptoms are likely to include feeling thirsty, passing large amounts of urine frequently, losing weight, loss of appetite and feeling or being sick, breath that smells of pear drops (indicating the presence of ketones), and increasing drowsiness or unconsciousness. When the acidosis caused by the ketones becomes very severe, breathing becomes slow and laboured, often described as 'deep and sighing'. This is called **Kussmaul's respiration**, or acidotic respiration, and is a sign that urgent hospital treatment is required.

As well as assessing the physical signs of hyperglycaemia, blood tests may be taken to assess how serious it is, and how acidic the blood has become. The body is not able to function very well if the blood becomes too acidic and hospital admission will be needed to correct the condition.

7.2.4 Treating hyperglycaemia

The aim of any treatment of hyperglycaemia is to correct the blood glucose to a normal level and adjust any other imbalances that have occurred in the body, for example, dehydration.

Treatment of hyperglycaemia depends on what is causing the high blood glucose level, but the aim of treatment is always the same. You have considered the effects of illness and stress on glycaemic control, and prevention and treatment in these situations. However, many people have periods of high blood glucose without being ill.

People with diabetes are usually encouraged to monitor their diabetes control by testing their blood glucose level, or by measuring the presence or absence of glucose in their urine. If the test results are not within their agreed target range, they should be encouraged to do something about it, if only to report the results to their GP or nurse. However, many people can recognise the cause of the hyperglycaemia and take the necessary action to correct the condition. Consider the examples given in Case Study 7.4.

Case Study 7.4

Mrs Smith

Mrs Smith is 58 years old and has had Type 2 diabetes for four years. She takes metformin tablets to control her diabetes. She notices that her blood glucose readings have been higher than usual in the last week.
However, as the weather has been cold and wet for the past fortnight, she has not been going for the daily brisk walk she usually tries to take every day. As the weather continues to be cold, she decides to go swimming and to an exercise class with a friend at the local sports centre instead.
Exercise helps her body to be more sensitive to the limited insulin supply she is able to produce. Stopping exercise means she needed to produce more insulin to control her blood glucose level. As she is unable to produce more, her blood glucose rose. Resuming exercise means her own amounts of insulin are sufficient again for her needs.

James

James is 48 years old and has had Type 1 diabetes for 22 years. It is 2 January and he has noticed his blood glucose level has been running high for the last week. He feels well and is not ill.
He realises that although he has been taking his usual amount of insulin, he has been eating far more than usual over the Christmas period. He therefore has insufficient insulin for the amount of sugar he is putting into his body. He knows he could increase his insulin and continue eating the same amount of food, but although this will bring his blood glucose level down to normal again, he is likely to gain weight. He decides to get back to his usual eating pattern, and reduce his food intake to match his insulin supply.

Ahmed

Ahmed has had Type 2 diabetes for seven years. He is on 1g metformin and 160 mg gliclazide twice a day. He is doing his best with his diet, and in fact has started to lose a bit of weight without really trying. However, he has noticed over the last six months that it is getting harder to keep his blood glucose level within the target he agreed with his diabetes team. Type 2 diabetes is progressive and Ahmed has now had the condition for a long time. He is on a large dose of tablets, but is not producing enough insulin for his needs. His GP suggests that he needs to change to insulin injections to control his blood glucose level.

Emma

Emma is 15 years old and has Type 1 diabetes. By lunchtime she feels very thirsty and keeps having to visit the loo. Her blood glucose is 22 mmol/l. She realises that she has forgotten her morning insulin injection. Although she does not normally inject in the middle of the day, she decides to give herself a dose of quick-acting insulin, to bring the blood glucose down during the afternoon, and to then resume her usual injection regime with her evening meal.

So far in this chapter you've considered high blood glucose – hyperglycaemia – how to recognise the condition and ways of treating it. We will now consider hypoglycaemia – that is, low blood glucose.

7.3 Hypoglycaemia

Start this section by reading David's story in Case Study 7.5.

Case Study 7.5

David is aged 19, and has had Type 1 diabetes for 12 years. He controls his blood glucose with two injections of insulin a day, one before breakfast and one before his evening meal. It is 2 pm and he has had a busy morning. He has not had time to have his usual mid-morning snack and he is late for lunch. He is finding it very difficult to concentrate, and has a terrible headache. His hands keep trembling, he keeps staggering, and he is sweating profusely. His workmate John notices David is unwell and gets him a sugary drink. After about 10 minutes, David feels better.

- What is wrong with David?
- He has hypoglycaemia, which is when the blood glucose level drops below the normal lower limit of about 4 mmol/l (see Section 2.3.4).

How do you think David felt about this happening? You may have thought he felt embarrassed at needing help from a workmate. Sometimes someone with hypoglycaemia can behave very differently from usual, as if they are drunk, for example. If the condition is not treated, the blood glucose level can drop so low that the person can lose consciousness, which is very frightening for those around them as well as for the person with diabetes. In certain situations, it can also be very dangerous.

- Can you think of a situation when low blood glucose can be dangerous?

- Hypoglycaemia can be dangerous if it occurs while the person is driving a car or using machinery.

As the term hypoglycaemia is a bit of a mouthful, it is usually referred to as 'hypo' for short. Although generally a blood glucose level of 3 mmol/l or less is usually defined as hypoglycaemia, in reality subtle signs and symptoms of low blood glucose can occur at a level of 3.9 mmol/l or less. Diabetes UK suggested the phrase 'make 4 the floor' for this reason, and so people with diabetes, while being encouraged to keep as near to normal blood glucose level as possible, are discouraged from regularly letting the level fall to 3.9 mmol/l or less. Hypoglycaemia is caused by too much insulin in the blood for the body's needs, which results in the blood glucose level falling to below normal limits. This excess of insulin may be from injections. As discussed in Section 4.5.1, insulin can be divided into three groups – short-acting, intermediate-acting and long-acting. All these types of insulin, if given in excessive amounts or without sufficient starchy food, can cause hypoglycaemia. An excess of insulin can also be caused by tablets that stimulate the pancreas to produce more insulin.

Activity 7.4 Medication that can cause hypos

Suggested study time 30 minutes

Go to the Diabetes UK website and find the information on 'Tablets available in the UK' (you will find a link to this article on the course website). If you can, print this document for further reference. If this is not possible, read the information carefully and make some notes of your own about the various drugs. Find the names of the common diabetes tablets that can cause hypos. If you are someone who has diabetes, are you taking diabetes medication that can cause low blood glucose?

Comment

The sorts of diabetes tablet that can cause low blood glucose are those that stimulate the insulin-producing β cells in the pancreas. These tablets are called sulphonylureas, and examples are glibenclamide, gliclazide, tolbutamide and glimepiride. There is another class of tablets called post-prandial regulators which are given just before meals and examples are repaglinide and nateglinide. (These two are more commonly known by their trade names NovoNorm® and Starlix®.) They stimulate the β cells to produce a short burst of insulin to cover that meal. Sometimes they can also cause hypoglycaemia, especially if they are taken without eating carbohydrate-containing food.

Case Study 7.6

Mr Shah is 78 years old. He has Type 2 diabetes treated by glibenclamide tablets. He is attending the day centre today, but lunch is late because a new cook has started who does not know the routine. Staff notice that Mr Shah is shouting at the lady sitting next to him, and staggering about.

Activity 7.5 What's wrong with Mr Shah?

Suggested study time 10 minutes

What is wrong with Mr Shah (as described in Case Study 7.6) and why has it happened?

Comment

It sounds as if Mr Shah has hypoglycaemia. Changes in behaviour, with people appearing as if they are drunk, can be a sign of low blood glucose. Mr Shah is taking a sulphonylurea called glibenclamide which can cause hypoglycaemia. The most obvious cause for Mr Shah's hypo is that his lunch has been delayed and the tablet is making his body produce insulin when it is not required. This particular tablet has a long action period, which can be a problem in older people as their kidneys do not clear drugs out of their body at the usual rate. This means that drugs may accumulate in the body over time.

Although many people are frightened about having a low blood glucose level (being hypo), and sometimes try to keep their blood glucose level higher than the recommended target range to avoid it, in general, hypos are less dangerous than a high glucose level. There are some exceptions to this, such as repeated severe hypos, and hypos following heavy alcohol intake, where the liver function may be affected. However, although in medical terms hypos may be less severe than high blood glucose, they may cause people to feel embarrassed and distressed if they occur in public, and may be dangerous for those driving a vehicle or operating machinery at the time. Many people with diabetes dread having a hypo, and fear this more than the development of diabetes complications from long-term hyperglycaemia. This is how one person described her hypos.

'Always at the back of my mind I am waiting for hypoglycaemia. And I wait for it with dread … Some hypos are mainly physical, some are mainly mental and some are both. They share a common core of ghastliness, but the ones I hate most are the mental ones … I am not violent or aggressive when hypo. Instead, I am without personality; a corpse performing a malignant parody of myself'

(Theresa McLean quoted in Tattersall, 2000)

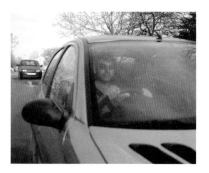

Figure 7.2 We take our right to drive for granted but it is important to be aware of our responsibilities.

There are some restrictions in relation to driving (Figure 7.2) and hypoglycaemia. As you can imagine, someone driving a vehicle while hypoglycaemic is extremely dangerous. Advice to stop driving temporarily (or in some cases, permanently) is given to those in the following situations:

- Anyone who is newly diagnosed with Type 1 diabetes or who is commencing insulin treatment should stop driving until his or her blood glucose level is stable, particularly if their eyesight is affected. In reality, it can take weeks to stabilise the blood glucose level when first starting insulin but this is usually due to a high, not low glucose level, so many people continue to drive.

- Anyone who is having recurrent hypos, especially if they are severe, should not drive.

- Anyone who has reduced or absent hypoglycaemic awareness should also avoid driving as they would be unable to detect a hypo developing while they are driving.

If a driver is having recurrent episodes of hypoglycaemia, especially if they have no awareness of the hypo developing, the DVLA will revoke their licence. This is in the interest of public safety as well as for their own safety. A doctor who is aware that someone is still driving despite having regular hypos or having lost their ability to spot the warning signs is obliged to inform the DVLA on the patient's behalf. They should, of course, always discuss this with the patient before doing so.

Drivers who have diabetes treated by insulin (or tablets that stimulate insulin production) must be warned about hypoglycaemia, and how to prevent it while driving. Drivers should follow a few basic rules.

- They should always keep fast-acting carbohydrate (for example, dextrose tablets) in the car, along with some biscuits or something similar. This is particularly useful if stuck in a motorway traffic jam!

- They should always carry some form of identification (such as is shown in Figure 7.3) indicating that they have diabetes.

- If they begin to feel hypo, they should stop the car as soon as possible, and get out of the driver's seat (to demonstrate they are not in charge of the car while unable to safely drive it).

- They should not drive for at least 45 minutes after a hypo, as it takes this long for brain function to be restored.

- They should always be prepared when driving – never drive when due for a meal or after drinking alcohol, stop for regular meals and snacks, and check blood glucose level regularly. Diabetes UK recommends drivers test their glucose level every 90 minutes on long journeys, as it is an offence to drive a vehicle while hypo and is likely to lead to prosecution and loss of driving licence.

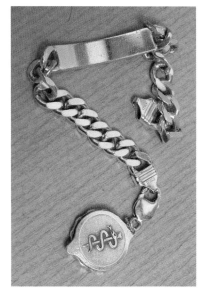

Figure 7.3 A medical alert bracelet to show that the wearer has diabetes.

7.3.1 Causes of hypoglycaemia

You now know about the symptoms and effects of hypoglycaemia, but what causes it to happen? Think about this in Activity 7.6.

Activity 7.6 Causes of hypos

Suggested study time 20 minutes

As hypoglycaemia occurs as a result of too much insulin in the blood, in excess of the body's immediate requirements, try to think of some reasons why this situation may occur. (You have already read in Activity 7.4 that some medication can cause hypos.) You may have personal experience, or be able to talk to people with diabetes who have experienced hypos.

Comment

Hypoglycaemia may occur if any of the following have happened.

- Too much insulin has been prescribed.

- There has been an accidental or deliberate overdose of insulin or insulin-producing diabetes tablets.

- The amount of exercise has been increased. Be aware that although exercise more commonly leads to hypoglycaemia, occasionally high blood glucose occurs. Regular monitoring can help the person know what is happening.

- Not enough foods containing carbohydrate have been eaten.

- Meals or snacks have been delayed or missed.

- The person is under stress. (Although this usually causes an increase in blood glucose level, some people experience a decrease when under stress.)

- The person has renal problems. (This causes insulin or tablets to accumulate in the blood for longer than normal because the kidneys are not disposing of them effectively.)

- The person has lost a significant amount of weight, whether intentionally from a weight-reducing diet, or unintentionally through ill health, for example, cancer. A dose reduction of insulin or tablets for diabetes is commonly required, since sensitivity to insulin increases with weight loss. However it is important to remember that a high blood glucose level can itself cause weight loss.

- The effect of excessive heat or hot weather can cause insulin to be absorbed more quickly, resulting in an overdose effect.

- A change to a new injection site from a previous area that had been used excessively can mean insulin is absorbed more readily. (Insulin is not absorbed well from over-used areas.)

- The injection technique is poor, for example where insulin is injected into a muscle instead of fat. Muscle has a much richer blood supply than fat and therefore the insulin dose is absorbed very rapidly, giving an overdose effect.

- During the early stages of pregnancy, especially when a woman has morning sickness and is not eating as much as usual. The hormones of early pregnancy can produce a hypoglycaemic effect, even in someone who does not have diabetes.

- The person has got drunk – alcohol has a blood glucose-lowering effect.

Insulin allows glucose to enter cells, for example muscle, liver and fat cells, where it is a source of energy, and also suppresses glucose release from the liver. All this has the effect of keeping the blood glucose level low. The body tries to correct a low blood glucose level by releasing other substances (hormones) including adrenaline, steroids and glucagon. (See Section 2.3.7.) All these substances raise the blood glucose level naturally. This is why people usually recover spontaneously from a hypo (albeit very slowly over several hours). Some people may go hypo while they are asleep, and wake up the next morning without being aware of the hypo. In these circumstances the blood glucose level is higher in the morning because of the hormones that were produced in an attempt to rectify the low blood glucose level.

7.3.2 Prevention of hypoglycaemia

Hypoglycaemia is prevented by making sure that the body does not have an excess of insulin, or alternatively has sufficient carbohydrate to match the energy needs of the body. This may mean reducing the amount of injected insulin, or increasing the amount of carbohydrate-containing foods in certain situations, for example before exercise. Case Study 7.7 illustrates various ways people manage their diet and insulin treatment to avoid hypoglycaemia.

Case Study 7.7

Jane

Jane has Type 1 diabetes. She injects quick-acting insulin with each meal and long-acting insulin at bedtime. She adjusts the units of quick-acting insulin according to the amount of carbohydrate she is having with her meal. Usually she takes four units of insulin with her breakfast of two slices of toast. Today, however, she only injects two units because she has got up late and only has time to eat one slice of toast.

Steve

Steve has Type 2 diabetes treated with insulin. He has an injection with breakfast which controls his blood glucose level during the day, and an injection with his evening meal which controls the blood glucose in the evening and during the night.

He has taken up jogging at the weekends and runs for four miles in the mornings. On Saturday and Sunday, therefore, he reduces his morning insulin by a third, because he knows the exercise will make his insulin work more effectively and so he is at risk of having a hypo while out running if he has his usual weekday dose. Also, the exercising muscles are taking up glucose very readily. He could eat extra food instead, to prevent the hypo happening, but he does not like to run with a full stomach.

Julie

Julie has Type 1 diabetes. She is visiting friends for an evening meal, which was supposed to be served at 7 pm. She had her insulin at 6.40 pm in preparation for this, but it is now 7.30 pm and there is no sign of the meal appearing. She eats three of the dextrose tablets she keeps in her handbag to keep her blood glucose level above 4 mmol/l and so avoids having a hypo.

7.3.3 Recognising hypoglycaemia

Experience of hypoglycaemia varies from person to person. Some people have no awareness of becoming hypo, so it is very important that they monitor their blood glucose level regularly, and in particular before driving or using machinery.

Activity 7.7 Experiencing hypoglycaemia

Suggested study time 20 minutes

Think of a time when you have been hypo, or talk to people you know who have. What symptoms have you experienced or had described to you?

Comment

Symptoms of hypoglycaemia come on quite quickly, usually within a period of minutes, and fall into two groups. There are those that occur as a result of stimulation of the peripheral nervous system, and those that occur because the functioning of the brain is affected.

If you have experienced or been told about symptoms such as feeling shaky, sweaty, clammy, having palpitations, feeling very hungry and irritable, these are likely to be due to stimulation of the nervous system by hormones such as adrenalin being released. If the symptoms are of feeling very lethargic and drowsy, being unable to focus or concentrate and being a bit vague, or other people commenting that you have a 'glazed expression', these are likely to be due to the brain's response to a low blood glucose level. Quite often, the first set of symptoms appears before the second, but this is not always the case. If the hypo is not treated, loss of consciousness may occur, but remember that people usually recover spontaneously. However, this may take several hours and the person with diabetes will feel unwell afterwards. Some people describe it as feeling as if they have a hangover, or they feel as if they have had a nightmare or disturbed sleep. Sometimes, the symptoms of hypoglycaemia are mistaken for those of being drunk, so if there is any doubt the person should be treated as if they are hypoglycaemic.

7.3.4 Treating hypoglycaemia

The aim of treating a hypo is to raise the blood glucose level to within normal limits and to relieve symptoms. This involves giving glucose by mouth or injecting glucagon intramuscularly. In some cases glucose is injected intravenously in a hospital, but this is rarely necessary.

All people treated with insulin or tablets that stimulate insulin production must be advised about how to treat hypoglycaemia. By recognising the early symptoms of a hypo, the progression to more disabling signs and symptoms can often be avoided by immediate treatment with rapid-acting carbohydrate.

Activity 7.8 Treating hypos

Suggested study time 10 minutes

If you have diabetes, and are at risk of hypoglycaemia, what do you use to treat the onset of a hypo? If you work with people who have diabetes, or know other people with diabetes, ask them the same question.

Comment

You should find that people use one or some of the following (see Figure 7.4):

*   three dextrose (glucose) tablets
*   Lucozade®
*   non-diet fizzy drinks
*   two or three spoons of sugar in a small amount of a warm drink
*   two or three barley sugar sweets or fruit pastilles.

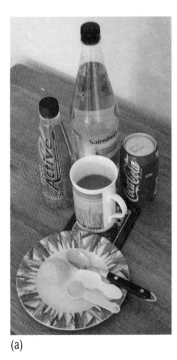

(a)

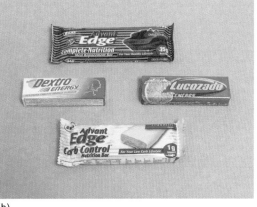

(b)

Figure 7.4 (a) Examples of some sugary foods and drinks and (b) energy bars and dextrose tablets that will help raise the blood glucose level rapidly.

Although these treatments cause a rapid rise in blood glucose, the effect is relatively short-lived. The treatments are repeated until the blood glucose has returned to normal and the symptoms have improved. A snack or meal containing starchy carbohydrate should then be consumed, to maintain the blood glucose and prevent a further episode of hypoglycaemia.

People at risk of hypos should carry rapid-acting carbohydrate (for example, dextrose tablets, Figure 7.4b) with them at all times, along with an identification card detailing their condition or a medical alert bracelet (Figure 7.3). A supply of hypo treatments should always be available in diabetes clinics.

If the early signs and symptoms of hypoglycaemia are ignored or not noticed, the person will become more uncoordinated and less capable of rational thought and action. They may not be able to treat the hypo themselves. Partners or carers of people at risk of hypoglycaemia should be advised on how to identify hypoglycaemia, and how to treat it. If the person with diabetes is refusing to drink a sugary drink, a sugary gel called Hypostop can be squirted into the person's mouth. This will either be swallowed, or it can be massaged into the inside of the cheeks. However, if the person is unconscious, nothing should be put into their mouth, to avoid choking. In such cases, a severe hypo is treated by intravenous injection of glucose, or by giving an intramuscular injection of glucagon. (This is the hormone that has the opposite effect to insulin, and it allows the liver to release glucose into the blood.) The partners or carers of people with diabetes who have frequent severe hypos may learn how to administer glucagon (Figure 7.5), rather than always having to call paramedic help.

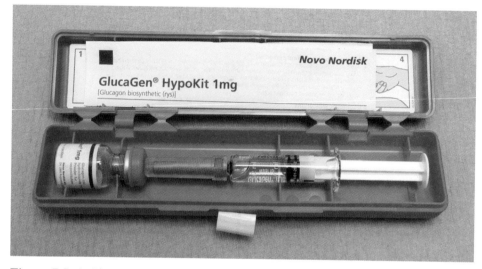

Figure 7.5 A GlucaGen® Kit for treating severe hypoglycaemia.

7.4 Summary of Chapter 7

This chapter has focused on hyperglycaemia and hypoglycaemia. The causes, prevention, recognition and treatment relating to the two conditions have been discussed. Many people with diabetes experience hyperglycaemia and hypoglycaemia at some time in their lives, but they are not inevitable and can occur to varying degrees. In general, hyperglycaemia is the more serious of the two in the long term (or the short term if diabetic ketoacidosis develops in people with Type 1 diabetes) and may be life threatening if left untreated. Education and blood glucose monitoring play an important role in their prevention. It is important to be sure that you can recognise the difference between hyperglycaemia and hypoglycaemia and know what to do in each case.

> It is vital that insulin is never stopped without first discussing it with a specialist health care professional in the diabetes team.

Table 7.1 summarises the differences between the symptoms of hyperglycaemia and hypoglycaemia.

Table 7.1 Symptoms of hyperglycaemia and hypoglycaemia.

Hyperglycaemia		Hypoglycaemia
Type 1 diabetes	**Type 2 diabetes**	**Type 1 and Type 2 diabetes**
thirst	thirst	headache
passing large amounts of urine	passing large amounts of urine	trembling hands
blurred vision	blurred vision	unsteadiness
tiredness	tiredness	sweatiness
weight loss (sudden)	weight gain (gradual)	clamminess
feeling/being sick		palpitations
breath smells of pear drops presence of ketones in urine		hunger
		irritability
		lack of concentration
		lethargy
		drowsiness
		glazed expression

Questions for Chapter 7

Question 7.1 (Learning Outcome 7.5)

Describe the signs and symptoms of hyperglycaemia.

Question 7.2 (Learning Outcome 7.4)

Who is at risk of developing hyperglycaemia?

Question 7.3 (Learning Outcome 7.3)

Explain why the signs and symptoms of hyperglycaemia occur.

Question 7.4 (Learning Outcomes 7.2 and 7.7)

How would someone with Type 1 diabetes avoid developing hypoglycaemia?

Question 7.5 (Learning Outcomes 7.6 and 7.7)

Which of the following treatments would not be suitable for hypoglycaemia?

Lucozade, cola, diet lemonade, honey, hypostop, glucagon injection, a sandwich.

Question 7.6 (Learning Outcome 7.8)

James has Type 1 diabetes and has woken up this morning feeling sick. What advice would you give him?

References

Diabetes Control and Complications Trial Research Group (DCCT) (1993) 'The effects of intensive treatment of diabetes on the development and progression of long-term complications in insulin-dependent diabetes mellitus', *New England Journal of Medicine*, **329** (14), pp. 977–986.

Diabetes UK (2003) 'When you are ill', *Balance*, January/February 2003 [online] Available from: http://www.diabetes.org.uk/balance/191/191ill.htm (Accessed April 2005).

Diabetes UK (2005) *Tablets available in the UK* [online] Available from: http://www.diabetes.org.uk/products/tablets.htm (Accessed April 2005).

Tattersall, R. B. (2000) Frequency, causes and treatment of hypoglycaemia, in *Hypoglycaemia in Clinical Diabetes*, Chapter 3, Chichester, Wiley.

UK Prospective Diabetes Study (UKPDS) (1998) 'Group Intensive blood glucose control with Sulphonylureas or insulin compared with conventional treatment and risk of complications in patients with type 2 diabetes (UKPDS 33)', *Lancet*, **352**, pp. 837–853.

CHAPTER 8

PSYCHOSOCIAL ASPECTS OF DIABETES

Learning Outcomes

When you have completed this chapter you should be able to:

8.1 Define and use, or recognise definitions and applications of, each of the terms printed in **bold** in the text.

8.2 Describe some of the different types of beliefs about diabetes.

8.3 Discuss how beliefs about diabetes can impact on diabetes self-management.

8.4 Describe how illness beliefs are shaped by emotions and experience.

8.5 List the guidance on conveying the diagnosis of diabetes.

8.6 Describe how emotions (including depression) affect diabetes and how people can manage their emotions.

8.1 Introduction

Although this chapter is titled 'Psychosocial aspects of diabetes', it would be wrong to assume that this is the only place in this book where you consider these issues. As you have read in the previous chapters, psychosocial aspects are not an 'add on' when thinking about diabetes, but are a constant thread running through the everyday experience of this condition. However, to aid your study and to bring certain issues to the forefront, we will focus in this chapter specifically on the psychosocial, that is, the psychological and the social consequences of diabetes. You start here by reading quite a lengthy story (Case Study 8.1) provided by an anonymous young adult in response to a survey study looking at how beliefs about diabetes affect the way people manage their diabetes. There are a lot of valuable insights and lessons to be learned from this narrative, but you should focus on three main themes: how people think about their diabetes, how people feel about their diabetes, and how people cope with their diabetes.

Case Study 8.1

About eight years ago, somebody dumped a big, awkward parcel in my arms, and told me that I had to carry it … until the end of my life. No warning, no explanation, and no escape route. I didn't see who did it to me, and I didn't even know what was in the parcel.

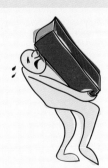

The immediate impact was that I had to walk incredibly carefully, because I couldn't see over or around it. It was so big that I had to carry it with both hands.

I was terrified of dropping it. I didn't know what the consequences would be, and anyone I asked gave me alarming replies; I was 'frightened into' carrying it carefully.

A few months on, I became sick of being only able to see the big parcel in front of me, with all my attention focused on it. I was unable to enjoy what was going on around me. Why *should* I carry it, I asked, but no one would answer. Then I started thinking, if this was how it was going to be, forever, I didn't want any more of it.

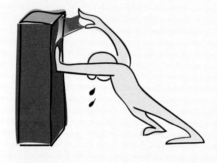

I tried to put it down, but couldn't. I tried *throwing* it down, but it was attached to me. I then tried every way I could think of to get rid of it; kicking, pushing, even getting my friends to try and pull it away, everything failed. I then tried to totally destroy it, but it was *me* who suffered from the repercussions.

I started missing my 'old self'. The happy, carefree (parcel free) person. It was like someone had stolen my identity, and replaced it with this stranger. I missed the old me terribly. The fact that I knew the parcel was a life sentence made me feel like the old me had not just been taken away, but killed too, and now I'd never get it back. What made it worse too is that no one talked about my former identity.

After failing to get rid of it, I became angry. None of my friends had to carry one, and there was just no logic to why it had happened to me. Had I done something really bad, to deserve it? I even started wondering if perhaps it was my fault, somehow I'd brought it all on myself. What if I had inadvertently asked for it?

I have to admit, though, that while I was feeling so angry, I did turn nasty on anyone who tried to tell me that it was *forever*, and that I'd better stop fighting and get used to it. Anyone who tried to enforce my order to carry it became a tangible, visible face to the problem, and I turned my anger on them. Unfortunately, it was usually my family and close friends just trying to help me, or give suggestions.

Then I dug my heels in and stopped walking, partly by way of protest, and partly because I could not face the struggling anymore. I would refuse to carry it by refusing to go on.

But I just got so left behind.

So I determined to ignore it. I battled on, pretending not to notice it dragging behind me, and more importantly, *I pretended not to care.*

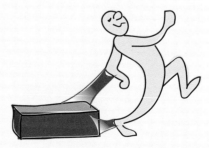

I managed for a little while, and it even seemed like I was enjoying myself, but it was dragging so heavily that it had pulled me out of shape, and I was really suffering. I had to admit that denial did not work either.

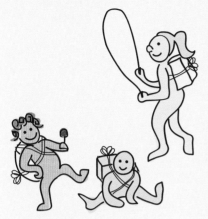

I had to find a comfortable way of carrying it, a reasonable and practical way, where I didn't neglect it, but neither would it be the centre of my life.

It was then that I noticed many young children with parcels, only theirs had been attached to them with special string, like back-packs. They weren't worrying about theirs at all. What was wrong with me? Why couldn't I manage mine? Where could I get some string? Could I make some?

Then I noticed the children's *parents* had been given the parcels, along with string, to attach them to the children. The difference was their parents had been given the responsibility.

Mine was given to *me* though, not to my parents, and no string came with it.

I had to get brave. It was a mixture of being brave enough to attempt it one-handed, and being too fed up to carry it with two anymore. I had to learn to balance it under one arm, and then my other hand was free to pick up all sorts of other exciting parcels; ones which I *wanted* to carry. As long as I kept hold, it worked OK.

But there came the times when I had a lot of important parcels which I had to carry all at the same time, and I couldn't drop any of them. It was then that I wanted to put down the awkward one more than ever; I hadn't ever *chosen* to carry that one in the first place. It was during these stressful times that it became even trickier still to carry it. It was the hardest one to carry, but of course, the only one I couldn't drop, even if I wanted to. I got exasperated that in the middle of such a hectic time, I was having to deal with all these negative emotions towards the parcel. I wanted to shout to the people in charge.

'Hey. Go easy on me, I've got one extra parcel than everyone else here … I'm struggling a bit.'

But I was far too frightened that if I drew attention to it – as a handicap, I would never be allowed to carry other parcels again. Some of the chosen parcels were good to carry, even if they did have responsibility with them.

I didn't want to say that *I couldn't do it* on account of my awkward one; just that I needed them to be understanding while I grappled to find a way of carrying them all at once whilst still balancing the awkward one satisfactorily. Even if it made me fall a few times whilst adjusting, I really wanted to succeed, given the chance.

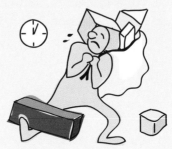

The thing is, there is no tried and proven solution. Nobody can give you 'the answer', and it's hard to take advice, because at the end of the day, it's you that has to carry it, not anyone else. Other people who also have parcels can tell you how *they* achieve it, but even if you followed their instructions verbatim, there's no guarantee it will work for you.

We may all have one parcel in common, but it's how you manage all the others in your armful along with it, and I think you have to keep adapting how you carry them all.

Some of life's parcels you get to put down after a valiant stint. Mine is not one of them. It's like an arranged marriage; there's a life-long commitment that I never agreed to take … I've stopped asking *why* because there is no answer, and I've tried to find ways of letting go of my anger, if it bubbles up; ways that don't involve hurting myself or pushing away the people who love me.

I do try to avoid feeling sorry for myself. (To be honest, I'm frightened of self pity, because it reminds me of the time when I stopped walking altogether for a while.) I try to keep the belief that if you can't change something, you have to make the best of it.

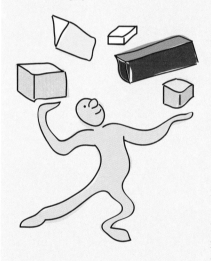

It's just a case of trying to find a satisfactory way of carrying it really. I can't see that I've found *the* way, which is going to work for me from now on. My other parcels keep changing all the time, and I continually have to readjust the weight-load and juggle things around. Sometime I do manage to forget the order of things and will rush on excitedly, forgetting the awkward parcel momentarily, and without having thought it through, it will end up falling on the floor, requiring picking up, sorting out, needing attention, and bringing to the foreground again.

But the one thing I can say is that I've been to both extremes; having it as my only focus, and ignoring it altogether. They're both unbearable. I need to stay somewhere in the 'middle of the road', that gives me the opportunity to carry as many other parcels as I want to, and as long as I give the 'awkward one' enough maintenance care for it not to slip, the road can be long and exciting!

(Anon)

8.2 How people think about diabetes – beliefs

What people think to be true, or believe about something, is an important factor in determining how they feel about and respond to it, and attempt to cope with it. This is true for diabetes: how and what we think about diabetes determines how we decide to respond to the task of managing it. In the narrative in Case Study 8.1 diabetes is perceived to be a 'big, awkward parcel' which then acts as a metaphor for the whole of their life so far with diabetes. Of course not everyone will think of their diabetes being like a parcel, for instance here are some quotes from a study looking at how people with Type 2 diabetes, all of whom have had diabetes for several years, think about their diabetes:

> '[You should] do things they tell you, if you're that bad … As long as I remain more or less as I am, it'll not bother me. I shall just carry on as I am.'

> 'I don't think I have [diabetes] … I don't suffer anything … I am a sensible enough person to know if anything was going wrong with me. If that happened I would make a move.'

> 'I know with my diet, like, if I eat anything I shouldn't do … I should get pains in my stomach and feel leggy.'

> 'Without sugar at all I get awful symptoms. I get very cold. A strict diet that a dietitian or a doctor gives me, I keep to it for about three weeks. I lose weight, but I feel really ill and I have to come off it.'

> 'It can be [serious] … I mean it's like cars. You can get a 600cc one or you can get a big 3000cc one … I'm the normal, standard family 1300 I should think.'

> (from Murphy and Kinmonth, 1995)

As these quotes illustrate, each person thinks about their diabetes somewhat differently, and some may not even be clear about what they think about their diabetes. Getting to grips with our thoughts about diabetes can help both the person with diabetes and their health care team make sense of what is happening in terms of diabetes management. How each of those people quoted above manages their diabetes will depend on the combination of beliefs they hold. At its simplest level, a person's beliefs can be divided into three broad categories:

- beliefs about diabetes
- beliefs about treatments for diabetes
- beliefs about self.

We will first look at people's beliefs about diabetes.

8.2.1 Beliefs about diabetes

If you were reading all the different studies that have been conducted on people's beliefs about diabetes, you'd come to realise that researchers have used a wide variety of terms or labels to try to understand what people think about their diabetes. People's beliefs about illness can be categorised into four broad groupings:

- beliefs about what the illness *is* (identity)

- beliefs about how long the illness will *last* (duration or chronicity)

- beliefs about the *cause* of the illness (cause)

- beliefs about how the illness will *affect* their life (consequences).

(Kleinman et al., 1978; Leventhal et al., 1984)

It is important to remember that a person may believe something is true generally, but at the same time believe that this does not necessarily apply to them. For instance someone may believe that smoking is bad for one's health, it may cause cancer or lung problems, but they may also believe that this does not apply to them. They may have parents who smoked for years but never had cancer or breathing problems, so they think they have protective genes, or they may do lots of exercise and so think this will prevent the smoking doing them any harm, or an abundance of other rationalisations (that is, a reason for believing something that is generally true is not true for them). The key point here is that everyone's beliefs are different, not necessarily right or wrong, and it's important to find out about them in order to promote better self-care.

Activity 8.1 Illness beliefs

Suggested study time 45 minutes

Read the two stories in Case Study 8.2 about how Elizabeth and David responded to having diabetes. As you read the stories, make notes on the following questions before reading the comment below.

- What does Elizabeth believe caused her diabetes?

- What do you think she thought were the consequences of diabetes?

- For how long does Elizabeth think she will have diabetes?

- What does David think is wrong with him?

- What do you think David thinks the consequences of diabetes are?

Comment

Elizabeth and David's stories are really quite striking in their contrast to each other. They each hold rather different beliefs, based upon different prior experiences and knowledge, and these beliefs have influenced how they have responded to their diagnosis. As one of the course team suggested, 'Elizabeth seems to be so much more proactive than David and also more open to learning about diabetes from different sources. Although we don't know much about their relationships with their health care teams, this might be a factor.'

Case Study 8.2

Elizabeth

Elizabeth is 65 years old, of African–American origin, and was diagnosed with Type 2 diabetes when she was 57. She takes oral hypoglycaemic agents, and currently her HbA_{1c} is 6.1%.

Elizabeth raised six children alone while working as a teacher's aide. Now living alone, her children, 17 grandchildren, and a number of great grandchildren continue to be the centre of her life. Aware of an extensive family history of diabetes, she expected to develop the disease. About eight years ago, she began to experience symptoms and sought a diabetes test. Once diagnosed, she believed that family history and weight gain were the cause and immediately changed her diet habits and added exercise to her activities.

Elizabeth devised her own diabetes self-management plan. 'First of all I did it myself. I just thought that maybe I could eat a lot of vegetables, a lot of fruit, not eat a lot of sweets and starches. I got that right, that's kind of related to sugar.' Elizabeth had never exercised before her diagnosis. She added walking to her schedule and three days a week went to a fitness centre offering memberships to people with a low income. Elizabeth learned from many sources – newspapers, television, and diabetes seminars offered by the public health department. Elizabeth attributed her dedication to self-management to watching family members endure painful deaths from diabetes. Her sister's legs were amputated and she had heart attacks and strokes. Her sister's sons died from heart attacks while in their 30s. She said: 'they just didn't seem to care, and they were all overweight. And they would anger me because there was nothing I could tell them. I was learning from their mistakes all the time.'

Elizabeth valued her family's support and encouraged her children to have healthy lifestyles. She had a straightforward belief about her own health. 'When it came to me, nobody needs to tell me, because I love me. I am going to do what I think is right by me.' (Savoca et al., 2004)

David

David is 51 years old, of African–American origin, and was diagnosed with diabetes at the age of 33. He takes insulin, and his HbA_{1c} is 10.9%.

David was not surprised when he was diagnosed with diabetes in his 30s because his mother had the condition. His initial reaction was that his lifestyle would change dramatically. He had been active in many sports and believed then, and now, that people with diabetes were unable to engage in these activities. David lived with his wife; his children lived on their own. His work required four 12-hour days per week; a schedule he believed complicated his diabetes care.

David described these early years: 'I knew about diabetes and read about diabetes but I was 33 and age and youth has a lot to do with it. I had diabetes and I was feeling good. If there was a piece of cake on the table, I ate the cake.' Now, more conscious of his eating, he tried to eliminate all sweets, a practice supported by his understanding of the fundamental cause of the condition: 'Basically what diabetes is, is the pancreas' inability to process artificial (added) sugars.' He eats what is available and tries not to 'go overboard'. He sees his doctor every 90 days and consulted with a dietitian each time. Despite nutritional counselling, he said he was never told to limit portion sizes of food and did not believe that high fat foods were a factor in the management of the condition. Instructed to count carbohydrates, he described the practice as 'Not practical. Not interesting.'

Long workdays made it difficult to get enough sleep, keep up with his church activities, and maintain a regular exercise program. David enjoyed exercise and knew he felt better when he walked two miles a day. Because of the hypoglycaemic risk, he believed that vigorous exercise was off limits to him. David often felt lethargic and unable to do anything. Because he frequently felt poorly, he appreciated his wife's concern for his condition. 'The easiest part of managing my diabetes is an understanding mate.' He had few friends and limited support from co-workers. David described the important elements of self-management as 'Stay away from sugar, eat a balanced diet and every four or five hours, do your exercise, and don't worry,' he said. 'And for most people that's very difficult to do.' Despite his doctor's concern that his blood glucose was too high, when asked if there was anything he would like to improve about any aspect of his care, his reply was 'No, not really.' (Savoca et al., 2004).

When considering the four broad groupings of diabetes beliefs stated above, little is generally known about what people believe diabetes actually is (identity). However, if you talk to health care professionals who specialise in diabetes care, a number of common issues are evident.

First, many people with Type 2 diabetes do not report any symptoms of having diabetes. They do not sense there is anything wrong with their bodies. This can happen for a number of reasons. They may not actually experience any symptoms, because their diabetes was picked up very early or they are managing it effectively. As Type 2 diabetes develops slowly over time and the symptoms may not arise quickly, the symptoms are often attributed to other factors. For instance, it is not uncommon for symptoms to be attributed to just generally getting older. Alternatively, some people may think any symptoms they have are caused by stress. This belief will be maintained until either the stress goes away, but the symptoms remain, or the symptoms become so severe that medical advice is sought.

Although many people may be aware that diabetes is a long-term condition, for which there is currently no cure, this does not mean that everyone with diabetes believes this to be the case. The media is full of stories of breakthroughs and potential cures for diabetes. This can create a false sense of hope for people who might believe that it won't be long before the cure comes, so they don't have to worry too much about it. As one 14-year-old, who had Type 1 diabetes for just over a year said:

'Well it is so hard, I don't see I need to bother so much as they will have a cure before I will get complications.'

Unfortunately for this girl, who had consistently poor control, this is simply not the case. Clearly this belief was one of the many factors that kept her from taking control of her diabetes. In one recent study, using anonymous questionnaires, around 10–14% of the young people (aged 12–18) and their parents who were surveyed did not think that they would have Type 1 diabetes for the rest of their life (Skinner et al., 2003).

The same may be true for people with Type 2 diabetes. Also if they make the necessary lifestyle changes, and bring their blood glucose level down, many people with Type 2 diabetes may feel they have beaten it or cured their diabetes.

'After diabetes counselling, Joan began to follow the dietary guidelines and monitor her blood glucose three times a day. "I was real good right away. I lost thirteen pounds, and I gained them back and more." After 6 months, she began working part time and reduced monitoring to once a day or less. "I think I thought I had it under control. I had thought I had changed my eating habits enough that I was fine and then I didn't need to take it." '

(Savoca et al., 2004)

In one study of people newly diagnosed with Type 2 diabetes, only two-thirds of individuals agreed that you have diabetes for the rest of your life. In another study of people who had had diabetes for several years, a quarter of participants did not agree that they would have diabetes for the rest of their life (Skinner and Hampson, 2001; Skinner et al., 2002, 2003). These two studies illustrate the importance of effective self-management education, so that individuals can make informed choices about how they want to respond to and manage their diabetes.

There are two sets of consequences to having diabetes. There is the immediate, short-term impact that diabetes has on day-to-day life. Then there are the long-term complications of diabetes (as discussed in Chapter 6), and the impact they or the fear of developing them may have on people.

It is important to make the distinction between these two elements of the consequences of diabetes, as they seem to play very different roles in relation to how people respond to living with diabetes. Both Type 1 and Type 2 diabetes have a substantial effect on people's lives. The nature of these effects is different, but this does not mean the impact is any less. In Type 1 diabetes, hypoglycaemia, or rather the fear of hypoglycaemia, is the most commonly reported negative impact of diabetes. This fear may stem from the experience of frequent and or severe hypos, or the fear of the unknown, especially in people who have been recently diagnosed with diabetes. However, it is not the anxiety that is the problem, but rather how an individual responds to it. It is not uncommon, especially in those who struggle to detect the early signs of hypoglycaemia, that the fear of hypos leads either to a very restrictive or regimented lifestyle, or to the individual running their blood glucose level high to prevent them having hypos. Both of these approaches have a negative impact on quality of life, either in the short term with the negative mood that may result from such a restricted lifestyle, or the long-term consequences of a high blood glucose level. Either way, if someone is particularly anxious about hypos, it is important to encourage discussion with the diabetes care team, as there is much that can be done to increase a person's ability to manage their diabetes without hypos, and to increase their ability to detect the early warning signs of hypos.

For people with Type 2 diabetes, the impact of trying to make multiple lifestyle changes to control their condition can be substantial, and is one of the major barriers to people initiating change. Some people feel they have been told to make so many changes in their lives that they cannot manage all of them, so feel it is pointless or hopeless and do not do anything. It is important to remember that it is not how much the 'objective' impact that diabetes has on people, but what each person perceives the impact to be. Some people say that diabetes has changed their life, but they see the changes in lifestyle in a positive way, such as making them feel healthier. As a result they do not perceive the impact of lifestyle changes to be so great.

There has been much research on how people's beliefs about the long-term complications of diabetes relate to how they manage their condition. Many health care professionals have worked on the basis that the more severe people think the complications are, and the more likely they think they are to get these complications, the more proactive individuals will be in managing their diabetes. However, this does not always seem to be the case. Although some research shows that a greater perceived threat of complications (more serious, or more likely to get them) is associated with better self-management, there are as many studies that show no relationship, and even some that show that the greater perceived threat is associated with poorer self-management (Skinner et al., 2000).

One factor not always considered in research studies is how people feel about whether or not they can affect their chances of getting complications. If people feel they are highly likely to get complications, and they feel it is inevitable no matter what they do to manage their diabetes, then it might make sense to them not to follow the diet, activity, monitoring and medication recommendations. After all, what is the point of doing it all if it will not change things? Trying to scare people into following treatment recommendations is often counter-productive. A more positive approach is to help people to understand their diabetes and the possible complications. By encouraging people to think about the options available for preventing these problems, the health care team can help people reflect more accurately on their risks. In many cases this alone can have a substantial impact on people's quality of life.

As well as thinking about people's beliefs about diabetes, it's important to consider beliefs about treatment and management of diabetes, including how people feel about their ability to follow the recommendations they are given. These two aspects of beliefs are focused on in the next two sections of this chapter.

8.2.2 Beliefs about treatments for diabetes

We start by thinking about what people believe about treatment for diabetes, what the alternatives for treatment are and what they can do to control or manage their diabetes. The following quotes illustrate the range of beliefs held.

'I think diabetic patients should listen to doctors, take drugs on time, … and when you've run out of medicine, you have to go back to the hospital to get more.'

'If you've got diabetes, you have to take medicine, it's as simple as that …'

'I am not against taking medicine. It's just I'm afraid that there might be something wrong, you know, side effects … But I've to put my fears aside, I still take my medicine … People often tell that too much medicine will damage kidneys … I don't really know. It's bound to be bad if you take this (medicine) …

'Some people take medicine for a while, quit a while, and then start again when there are fewer toxins left in your body. Or you have to quit while you are taking medicine for a common cold.'

'… if I don't eat anything sweet today, why should I take so many drugs? A few are quite enough. I would just take it in the morning and evening.'

(Lai et al., 2005)

Treatment beliefs can be categorised into two groups: the benefits of a particular behaviour, and the costs or risk of carrying out the behaviour. Unsurprisingly, individuals who have a stronger belief in the benefit of a particular behaviour or treatment recommendation are more likely to follow that advice. Conversely, the more barriers, or risks that individuals attribute to a particular treatment or behaviour, the less likely they are to follow that treatment. However, it is the ratio of one to the other that is important, as people will have both positive and negative beliefs about any one treatment.

Quite often, people tend to act more on the short-term benefits and risks of a behaviour, rather than consider the long-term benefits. However, it is important to appreciate the complexity of people's beliefs about treatment and how these beliefs develop. Take, for instance, the common issue of people with Type 2 diabetes needing to start on insulin. Recent research suggests that both people with diabetes and doctors may have strong preconceptions about insulin. Some doctors, for example, use insulin with their patients as an indication that other forms of diabetes management have failed. In the words of one diabetologist:

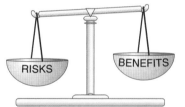

'I don't like initiating insulin at all, since it's a kind of surrender – that the previous therapy has failed.'

Health care professionals may unwittingly communicate to patients their own reluctance to prescribe insulin. Alternatively doctors may sometimes use the threat of insulin as a weapon to try to force patients to follow the advice they are giving them. These doctors' attitudes are likely to influence patients' attitudes to insulin, further reinforcing their negative preconceptions. A recent international study focused on this issue. 253 people with diabetes and health care professionals from Germany, France, Italy, the UK and the USA took part in a series of interviews and focus groups (The DAWN Study, 2002). This generated some interesting results, as you will read below.

Some GPs appeared to:
- lack detailed knowledge about Type 2 diabetes as a serious progressive disease
- lack detailed knowledge and first-hand experience of insulin therapy and pens
- believe that the most appropriate treatment for diabetes is diet and oral hypoglycaemic agents (OHAs)

- perceive starting insulin therapy as indicating failure
- communicate their own reluctance to start insulin therapy to their patients
- perceive typical Type 2 diabetes patients as elderly and obese.

Some GPs made misleading or confusing statements:

- 'non-insulin dependent diabetes'
- 'mild diabetes'
- 'a little sugar in the blood'.

Some GPs:

- failed to explain why patients needed to lose weight
- used insulin as a threat to help enforce patient compliance
- planned to inform patients more fully about Type 2 diabetes in a gradual way, but usually failed to follow through on these plans.

Some diabetologists believed that:

- GPs' over-reliance on oral hypoglycaemic agents and their avoidance of insulin were motivated by a misguided attempt to 'protect' the patient from insulin therapy.

The study showed that individuals with diabetes appeared to:

- have poor knowledge of Type 2 diabetes
- have little knowledge of the consequences of poor glycaemic (blood glucose) control
- feel that their GPs failed to give them enough information at diagnosis
- find out about diabetes from their own reading, or from diabetes associations and hospital clinics.

Patients who were taking tablets to control their diabetes appeared to:

- have a negative view of insulin therapy
- be reassured by seeing insulin pens and by positive feedback from patients on insulin therapy.

However, individuals who were using insulin appeared to:

- be more positive about the benefits on their lifestyle and general well-being.

Conclusions from the DAWN study

The study came to some conclusions, which included the following.

- One of the main obstacles to improved patient acceptance of insulin therapy may be the attitudes and perceptions of GPs.
- GPs' lack of acceptance and experience of insulin therapy and their perceptions of how best to manage treatment appeared to be the major source of patients' reluctance or anxieties about accepting insulin therapy.
- Once patients had begun insulin therapy, they became more positive about its benefits on their lifestyle and general well-being.

Activity 8.2   Quotes from a survey

Suggested study time 30 minutes

The quotes in Table 8.1 are taken from people taking part in the research survey you have just been reading about (The DAWN study, 2002). Note your reaction to each of the comments and consider what you might say to the person or do if they made these remarks to you.

Table 8.1 Quotes from people taking part in the DAWN study (2002).

I don't know if a normal GP is capable of giving you the information you require. Even the books give you a lot of contradictory information. *German patient*	You can go blind, lose limbs – I know that. What I am trying to control is my sugar level. *English patient*
The doctor told me not to worry, and to hope that a proper diet would be enough to control it. *Italian patient*	It's a major problem, being confronted with the fear of constantly injuring, hurting myself. *German patient*
I was told that it was very important to stick to the diet and to eat at very strict times – they must have said why, but I've forgotten. *French patient*	[Insulin therapy] means that the illness has got worse. Then you become a slave to the little black box – you've got to carry it in your pocket all the time. *Italian patient*
I wasn't doing what I was told, and he said 'if you don't do this properly, you are going to die.' *American patient*	Insulin is the final step that forces you to face the whole disease much more intensely. Taking pills makes diabetes seem not too serious. *German patient*
I didn't understand very well in the beginning. My doctor probably did not want to worry me. That is probably why he did not explain anything to me. *Italian patient*	You're no longer as independent as before. When you go out, you'll be constantly worrying about having forgotten something. *German patient*

Comment

As you have seen, although the people quoted above come from different countries there appear to be common worries and anxieties, and in particular these quotes suggest difficulties in the communication between the doctor and patient. By this point in the course you've probably realised that a supportive, open and positive relationship between the person with diabetes and the other members of the diabetes care team is vital, and this hinges on good communication between all parties. (Communication was discussed in Section 1.5.)

You now move on to the final category of beliefs, where you think about people's beliefs about themselves.

8.2.3 Beliefs about self

So far you've thought about beliefs about diabetes and beliefs about treatment; you now move on to consider the beliefs that people hold about themselves and their abilities. There are a number of different ways of looking at how we think about ourselves, for example, how much we value ourselves, how we describe ourselves, and how good we think we are at doing things. The first two of these relate to our self-esteem or our self-concepts. The third example is often termed 'self-capacity' beliefs or self-efficacy, and refers to people's belief in their ability to perform a task. It is similar to the concept of confidence and is an important predictor of how well people manage their diabetes. Self-efficacy is not a general belief someone has about themselves, but is different for different behaviours. For instance someone may have low self-efficacy/confidence in their ability to eat a healthy diet, but have a high self efficacy/confidence in their ability to take their diabetes tablets every day.

Self-efficacy has been shown to be one of the most consistent predictors of people's self-care behaviour, with those who have a higher sense of self-efficacy for a particular behaviour being more likely to perform that behaviour. The importance of self-efficacy in influencing behaviour is highlighted by the fact that nearly all psychological models that attempt to predict or are designed to improve a person's self-care behaviour use this approach. There are four clear strategies that can be used to enhance self-efficacy. These are mastery experience, modelling, social persuasion and emotional regulation. We will consider each of them in turn.

Mastery experience

Mastery experience means the experience of success when performing a behaviour increases people's confidence in their ability to perform it a second time. This may seem obvious, but it is important to remember that many people seem to forget the successes they have and only remember the failures. People frequently make plans to change their behaviour (e.g. walk more, eat less) and stick to this plan for a few days. Then something happens and they are unable to do it for a day or two. People commonly interpret this as 'I can't do this' and stop. They seem to forget about all the days they did manage it, and the benefits they gained from that. So simply helping people to tune in to the times they did manage to do something and emphasising the benefit of this process can be very important. It also means that when people are taught new skills, they should be encouraged by the things they do well, and their desire to learn should be seen as a positive goal in itself. They may not learn a task first time, but they will have learnt something. This also means breaking complex activities down into different tasks and helping people to learn one step at a time.

For people who are finding it particularly difficult to learn a task it is sometimes worth starting with the last step and working the learning process backwards. This means that the person gains a positive boost from completing the task. For example, when learning about blood glucose monitoring, a person might start by learning how to put the strip with blood on it into the meter. The main point about mastery experience is that all of us sometimes need help to focus on the positives in ourselves and in others when we are learning something new or difficult.

Modelling

Modelling relates to the benefits of seeing someone else performing the behaviour or skill that a person is trying to learn. This can be a difficult strategy to use, for example in one-to-one consultations between a doctor and patient, as there are no other people around to model things. As a result, some people have tried using examples of people who have managed to achieve things and live their life with diabetes, such as famous athletes and actors. However, modelling only works if the person doing the modelling is perceived by the individual as being a similar person in a similar situation to themselves.

Social persuasion

Social persuasion relates to the strategies that may be used to develop someone's confidence or self-efficacy in managing their diabetes. There are a number of strategies that can be used but one of the most important is supporting people in making achievable goals for themselves. Ideally the agreed goal(s) need to be **SMART**, i.e.:

Specific

Measurable

Action-orientated (that is, tied to something they already do)

Realistic

Time-limited.

This approach is illustrated in the following example. Bill's goal to reduce his weight needs to be SMART (see Table 8.2).

Table 8.2 Example of a specific, measurable, action-orientated, realistic and time-limited (SMART) strategy.

Specific	Bill wants to reduce his weight
Measurable	By 5 kg
Action-orientated	By taking physical activity such as fast walks
Realistic	He needs to decide when, how far and how often he can manage to walk
Time-limited	He wants results in 3 months

Once Bill has been through this thought process, a behavioural goal can be agreed, for example:

> 'To walk fast for 40 minutes four times per week, on Tuesdays, Wednesdays, Saturdays and Sundays.'

Once a person has chosen to take action they have an intention to do something. For example, a person can intend to lose weight, diet, be more active (Figure 8.1), or stop smoking. However, these are much more generalised intentions; they are vague in terms of what exactly the person wishes to do or achieve. If we develop a strategy to implement these generalised intentions, for example, 'I am going to walk to work every day/I am going to change all the dairy products in my diet for low fat options/I am going to get nicotine patches from my GP and attend smoking cessation support groups', we have developed what is called an implementation intention.

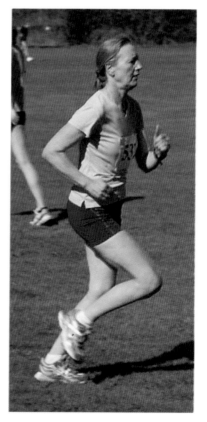

Figure 8.1 Increasing your level of activity, for example by running, can be one of your SMART goals.

Activity 8.3 Goals need to be SMART

Suggested study time 20 minutes

Complete Table 8.3 below. Your aim is to go through the same thought process as Bill in the example above, but your goal is to be more physically active.

Table 8.3 Your own SMART strategy.

Specific	You want to be more physically active
Measurable	
Action-orientated	
Realistic	
Time-limited	

Comment

There is no absolutely correct answer to this activity, but it is worth considering the following.

Recent research shows that if people actually plan how they will enact or implement their generalised intention, there is a substantial increase in the likelihood that they will follow through on their intentions. Therefore, by trying to set goals that are SMART, we are encouraging the development of an implementation intention.

It is important that these SMART goals are behaviours. For example, setting a lower blood glucose level as a goal will not work; people do not have complete control over this outcome, as it is influenced by their medication regimens, stress responses, etc.

Note that goals must be truly specific, for example; 'eating less fat' is not specific enough. The 'how', 'when' and 'where' (the 'realistic' points) are important if people are going to achieve their goals.

Once the goals are established, it's important to identify anything that might get in their way. If they are to commit to action, the person with diabetes has to drive the planning process.

Questions that could be asked when planning how to achieve goals include the following.

- What could the person do to change the situation?
- What are some steps the person could take to bring them closer to their goal?
- What are the main barriers preventing the person from achieving their goal?
- How can the person overcome these barriers?
- How can the health care team provide support and help identify solutions?

It is then important to consider any aspects of the person's physical, social, financial or personal life that might present a barrier to them achieving their behavioural goals. Once actual or potential barriers have been identified, they can be explored with other members of the health care team, for example:

> 'Now that you have decided to take these walks four times a week, can you think of situations when you will be tempted to stay at home and not take your walk?'

When people are prompted to consider the problems they may encounter, they start to prepare options for problem-solving. It's important that the health care team supports their efforts, as well as showing that they understand that what the person with diabetes is about to start is difficult and that it is natural for them to be tempted to relapse into old patterns of behaviour.

The health care team can help people with diabetes by teaching them how to problem solve using a simple four-step strategy:

1 define the problem

2 find solutions

3 choose solutions

4 describe the solution in terms of behaviour/actions.

1 Define the problem – The process starts by asking questions that help people to formulate their problem in specific terms. For example:

> 'When I come home late from work, I'm so hungry that most often I eat sandwiches instead of cooking food.'

2 Find solutions – There are many different ways of solving a problem. Often however, it is tempting to try the first solution that comes to mind and, if that does not work easily, to give up. To avoid failure people need to find several solutions to a problem. One way of doing this is through discussing ideas with other members of the health care team, and coming up with as many solutions as possible, without evaluating the suggestions.

Following on from the problem quoted above, possible solutions are to:

- stop working
- leave work earlier
- eat more at lunch time
- have snacks between meals
- have a piece of fruit on the way home

- prepare dinner the day before
- have sandwiches with less fat
- have all meals in restaurants
- have the partner – (who arrives home earlier) cook the dinners.

3 Choose solutions – The next step is to select one of the solutions to try. Remember that it is the person with diabetes who chooses from the suggested solutions. First, they can get rid of alternatives that are unrealistic, and then rank those which are left in terms of what they think they can feasibly do. Finally, they need to choose two of those with the highest rankings. In the example given, the person with diabetes deletes unsuitable solutions, and then ranks the remaining items as given below:

- leave work earlier (3)
- have snacks between meals (2)
- have a piece of fruit on the way home (1)
- prepare dinner the day before (5)
- have sandwiches with less fat (4).

They then choose to try the two solutions with the highest ranking (that is, having fruit on the way home and snacks between meals).

4 Describe the solution in terms of behaviours/actions – The next step is to turn the solution into behaviours that are specific and measurable. So, for the example above, the person might write:

> 'I will bring two pieces of fruit to work each morning, and save one for the bus back home. I will have one piece of fruit with the afternoon coffee at work in addition to the biscuits I usually have. I will do this at least four of the five days of the week. I will start on Monday.'

The description above is one necessarily simplified account of how social persuasion might work. You now move on, however, to the final strategy used to enhance self-efficacy.

Emotional regulation

The fourth strategy to enhance self-efficacy is emotional regulation. Emotions such as depression and anxiety lower people's self-efficacy, and so helping people to manage them will boost their self-efficacy. This is such an important issue that the next two sections of this chapter focus on the role of emotions in diabetes.

8.3 Emotions

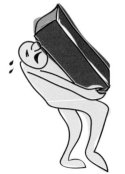

One striking feature of the narrative at the start of this chapter (Case Study 8.1) is its emotional content. Throughout, the author is attempting two tasks, it seems: one is to actually carry the parcel as they walk through life (made difficult by the shape and size of the parcel), the second task is to carry the emotional weight that is contained in the parcel. Throughout the story, as the author moved through different emotional responses, the emotional weight changed but it was always there. At times it seemed that this emotional weight was what they needed the most help with, but seemed to have the least assistance with.

'What made it worse too, is that no one talked about my former identity.'

'… I did turn nasty on anyone who tried to tell me that it was forever, and that I'd better stop fighting and get used to it. Anyone who tried to enforce my order to carry it became a tangible, visible face to the problem, and I turned my anger on them.'

(Anon)

The person quoted above appreciated that the people around them, whether personal or professional, were only trying to help. But how different would their experience of this help have been if it had focused on understanding, and helping them to understand what they were feeling? To gain from an experience we need to truly have the experience and understand it, and having others trying to understand it as well, is one of the most powerful forms of help we can have from another person.

The diagnosis of diabetes generates a wide range of emotions, from shock and disbelief through to relatively calm acceptance of the news. There is a range of factors that can influence how someone responds to the diagnosis of diabetes (Peel et al., 2004), and we turn to them now.

8.3.1 Experience and knowledge of diabetes

Already having a family member with diabetes does not necessarily mean that one's own diagnosis will be readily accepted. Much depends on the nature of the individuals' experience of diabetes in the family. Consider the different responses given below.

'Quite a few of my relatives were diabetic so when I realised I was, it didn't matter. I didn't accept diabetes gracefully but I did accept it and I did as I was directed.'

(Woman with Type 2 diabetes)

'I was angry when I was told as I have a sister who is diabetic so I have seen what she has to do. I couldn't come to terms with it because of having to give up the things I love to eat most.'

(Woman with Type 2 diabetes)

Although both these women have close relatives with diabetes, their different experiences have led to very different responses to being diagnosed with diabetes. However, it is also important to note that this does not mean that the response of the first person is somehow better than that of the second.

Where people are unfamiliar with the condition the diagnosis could act as a profound shock, regardless of which type of diabetes they are diagnosed with.

'I was on my own and when I was told, I just felt numb. You feel numb when you have just been told you have got diabetes.'

(Man with Type 2 diabetes)

'I was diagnosed 5 years ago. It was like a life sentence when I heard the news. The doctor had casually mentioned having a blood test but the result was so unexpected as there is no history of diabetes in the family.'

(Woman with Type 1 diabetes)

It can be a relief to be diagnosed with diabetes, however, especially when people are anticipating something else, such as cancer.

'When I was diagnosed, I just felt relief that it was that and nothing else. I felt instantly better – incredible. Although I was in shock, it was such a relief to find out what was wrong.'

(Woman with Type 1 diabetes)

8.3.2 Conveying the diagnosis

The way in which health care professionals break the news can have a substantial impact on the short-term and long-term process of adjusting to living with diabetes.

Activity 8.4 Conveying the diagnosis

Suggested study time 45 minutes

Take a few moments to think about how you would prefer to be told that you have diabetes – what would you want the health professional to be like with you, what kinds of words would you like them to use? If you have diabetes, reflect on your own moment of diagnosis and try and remember what happened.

Now read the guidance in Box 8.1 for giving a diagnosis of Type 2 diabetes.

Having read the guidance, what similarities and differences are there between the guidance and what you imagined you would like or what really happened? If there are differences, which approach would you prefer?

Comment

Did you find that you didn't change anything you would like the GP to say, or perhaps you made a number of changes? Of course it's easier to carry out this sort of activity when you are not in the actual situation, where you might be faced with someone who is upset or does not want to accept their diagnosis. The point of this exercise, however, is to help you become aware, from both the patient's and the health care professional's point of view, how important sensitivity and clarity of information are at times like these.

Box 8.1 Giving patients a diagnosis of Type 2 diabetes – good practice guidance

1 Elicit patient views (start with what they know)

'Do you have any suspicions as to what is happening to you medically at the moment?' or paraphrase. Start with what they know or suspect.

2 Prompt that serious news is to be given (this lessens the shock)

'Well unfortunately it is serious news from the blood tests we have been doing (as you suspected/that you weren't expecting)' or paraphrase.

3 Give the news without jargon

'You do have Type 2 diabetes' or paraphrase.

Avoid confusion – do not say that this is 'mild' or 'the type that does not need insulin'. Talk about the high blood glucose level and its need to be controlled. Then give the following information:

'This means you have high glucose levels in your blood.'

'This is because your body's machinery for using glucose, which involves insulin, is not working properly.'

'This is serious because high glucose is harming your body, and could lead to serious health problems in the future.'

'The implications for you are that you now need to find ways of reducing your glucose level (perhaps with lifestyle and medication).'

'You also need to take more care of your health by looking at your diet to reduce the amount of sugar, fat and salt in your diet, being more active, and stopping smoking.'

'The good news is that there is a lot we know and a lot of help available to help you reduce the risks that come with diabetes.'

This may start with an education programme within the first few weeks following diagnosis – which will be explained in the leaflet, if one is provided, so that they will know about diabetes and its implications. 'It will help you to develop your way of dealing with your diabetes' or paraphrase.

4 Elicit reactions to encourage emotional expression

'What are your reactions to this news?' *or* 'I wonder how you are feeling after this news?'

'What are your thoughts at the moment?' *or* 'What concerns you about this?'

'What questions do you have?'

5 Give reassurance and hope (positive attitude)

'You are one of many with Type 2 diabetes (1 in every 10 people over the age of 45).'

'There is now a lot that can be done to reduce the problems that come with diabetes.'

'You can have the same or improved quality of life, but you need to decide how to look after yourself.'

6 Explain support and answer questions

Explain that the patient leaflet (such as mentioned in point 3 above) provides information about diabetes and suggests where to get further information.

Write down the name of the contact person from the practice.

Explain that there may be a diabetes education programme (mentioned above), and how to get booked on to it, and explain that the course is informal.

Ask if they have any immediate questions.

7 Summary, reflection and caring statement to help recollection and attitude

'So you have Type 2 diabetes.'

'You're shocked/not shocked, your thoughts were …' (reflection of what was said)

The next step is to go on the diabetes education programme which will:

- let you know what is happening

- give you options for what to do

- help and support you with your plans to manage your diabetes

- be relaxed and friendly so don't worry about it.

'Contact the named nurse here if you have any difficulties.'

'There will then be regular support to help you manage your diabetes.'

REMEMBER: The quality of this consultation will be remembered forever!

When health professionals appreciate the vulnerable nature of patients at times like this, and act accordingly, the process of adjustment and adaptation can be aided. However, when this process of supporting people through diagnosis is absent unnecessary distress is common. This can be particularly problematic for people with Type 1 diabetes, as professionals frequently want to start patients on insulin urgently and the emotional aspects of care can be easily forgotten.

> 'The doctor just phoned me and said, "I think I had better talk to you. You are very seriously ill and you don't know it". I was in total shock thinking, "Oh my God, I have either got cancer or Aids".'

'I took my daughter's sample to the doctor and was told within the space of 5 minutes to go up to the hospital as she had diabetes. I was shocked.'

'I couldn't believe the urgency … I couldn't understand why the prognosis (sic) was so rushed, and why she had to become an insulin diabetic that night. Why couldn't it wait a week? Why couldn't we see how she went? I felt I was losing control I suppose. I felt like saying, now wait. Let's all calm down now … but it all seemed to be railroaded on so fast.'

(parent of girl newly diagnosed)

(Lowes et al., 2004)

It is vital for health professionals to understand the psychological impact of learning that one has a serious health problem (Peel et al., 2004). People commonly described being in shock immediately after hearing the news and felt that they first needed to deal with the complex emotions this evoked. Some form of emotional support was therefore viewed as the primary need at this point. Without addressing the varied emotional responses people may be going through, information provision and education may prove ineffectual, as anxiety is a significant barrier to attention, processing and recall of information.

'When you are diagnosed is the wrong time to ask questions as you are on another planet. Your brain doesn't want to take it in as part of your brain has died or gone to sleep.'

(Man with Type 2 diabetes)

All these points are equally applicable when people are being told about the development of complications, such as retinopathy. These complications can generate as much if not more distress than the original diagnosis.

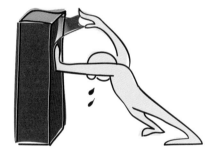

'I tried to put it down, but couldn't. I tried *throwing* it down, but it was attached to me. I then tried every way I could think of to get rid of it; kicking, pushing, even getting my friends to try and pull it away, everything failed. I then tried to totally destroy it, …'

(Anon)

This is denial, an active attempt to convince the self that one does not have diabetes, in this case by getting rid of it. This is very different from ignoring that you have it, which is the next approach the author of the narrative in Case Study 8.1 takes to managing diabetes. However, this just makes the parcel a drag; instead of being carried forward it pulls them back 'dragging them out of shape'. The author seems to have reflected on the consequences of these coping strategies and moved on from there. Sadly, some individuals with diabetes do not seem to move on from here, but this narrative gives us some clues as to how people can move on and try out different ways of coping.

Learning to see how much energy is being used to deny the existence of diabetes, and reflecting on whether this is an appropriate use of energy, is fundamental to moving forward.

It is important to consider that there may be other parcels the individual is carrying that may be bigger, heavier or more awkward to carry than the one labelled diabetes. Some of these parcels may have been given to the individual before the diabetes one, and they cannot be put down either. Unless the other parcels are opened and what is inside explored, and possibly re-packaged, it can be difficult, if not impossible, to move on.

When the parcel is ignored, it does not detach itself but keeps dragging along behind the person. The insight comes from thinking about why dragging it along makes it that much more difficult. Not only is there the emotional weight of the parcel, but all the friction that the parcel encounters as it is pulled along the ground making it an even heavier burden. Simply exploring the experience of ignoring diabetes can help people reflect on how this affects them and helps them decide if that is the way they wish to remain attached to their diabetes.

8.4 Depression and diabetes

Although a depressed mood is a common occurrence in people both with and without diabetes, research has shown that it is more common among people with diabetes (Lustman et al., 1996). In the general population 5–8% of people are experiencing a major depressive episode at any point in time, but it is two to three times more common in people with diabetes compared with those without diabetes, and so can be found in about 15–20% of people with diabetes (Anderson et al., 2001). In one study in the UK, just under 38% of adults attending diabetes outpatients in one hospital reported moderate to severe levels of anxiety or depression, or both (Lloyd et al., 2000).

8.4.1 Effects of depression

Depression is a serious condition that can have a devastating effect on people's quality of life. It also affects diabetes in several ways. Firstly, depressed people often lack the motivation for self-management, which leads to poor dietary care, lack of physical activity, and infrequent monitoring, which in turn can lead to further feelings of failure and hopelessness. This is then frequently managed by comfort eating or drinking, and for those who smoke, increased smoking. This is often referred to as the indirect effect of depression on diabetes, but there is also thought to be a direct effect. That is, depression is associated with an increased level of a hormone called cortisol, which acts in a number of ways (stimulating glucose release from the liver, and blocking the action of insulin) to increase the blood glucose level (Figure 8.2). For these two reasons depression in people with diabetes is linked to poorer control, earlier onset of complications, more rapid progression of diabetes, and is particularly predictive of the onset of coronary heart disease.

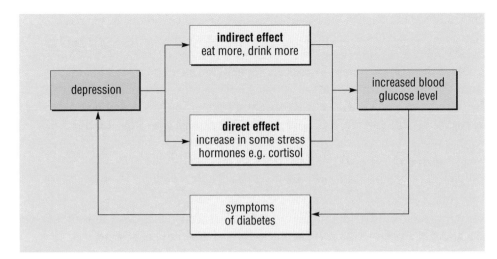

Figure 8.2 Direct and indirect effects of depression.

8.4.2 Causes of depression in diabetes

There are a number of possible reasons why depression is more common in people with diabetes. One frequent explanation is the demands of managing a serious long-term condition (whether this is diabetes or another condition) becomes too much for some people. When people do not have, or perceive they don't have, the resources they need to manage the challenge of diabetes, they may feel overwhelmed, feel useless and hopeless for the future resulting in the development of symptoms of depression.

A second explanation is that diabetes causes a number of physiological changes, including changes in our bodily systems that are also linked to feelings of depression (Lustman et al., 1996). However, recent research (Talbot and Nouwen, 2000) suggests that the link between depression and diabetes works the other way round for Type 2 diabetes. That is, depression acts as a risk factor for the development of diabetes, which would also explain why people newly diagnosed with Type 2 diabetes already report feelings of depression.

8.4.3 Detection of symptoms of depression

Given the scale of the problem and the serious consequences of depression in diabetes, it may be surprising that it largely goes undiagnosed (Rubin and Peyrot, 2002) and is treated in only one-third of cases (Lustman et al., 1996). This is thought to be due to the fact that many health care professionals view depression as secondary to the serious medical condition of diabetes and hence not of independent importance. Some health care professionals may feel that they do not have the time or training necessary to detect and diagnose depression. Added to this there are concerns about the accuracy of diagnosis, as various symptoms of depression are similar to symptoms of hyperglycaemia, such as fatigue and weight changes (Rubin and Peyrot, 2002).

There are various methods that can be used to detect depression, the least structured of which is to ask patients how they are feeling. As many symptoms of depression can also be symptoms of a high blood glucose level, it can be difficult to know what is the cause of symptoms such as tiredness, or weight changes. However, one important symptom to look out for is people reporting a loss of interest in things they always used to find interesting. Another alternative is to use short questionnaires to assess depression or emotional well-being. Although there are many measures that assess depression (such as the Beck Depression Inventory, the Zung Self Rating Depression Scale and the Centre for Epidemiological Studies Depression scale), people can get worried about using them, as they do not know how to interpret the results. As an alternative to assessing depression, it is possible to use questionnaires that measure more general well-being, such as the one recently developed by the World Health Organization, the WHO 5 Well-Being Measure (see Box 8.2).

These questions assess emotional well-being generally, and because the items ask about positive mood states, people with diabetes and health care professionals can find it easier to talk about the results. If someone scores low on this measure (that is, less than 13) this does not mean they are depressed, but it is an indicator that someone in the team should discuss the results with the person concerned.

Box 8.2 WHO 5 Well-Being Measure

Please indicate for each of the five statements which is closest to how you have been feeling over the last two weeks. Notice that higher numbers indicate better well-being.

For example, if you have felt cheerful and in good spirits more than half of the time during the last two weeks, put a tick in the box with the number three at the top of the column. Finally add up your score.

Over the last two weeks	scores					
	All of the time 5	Most of the time 4	More than half of the time 3	Less than half of the time 2	Some of the time 1	At no time 0
1 I have felt cheerful and in good spirits	☐	☐	☐	☐	☐	☐
2 I have felt calm and relaxed	☐	☐	☐	☐	☐	☐
3 I have felt active and vigorous	☐	☐	☐	☐	☐	☐
4 I woke up feeling fresh and rested	☐	☐	☐	☐	☐	☐
5 My daily life has been filled with things that interest me	☐	☐	☐	☐	☐	☐

8.4.4 Treatment of depression

There are two general methods for treating depression: medication and interpersonal therapy. People can be prescribed antidepressants, with the current trend (2005) being to use a class of antidepressant drugs known as **selective serotonin reuptake inhibitors (SSRIs)**, which have less-severe side-effects for people with diabetes than do alternative antidepressants, and have been found to be effective in reducing depressive symptoms in people with diabetes (Lustman et al., 1998). Medication alone only really addresses the symptoms of depression and does not treat the underlying cause. It should also be noted that medications can take two to three weeks before they have their effect, and are only a short-term treatment.

Interpersonal therapy covers a diverse range of one-to-one or group counselling approaches used to help people identify and address the causes of depression. At the time of writing, the main approach to treatment in the UK is **cognitive behavioural therapy (CBT)**. CBT is based on trying to address the negative and stereotypical ways people with depression tend to think. Negative thoughts and actions are identified and efforts are made to replace them with more accurate and positive thoughts and actions (Rubin and Peyrot, 2002). In the only controlled study to evaluate the effectiveness of psychotherapy in people with diabetes and depression, Lustman and colleagues (1998) found CBT to be effective in the treatment of depression in people with diabetes (Type 2) by reducing depressive symptoms and HbA_{1c} values (see Figure 8.2). Ideally, current recommendations would suggest that a combination of interpersonal therapy and medication provides the optimal outcome of early remission of symptoms of depression.

8.4.5 Coping with the emotional reactions to diabetes

Coping refers to the different things a person does to manage a problem. This is illustrated in Case Study 8.1 in the way the person learns how to manage their diabetes. Coping can also refer to how people manage their emotions, as they adjust to living with a long-term condition. This is important because, although health care professionals can tell people with diabetes how to manage the condition, this is not enough. The person with the diabetes has to learn for themselves (diabetes self-management) and at the same time deal with their emotional reactions. There are usually lots of other parcels that need carrying, and these parcels are different for every individual with diabetes.

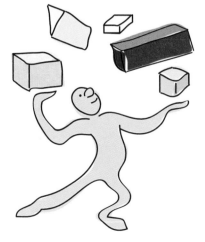

> 'We may all have one parcel in common, but it's how you manage all the others in your armful along with it, and I think you have to keep adapting how you carry them all.'

> (Anon)

It is striking the balance and juggling all the parcels together that is important, with each person with diabetes having their own particular set and having to learn to find ways of living with the extra parcel. The diabetes care team can support the person as they find a sense of balance with all the parcels, including the one with diabetes.

8.5 Summary of Chapter 8

In this chapter you have read how beliefs about diabetes can be divided into three broad categories, and how these different beliefs can impact on diabetes self-management. Coping with diabetes, depending on what form this takes, can assist self-management and can help people juggle all their 'parcels'. Currently the emotional and psychosocial aspects of diabetes are receiving more attention than ever before, both in terms of national strategies for diabetes care (for example, the National Service Framework for Diabetes), and also in the research world. We will delve further into the psychosocial aspects of diabetes in the final two chapters of this course.

Questions for Chapter 8

Question 8.1 (Learning Outcomes 8.3 and 8.4)

What are the strategies that can be used to enhance self-efficacy?

Question 8.2 (Learning Outcome 8.6)

What are the two means by which depression may influence diabetes control?

Question 8.3 (Learning Outcome 8.2)

What are the categories of beliefs that make up an individual's personal model of diabetes?

Question 8.4 (Learning Outcome 8.5)

What are the six steps to giving a diagnosis of diabetes to someone?

References

Anderson, R. J., Freedland, K. E., Clouse, R. E. and Lustman, P. J. (2001) 'The prevalence of comorbid depression in adults with diabetes: a meta-analysis', *Diabetes Care*, **24** (6), pp.1069–1078.

Kleinman, A., Eisenberg, L. and Good, B. (1978) 'Culture, illness and care: clinical lessons from anthropologic and cross-cultural research', *Annals of Internal Medicine*, **88**, pp. 251–258.

Lai, W. A., Lew-Ting, C. Y. and Chie, W. C. (2005) 'How diabetic patients think about and manage their illness in Taiwan', *Diabetic Medicine*, **2** (3), pp. 286–292.

Leventhal, H., Nerenz, D. R. and Steele, D. J. (1984) 'Illness representation and coping with health threats', in Baum, A., Taylor, S. E. and Singer, J. E. (eds) *Handbook of Psychology and Health*, (pp. 219–252), Hillsdale, New Jersey L. Erlbaum Associates Inc.

Lloyd, C. E., Dyer, P. H. and Barnett, A. H. (2000) 'Prevalence of symptoms of depression and anxiety in a diabetes clinic population', *Diabetic Medicine*, **17** (3), pp. 198–202.

Lowes, L., Lyne, P. and Gregory, J. W. (2004) 'Childhood diabetes: parents' experience of home management and the first year following diagnosis', *Diabetic Medicine*, 21 (6), pp. 531–538.

Lustman, P. J., Griffith, L. S. and Clouse, R. E. (1996) 'Recognizing and managing depression in patients with diabetes', in Rubin, R. R. and Anderson, B. J. (eds) *Practical Psychology for Diabetes Clinicians*, Alexandria, American Diabetes Association.

Lustman, P. J., Griffith, L. S., Freedland, K. E., Kissel, S. S. and Clouse, R. E. (1998) 'Cognitive behavior therapy for depression in type 2 diabetes mellitus. A randomized, controlled trial', *Annals of Internal Medicine*, 129 (8), pp. 613–621.

Murphy, E. and Kinmonth, A. L. (1995) 'No symptoms, no problem – patients' understandings of non-insulin dependent diabetes', *Family Practioner*, 12 (2), pp. 184–192.

Peel, E., Parry, O., Douglas, M., and Lawton, J. (2004) 'Diagnosis of type 2 diabetes: a qualitative analysis of patients' emotional reactions and views about information provision', *Patient Education and Counselling*, 53 (3), pp. 269–275.

Rubin, R. R. and Peyrot, M. (2002) 'Emotional responses to diagnosis', in Rubin, R. R. and Anderson, B. J. (eds) *Practical Psychology for Diabetes Clinicians*, 2nd edn, Alexandria, American Diabetes Association.

Savoca, M. R., Miller, C. K. and Quandt, S. A. (2004) 'Profiles of people with type 2 diabetes mellitus: the extremes of glycemic control', *Social Science and Medicine*, 58 (12), pp. 2655–2666.

Skinner, T. C. and Hampson, S. E. (2001) 'Personal models of diabetes in relation to self-care, well-being and glycemic control: a prospective study in adolescence', *Diabetes Care*, 24 (5), pp. 828–833.

Skinner, T. C., Howells, L., Chanon, S. and McEvilly, A. (2000) 'Diabetes in adolescents', in Snoek, F. and Skinner T. C. (eds) *Psychology in Diabetes Care*, Chichester, John Wiley and Sons Ltd.

Skinner, T. C., Howells, L., Greene, S., Edgar, K., McEvilly, A. and Johansson, A. (2003) 'Development, reliability and validity of the diabetes illness representations questionnaire: four studies with adolescents', *Diabetic Medicine*, 20 (4), pp. 283–289.

Skinner, T. C., Tantam, L., Purchon, A. and John, M. (2002) 'Do illness beliefs explain poorer outcomes for ethnic minority populations: a pilot study', *Diabetic Medicine*, 19 (s4) (suppl. 2), Poster 274, pp. 96–97.

Talbot, F. and Nouwen, A. (2000) 'A review of the relationship between depession and diabetes in adults: Is there a link?', *Diabetes Care*, 23, pp. 1556–1562.

The DAWN (Diabetes Attitudes, Wishes and Needs) study, (2002) *Practical Diabetes International*, 19 (1), January/February, pp. 22–24.

World Health Organization (WHO) Information Package (1998) *Mastering depression in primary care*, Frederiksborg, World Health Organization Regional Office for Europe, Psychiatric Research Unit.

CHAPTER 9

EDUCATION FOR EFFECTIVE SELF-MANAGEMENT

Learning Outcomes

When you have completed this chapter you should be able to:

9.1 Define and use, or recognise definitions and applications of, each of the terms printed in **bold** in the text.

9.2 Discuss self-management, including the reality of who is in control and the role of professionals and carers and people with diabetes.

9.3 Describe the difference between compliance, concordance and empowerment in relation to diabetes self-care.

9.4 Outline the elements of effective self-management including dietary changes, activity, self-monitoring, taking medication and adjustment.

9.5 Identify common barriers to effective self-management (including professional–patient communication).

9.6 State how good communication between health care professionals and people with diabetes can optimise self-care.

9.1 Introduction

When someone develops diabetes there soon follows a realisation that there is no cure and that there are 'tasks' that will need to be performed to help them control their diabetes in such a way that their health and quality of life is maintained as much as possible. Health care services are set up to help people with diabetes learn how to manage these tasks from day to day. It is important to remember that the work of health care professionals is not limited to making a diagnosis and supplying information regarding health status and possible strategies for health maintenance or improvement. In addition, health care professionals assist people with diabetes in the understanding of that information, the setting of goals and incorporation of these negotiated strategies into their daily life. This is an ongoing process, the aim of which is to improve people's quality of physical, mental and social life. This chapter focuses on diabetes self-management: what it means for people with diabetes and how it can be aided by those people around them, especially the health care professionals in the diabetes care team, and considers the 'how' of behaviour change.

You may find the ideas and language from psychology in this chapter quite new and different, even from the medical language in earlier sections. As you work through the chapter, this terminology will become more familiar and the glossary will also help you get to grips with it.

9.1.1 Diabetes: a self-managed condition

Diabetes is now recognised as one of Europe's increasing health burdens both for those who live with the condition daily and for those who care for them. As you read in earlier chapters, there is now evidence that controlling blood glucose level, blood pressure and blood lipid level can reduce the personal risk of developing microvascular and macrovascular complications. Yet, even with increasingly effective medication and specialist services developing both in primary (community) and secondary (hospital) care services, there is recognition that improving outcomes for people with diabetes requires the *individual themself* to be skilled in active self-care management. Increasingly, research studies are showing us that current health care services are not supporting people to effectively self-manage through behaviour change. It is now clear that successful behaviour change by an individual is related to good communication with the health care professional. In addition to this, health care professionals are becoming increasingly challenged (and frustrated) by the need to provide such care within the current health care framework. Health care policies are beginning to identify the need for partnership-working with people with chronic conditions such as diabetes. This requires health care professionals to reflect on their changing role with people with diabetes, from that of carer, decision-maker and prescriber of care to that of facilitator and 'coach' of self-care.

> 'Diabetes is a self-managed illness. It has to be. Diabetes self-management is the responsibility of the patient, so it requires new roles for both the patient and the professional and a completely new vision of patient education. It took us many years to fully appreciate this and to understand the fundamental changes it required in our philosophy of diabetes education.'

> (Anderson and Funnell, 2001)

To consider the fundamental changes required, we need to consider a few 'truths' about humans and their responses to health and self-care.

Truth 1: Every human is seen as basically striving for health and well-being.

Health care professionals often ask: 'If this is true why don't patients quit smoking, take their medication or lose weight?'

These so-called 'self-destructive behaviours' can be seen as a result of internal or external barriers to change to a more healthy way of living. We all live with such barriers that influence the decisions we make.

People's attitudes towards diabetes, and their understanding of the importance of taking care of themselves, are the cornerstones of their actions; for example, if a person believes that their diabetes is not serious (and by this they mean that it will do them no harm) then it is not surprising that they do not see losing weight as a priority.

However, people are often not fully aware of the sets of values (personal reasons) behind their behaviours. For behaviour change to be successful, therefore, an increase in awareness and understanding of self, values and emotions regarding diabetes and self-care is required; for example, why do they do what they do? Or why do they not do what they could do?

Truth 2: Diabetes self-care is the responsibility of the individual with diabetes.

Typical health care professional responses: 'But they are my patients and my responsibility'; 'I am the one that gets audited, not them.'

Every day people with diabetes make decisions about what they eat, how active they are, stress management, blood glucose monitoring and taking medication.

Six times a year (at most) they make decisions with health care professionals about their treatment. So which set of decisions has the greatest impact on their metabolic control and quality of life?

People with diabetes can veto any recommendation a health care professional makes, no matter how important or relevant the provider believes that recommendation to be.

The consequences of these choices accrue first and foremost to the person with diabetes.

Health care professionals may be audited and evaluated to ensure they are delivering good care, but they cannot share in the experience of developing retinopathy, neuropathy or cardiovascular disease.

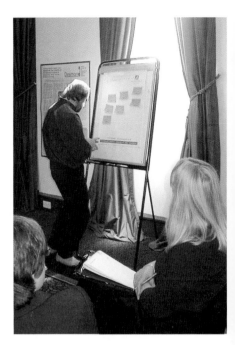

Figure 9.1 Participants of a DESMOND group discussing effective communication skills.

Truth 3: Problems related to self-care are often found in the domain of the patient's everyday life.

What stops the person with diabetes from following all the current healthy living guidelines?

Poor self-care is seldom strictly a result of medical problems or lack of knowledge.

The giving-up of old habits and/or the development of new ones has to be a very conscious, step-by-step process with thoroughly planned actions. The person's resources and expertise regarding their situation and way of living must be acknowledged and developed if changes in behaviour are to be achieved.

Who is the expert then?

The person with diabetes *and* the health care professional are both experts – the person with diabetes on their experience of diabetes and their lifestyle, social and personal resources; the health care professional on the effects of diabetes and general recommendations regarding lifestyle issues.

Who knows what is best for the management of an individual's diabetes?

If the person with diabetes and the health care professional are both experts and working together, then *no one person* knows what is best!

The DESMOND (Diabetes Education and Self-Management for Ongoing and Newly Diagnosed) Collaborative (Figure 9.1), supported by Diabetes UK, derived its educational approach from these key principles (DESMOND Collaborative, 2004).

Working from this start point the Collaborative identified a number of responsibilities of health care professionals, as shown in Box 9.1.

Box 9.1 Responsibilities of health care professionals

1   For ensuring that individuals with diabetes and their carers are provided with honest, up-to-date, evidence-based information regarding the causes, effects and options for the management of Type 2 diabetes.

2   For ensuring that those living with Type 2 diabetes are aware of their specific individual ongoing health risks for developing the complications of diabetes.

3   For providing an expert forum for individuals to discuss methods of reducing their identified risk factors.

4   For ensuring individuals are supported in developing their own diabetes management plan.

5   For providing systems of care that are accessible to everyone.

6   For ensuring individuals with diabetes are supported in processing and understanding the information provided to them.

7   For ensuring that everyone, regardless of how they decide to manage their diabetes, is treated with the utmost respect and unconditional positive regard.

8   For ensuring that everyone, regardless of how they decide to manage their diabetes, is offered the same pharmaceutical and technological resources to do so and the same equitable access and quality of care.

9   For ensuring that although an individual's readiness to be an active self-manager will vary with time and life circumstances, no-one will ever be excluded from any education or care activity should they choose not to self-manage at any time.

10 For ensuring that empathy and warmth typify all clinical and educational interactions.

11 For ensuring that people with Type 2 diabetes are given the opportunity to reflect on their day-to-day self-management in relation to possible barriers to change.

12 For ensuring that individuals with diabetes are supported in the development of the general self-management skills (e.g. goal setting, action planning and problem solving) necessary for the effective management of a chronic condition.

13 For ensuring that individuals with diabetes are supported in the development of the general diabetes specific self-management (e.g. self-monitoring, management of hypo- and hyperglycaemia, foot care and cardiovascular risk, etc.) necessary for the effective management of Type 2 diabetes.

14 For ensuring that individuals with diabetes are provided with a forum in which to discuss and explore their experiences, frustrations and successes of living with the condition.

15   For ensuring that individuals are supported in managing their emotional responses to the diagnosis of diabetes, its impact on their life and the impact of complications.

16   For ensuring that individuals experiencing significant emotional distress are offered appropriate care to facilitate the management and alleviation of such distress.

Activity 9.1   Professional responsibilities

Suggested study time 30 minutes

Consider the list of professional responsibilities above. Choose five from the list. Then think back to a diabetes care consultation that you experienced or observed (this may be the video of the annual review on the course DVD). What did the professional do that fulfilled these responsibilities or contradicted them?

Comment

How did you get on? As one member of the course team said, this is a very comprehensive list of responsibilities and it's difficult to see how they can all be fulfilled in every consultation. Indeed, some of them may not need to be fulfilled every time; for example, if the person with diabetes is not experiencing significant emotional distress they do not need to be offered appropriate care (no. 16). The important point is that this list of professional responsibilities all come from the same ethos or way of working, one which is person-centred, supportive and equitable.

In spite of this way of working, which is becoming more generally accepted, there remain common misconceptions about diabetes self-management. Sometimes it is possible to recognise these misconceptions by the use of certain words or language in the diabetes care environment. You look at the use of some of these words in the next section.

9.2   Empowerment, compliance and concordance – what's in a word?

There are a number of words used to describe what people do or don't do as regards their health care advice and self-care: some of them are applied in relation to someone else's behaviours or judgements, including 'compliance', 'concordance' and 'adherence'.

Compliance (or non-compliance) is a concept that has generated a mass of literature, but it is a wholly inappropriate term when applied to diabetes care (or any other form of health care). One NHS website describes compliance as 'the act of following orders' (NHS UK Transplant, 2005).

We could tone this down and say compliance is the act of following treatment recommendations. This sounds reasonable, so why is it inappropriate, and what are the recommendations that people with diabetes are 'supposed' to follow?

1 Given the nature of diabetes, there is no single set of clear recommendations given to every patient. The way a person with Type 1 diabetes best manages their diet and lifestyle depends on which insulin regimen they are on. So the set of recommendations for one person may be very different from that for the next.

2 A person with diabetes is likely to see many different health care professionals: a doctor and nurse as a minimum. However, it is very unlikely that these different health care professionals will give exactly the same set of recommendations to the same individual. So which set of recommendations is the person with diabetes supposed to follow?

3 Even if we look at a single consultation we encounter the problem that what the patient recalls was recommended is frequently substantially different from what the professional recalls they said (for example, Page et al., 1981; Parkin and Skinner, 2003). So if the patient follows the recommendations they recall, they still may be accused of non-compliance by the professional next time they meet. Furthermore, when consultations have been recorded, the professional recall of what they said in the consultation does not always agree with what was actually said (Skinner et al., 2003).

There is also variation in how people comply or do not comply with recommendations.

1 Managing diabetes involves many different tasks, incorporating taking medication, monitoring blood glucose level, food choices and physical activity. Research literature shows clearly that how well a person follows recommendations in one part of their diabetes care, for example, taking their medication, is not related to how well they follow other recommendations, for example, eating a low-fat diet. So using the term compliant or non-compliant does not allow for the multi-faceted nature of diabetes management.

2 The same can also be said within a particular facet of diabetes management. The most obvious example is food choices. An individual may be very good at following recommendations on the quality of food, but might still eat more than is recommended.

3 In addition, many individuals engage in a range of activities to enhance their diabetes management, which are not directly recommended to them. For example, they may meditate to manage stress or they may take herbal remedies or other supplements. Compliance does not take these other attempts to manage diabetes into account.

In addition to these issues, compliance and adherence (which in effect mean the same thing) place the blame for poor control at the person's doorstep. It does not allow for the fact that the professional may not be the best person to judge which insulin regimen is going to work best for the patient. It also implies that the person with diabetes has no valid role in the decision-making process of treatment regimens and that they should just do what they are told. This is probably why the concept of non-compliance has been debated and researched for many years without finding a solution. However, over the last few years researchers have started to realise that a new approach is needed, and this is known as an 'empowerment approach'.

Empowerment is often a misunderstood term but its use is in relation to a different approach from the one outlined above and is founded on the recognition that people make the best choices for themselves given the situation that they find themselves in at the time.

Activity 9.2   Empowerment

Suggested study time 20 minutes

Look at Table 9.1, which is taken from an article on compliance and adherence (Anderson and Funnell, 2000). Compare the two models of care and identify whether it is the patient or the health professional who is the focus of the consultation in each of the models.

Table 9.1 Comparing the empowerment model with the traditional model.

The empowerment model	The traditional model
Diabetes is a bio-psychosocial illness.	Diabetes is a physical illness.
Relationship of provider and patient is democratic and based on shared expertise.	Relationship of provider and patient is authoritarian, based on provider expertise.
Problems and learning needs are usually identified by the patient.	Problems and learning needs are usually identified by the professional.
Patient is viewed as problem-solver and caregiver, i.e. professional acts as a resource and helps the patient set goals and develop a self-management plan.	Professional is viewed as problem-solver and caregiver, i.e. professional responsible for diagnosis, and outcome.
Goal is to enable patients to make informed choices. Behavioural strategies are used to help patients experiment with behaviour changes of their choosing. Behaviour changes that are not adopted are viewed as learning tools to provide new information that can be used to develop future plans and goals.	Goal is behaviour change. Behavioural strategies are used to increase compliance with recommended treatment. A lack of compliance is viewed as a failure of the patient.
Behaviour changes are internally motivated.	Behaviour changes are externally motivated.
Patient and professional are powerful.	Patient is powerless, professional is powerful.

Comment

As you can see, there is a different focus in each of the two models. Did you notice that in the traditional model the focus in the doctor–patient interaction is often on the professional, who leads the conversation, makes the decisions on treatment and so on? This is in stark contrast to the empowerment model, where the person with the diabetes is usually the focus and makes the decisions regarding their care, with the help of the health care professional. Given that most diabetes care occurs outside the consulting room, it is more important that the person with diabetes feels able to self-manage and make decisions, etc., independently, knowing that there is advice and support from the rest of the diabetes care team when they need it.

Within the UK, the word **concordance** is gaining popularity with NHS policy makers who are trying to increase the effective use of medications. Their approach is to use concordance instead of compliance. Box 9.2 looks at concordance in more detail (Medicines Partnership, 2005).

Box 9.2 What is concordance?

Concordance is a new way to define the process of successful prescribing and taking medicine, based on partnership. It has four essential elements as shown in Figure 9.2.

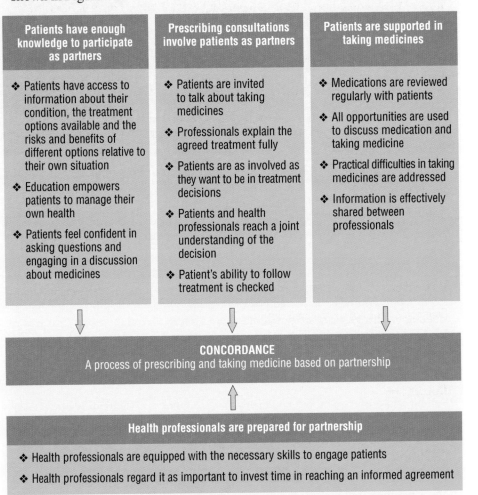

Patients have enough knowledge to participate as partners	Prescribing consultations involve patients as partners	Patients are supported in taking medicines
❖ Patients have access to information about their condition, the treatment options available and the risks and benefits of different options relative to their own situation ❖ Education empowers patients to manage their own health ❖ Patients feel confident in asking questions and engaging in a discussion about medicines	❖ Patients are invited to talk about taking medicines ❖ Professionals explain the agreed treatment fully ❖ Patients are as involved as they want to be in treatment decisions ❖ Patients and health professionals reach a joint understanding of the decision ❖ Patient's ability to follow treatment is checked	❖ Medications are reviewed regularly with patients ❖ All opportunities are used to discuss medication and taking medicine ❖ Practical difficulties in taking medicines are addressed ❖ Information is effectively shared between professionals

CONCORDANCE
A process of prescribing and taking medicine based on partnership

Health professionals are prepared for partnership

❖ Health professionals are equipped with the necessary skills to engage patients

❖ Health professionals regard it as important to invest time in reaching an informed agreement

Figure 9.2 The four elements of concordance.

Why is concordance needed?

There are many reasons why people do not take their medicines:

- lack of information about their condition and the importance of treatment
- practical difficulties, such as getting to a pharmacy, opening containers and remembering to take medicines

- problems with side effects
- interference with their daily lives
- beliefs about the medicine, or medicines in general – for example, that medicines are unnatural, harmful, addictive, or that their effects wear off over time.

Many compliance programmes have focused on the practical difficulties of taking medication. However, the differences between the patient's beliefs and understanding of the diagnosis and proposed treatment and those of the health care professional are crucially important. The health professional has a set of beliefs about the appropriateness of particular medicines, and about how they should be used based on a biomedical model. These beliefs are shaped by the content of professional training, and on the evidence from a large body of scientific research. The patient has their own equally cogent and coherent set of ideas about their illness, medicines in general and their own medicines in particular. These are based on their preferences, priorities, beliefs, attitudes and life experience.

It is important to recognise that the decision to take a medicine or not ultimately lies with the patient. A successful prescribing process is an agreement that builds on the experiences, beliefs and wishes of the patient to decide when, how and why to take medication. This agreement may not always be easy to reach, but without exploring and addressing these issues patients may not be able to get full benefit from the diagnosis and treatment of the illness (Medicines Partnership, 2005).

Activity 9.3 Defining terms

Suggested study time 30 minutes

In your own words, explain the difference between the words compliance and concordance.

Comment

How did you get on with this activity? However you described the difference between these two words, you should be able to recognise that compliance is about doing what you are told, whereas concordance is about having an agreed plan or approach to a problem.

Most of us participate in some kinds of self-care activities, regardless of whether or not we have a chronic condition such as diabetes. We wash ourselves, clean our teeth, eat and drink, sleep, etc. Caring for ourselves, and having a 'healthy lifestyle' has become more and more important recently, so much so that even the government has become involved. In the next section you consider healthy living and what it is that encourages or discourages you to maintain or develop aspects of a healthy lifestyle.

9.2.1 What are the barriers to effective self-care?

To consider this question, it is useful to start with your own barriers to change. In the following activities you reflect on your response to your own self-care activities in relation to your own health.

Lifestyle self-care

Diabetes requires individuals to change several aspects of their lifestyle (diet, physical activity, smoking, drinking) if they are to optimise their control of the condition and prevent or delay complications. (The guidelines for individuals with diabetes with no renal complications are no different from the recommendations for healthy living for the general population.)

Activity 9.4 Lifestyle self-care

Suggested study time 1 hour

(a) Complete Table 9.2 about what you think are the current recommendations for a healthy lifestyle.

Table 9.2 For use with Activity 9.4a.

What do you think are the current lifestyle recommendations for healthy living?	Your answer
What is the current recommended daily maximum intake of alcohol in units (1 unit = half a pint of beer, 1 glass of wine, 1 shot of spirit)?	
What are the current recommendations for the amount and intensity of physical activity recommended for protection against cardiovascular disease?	
What are the current recommendations for adding salt to your food?	
How many cigarettes a day do the current recommendations say you can have?	
How many portions of fresh fruit and vegetables should you be eating each day for a healthy diet?	
If a plate represents a whole meal, roughly what proportion of the plate should be covered by each of these three food types? Fruit and vegetables: Bread, cereals and potatoes: Meat, fish and alternatives, e.g. pulses:	

Now look at Table 9.4 overleaf and see whether your answers match.

(b) Now think back over the last week. For each guideline in Table 9.2, estimate the number of days on which you succeeded in achieving the recommendation. Complete Table 9.3.

Table 9.3 For use with Activity 9.4b.

Recommendation	Number of days in the last week
On how many days did you limit your alcohol intake to 2–3 units (females) or 3–4 units (males)?	
On how many days did you accumulate a total of 30 minutes of moderate intensity activity?	
On how many days did you only add salt once food was on the plate and you had tasted it?	
On how many days did you not smoke?	
On how many days did you manage to eat five portions of fruit and vegetables?	
On how many days did you have at least two meals that approached the Balance of Good Health example (Section 4.5.4)?	

Comment

How well did you do? If you were unable to meet the recommendations, why do you think that was?

Did you succeed in achieving all these goals for healthy living? If not, what stopped you achieving them?

Not everybody feels that it is important to live a healthy lifestyle, and some people feel that achieving all these goals would get in the way of living the life they want to. For example, achieving all of these goals might not be practicable given the type of job you do.

People diagnosed with Type 2 diabetes, particularly when associated with obesity, are amongst those living the least healthy lifestyles. Unfortunately we do not have large amounts of lifestyle data on people with diabetes in the UK. However, data from the USA indicate that people with Type 2 diabetes report following their dietary recommendations about 50% of the time, their exercise recommendations about 35% of time and their foot care recommendations 47% of time, there being no difference between the smoking rate of those with or without diabetes. You should remember that these data are all based on self-report data, and therefore may be overestimates. It is also worth noting that people with diabetes often report that diet is the hardest part of diabetes care, and it is to this that you turn in the next section.

Table 9.4 For use with Activity 9.4a.

What do you think are the current lifestyle recommendations for healthy living?	Recommendation
What is the current recommended daily maximum intake of alcohol in units (1 unit = half a pint of beer, 1 glass of wine, 1 shot of spirit)?	Females 2–3 units Males 3–4 units
What are the current recommendations for the amount and intensity of physical activity recommended for protection against cardiovascular disease?	30 minutes of moderate intensity activity at least five times a week (moderate intensity activity makes you slightly breathless, such that you can have a conversation but with difficulty)
What are the current recommendations for adding salt to your food?	Only add salt once food is on the plate and you have tasted it
How many cigarettes a day do the current recommendations say you can have?	None
How many portions of fresh fruit and vegetables should you be eating each day for a healthy diet?	Minimum of five portions (one portion equates to about a handful of fruit or vegetables; only one portion can be drunk in the form of juice each day)
If a plate represents a whole meal, roughly what proportion of the plate should be covered by each of these three food types?	Fruit and vegetables: 33% Bread, cereals and potatoes: 33% Meat, fish and alternatives, e.g. pulses: 12%

9.3 The challenge of dietary management

Regardless of the type of diabetes, dietary management is often reported to be the most demanding, difficult and frustrating part of living with diabetes. There are many reasons for this, as food is not just a means to reduce hunger and provide energy. Food serves many other functions (for example, it is used to celebrate and reward, to comfort and reassure, to alleviate boredom or to show how much you care or how good a host you are) and is linked with many activities in our cultures (Figure 9.3), such as weddings, funerals, birthdays, festivals and fasts. There is an abundance of social pressures to eat and drink certain foods. Furthermore, millions of pounds are spent on advertising by manufacturers trying to get people to eat their foods.

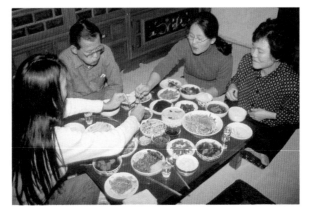

Figure 9.3 Mealtimes are often social occasions.

One of the other aspects that makes any dietary management difficult is that food is constantly visible. When you have taken your medication, or have done your 30-minute walk, you have done what you need to do and you don't have to think about it any more for that day. But food presents itself to you constantly throughout the day through meal times and snacks and drinks that accompany them.

So how can people with diabetes be supported to manage their food choices to optimise their physical health without making them feel deprived of food, or resenting their diabetes, and without taking away the pleasure of food? The first step is to help people understand how food fits into a lifestyle with diabetes; for example, if you take insulin-stimulating tablets or insulin for your diabetes, going too long without food will cause a hypo, and therefore missing meals, even if you are not hungry, will present difficulties.

Table 9.5 presents common lifestyle influences on dietary self-care. Each entry represents a type of everyday situation that makes dietary management difficult, and provides some key questions that can be used to help people identify where specific barriers or difficulties to dietary management are. You can try answering these questions for yourself about your lifestyle, to see what insights it may give you.

Table 9.5 Common lifestyle influences on dietary self-care (adapted from Schlundt et al., 1994).

Type of problem	Description	Interview questions
Negative emotions	The person overeats to cope with stress and negative feelings.	Are there any situations in your life that are currently causing you a lot of stress? Do you eat differently when you feel upset, depressed or stressed?
Resisting temptation	Food cues and cravings are tempting the person to eat inappropriate foods.	What foods or situations trigger cravings? What foods or situations tempt you to eat inappropriately?
Eating out	Eating away from home (e.g. restaurants) makes it hard for the person to control what and how much they eat.	How do the amounts or kinds of food you eat differ when you eat away from home or at a restaurant?
Feeling deprived	The person feels they cannot eat certain foods they enjoy and is tempted to give in.	How often do you feel like giving up on taking good care of your diabetes because it keeps you from eating the way you enjoy? What foods do you feel you should give up eating?
Time pressure	Having many demands on the person's time makes healthy eating difficult.	What kinds of social, family, or job pressures make it hard for you to find the time to eat the way you want to?
Tempted to relapse	The person feels discouraged or feels like a failure and no longer tries to eat healthily.	How often do you feel so discouraged about your eating plan that you want to just give up? Do you see your current plan as rigid or flexible?

Table 9.5 *continued*

Type of problem	Description	Interview questions
Planning	A hectic schedule makes it hard for the person to plan what and when to eat.	How difficult is it for you to plan when, where and what you will eat?
Competing priorities	Many responsibilities and obligations (e.g. family and job) interfere with the person's ability to make healthy food choices.	What important priorities in your life get in the way of making healthy food choices? Do you sometimes feel like you have to choose between good diabetes care and other important life goals?
Social events	The person overeats at parties, holidays, special occasions, and other social events that involve food.	How do the amounts or kinds of foods you eat differ when you eat at parties or social events?
Family support	The person's family does not support healthy food choices.	What things do your family do to support or hinder your efforts to eat the way you want to?
Food refusal	Someone offers an inappropriate food and the person finds it hard to refuse.	How hard is it for you to refuse food when someone offers it to you?
Friends' support	The person's friends do not support healthy food choices.	What things do your friends do to support or hinder your efforts to eat the way you want to?

Once people have identified their problem areas, they need to find a way to help them address the issues for themselves. The key for the diabetes care team is not to tell the person with diabetes how to solve things, but to support them in finding their own solutions to the challenges they face in managing their diet. However, Polonsky (1999) suggests there are seven key strategies that can be helpful in helping people manage their dietary self-care.

1 Develop a plan

Many people are not sure what changes they should make to their diet that would be most effective in managing their diabetes. Many people know they should eat less fat, but do not know how much fat is in particular products. So it is important that people with diabetes are supported in working out what their priorities for dietary management are, and the types of changes they need to make.

Once a broad objective is identified, use goal setting as described in Section 8.2.3 to help people set SMART goals, and establish how they are going to achieve these goals. Identifying barriers to change and providing information about food choices can make life easier. As there is a lot of confusing information about diet in the literature and on food products themselves, it can be helpful to ensure that people understand their options, and a dietetic consultation or group education session may be a valuable tool to help.

2 Modify environments

Many of our poor food choices result from unplanned decisions in response to temptations, or old habits that are difficult to break. Once a plan has been identified, it can be helpful to think about things in the environment that make it difficult to change. For example, if certain foods are kept in a cupboard and are visible each time the door is opened it can be very difficult to resist temptation. It may be helpful to move certain foods out of sight to reduce temptation and thereby eat less of them or even none at all.

Someone may have a habit that is difficult to break, for instance adding salt to food when cooking, almost automatically. Simply moving the salt will break the chain of habit and require the person to think; this act alone can be very productive in helping the person break the habit. Some people find prompts left in appropriate places helpful. The key is to think about what normally happens, and to support the person in finding strategies that will support efforts to achieve their plan.

3 Get perspective

This strategy also relates back to Section 8.2.3 on self-efficacy. Demanding 100% success with difficult changes is unrealistic; people need to develop plans that are realistic for them. Even so, there will be times when they don't follow through with the treatment plan. It only takes a number of pressures to coincide, and the plan is abandoned when the offer of tea and chocolate biscuits is presented. Furthermore, because the benefits of dietary change on blood glucose level are not always immediate or consistent, someone may follow their plan to the letter and yet still have a high blood glucose value on a particular day.

Therefore, supporting people in developing a longer term perspective can be very helpful. Here it is beneficial to set a date to review the plan to find out whether they have been able to follow it through and, in the longer term, to see how the changes have helped. It is also worth thinking about how to deal with those moments or days when the plan does not work. Many people may start thinking to themselves, 'I can't do this diet' or 'Oh blow it, I give up'. When learning to drive a car, people don't give up the first time they grind a gear, or hit a kerb. The perspective to remember is that changing behaviour or learning a new skill or way of making choices is hard.

4 Structured cheating

One of the biggest challenges with food is cutting something out altogether. This is particularly difficult, as it is often the case that the more you want to stop doing something, the more you find yourself thinking about it.

> Whatever you read next, whatever it says, you must not think about a pink elephant.

Most people find that when they read a statement like the one above, or are told not to think about a pink elephant, that the thought or image of one immediately pops into their head. This is the challenge of stopping something, whether it's smoking, eating chocolate or crisps or any other habit.

So it may be worth including some 'cheating'. For example, if someone wants to stop eating chocolate, it can help to build some chocolate into their plan; they may have something at a set time, or for achieving their plan. It is also worth helping people make the most of their cheating. Rather than just eating the chocolate as normal, some people find that making it a real treat actually makes the chocolate far more enjoyable than it ever was before.

5 New not old

This strategy also relates to the discussion on self-efficacy in Section 8.2.3. If we try to reduce or stop an old behaviour or food choice, then it is likely that we will have lapses. If our mindset is to keep track of these lapses and think, 'I can't do this, look what keeps happening', then this mantra can become a self-fulfilling prophecy. If we tell ourselves we can't do something, we will learn to believe that, and will not be able to do it.

A different approach is to focus on the success that a person has. When there is a lapse, finding ways to prompt the person to think of all the times they did follow their plan changes the internal dialogue. For example, 'if you have done something once, you can do it twice, etc…'. Focusing on the times they have enacted their plan helps them feel more positive and enables them to think differently about the lapses. This is why it is important for people to monitor their efforts, and to focus on the new changes that they see entering their life, and not on the old ways that may return to haunt them.

6 Address boredom

Boredom is a risk for many people trying to change their dietary choices and lifestyle. When nothing else is going on, the mind can easily wander, and find old familiar paths of behaviour. Whether it brings up negative emotions that need reassuring, or just the temptation of a really good take-away, then food is an easy, quick and satisfying solution.

In situations such as these, the key is to find a solution to the problem. However, it is easy for health care professionals to fall into the 'I know what you need' trap. It is amazing how many people are encouraged to join an evening class to help them manage their eating behaviours. There are many things that can alleviate boredom, and what people find interesting and stimulating varies so much from person to person, that it is not worth trying to guess what will work for each individual. It is also worth remembering that if the individual can't think of things they find interesting any more, especially if they have lost interest in activities they used to enjoy, then it is worth considering whether the individual is showing signs of depression rather than boredom.

7 Assertive strategies

These are particularly useful when social situations cause challenges to dietary management. Whether work requires a great deal of socialising, or a regular social life is associated with food and drink pressures, or food has strong cultural meanings that are difficult to manage, it is important to help people find productive, creative and positive ways to manage these pressures.

Assertiveness can sometimes be seen as a negative trait, but here it simply means using your ability to say no politely, while also putting forward a positive image of yourself. Whether people want to talk about their diabetes or not, being assertive does not have to be difficult. The following tips can help:

- Use 'I' statements. For example, consider the difference between 'Thanks, I don't want any potato skins right now' and 'Thanks, but potato skins really aren't good for me.' By beginning your sentences with 'I,' you are taking responsibility for your thoughts and feelings.

- When appropriate, acknowledge that you don't want to be rude. For instance, if your neighbour invites you for ice cream, don't be shy about stating the different aspects to your feelings. You might say, 'Thanks for the offer, but I don't eat ice cream. I hope I haven't offended you. We should get together anyway.' By communicating both parts of your message out loud (no ice cream for me *and* I don't want to hurt your feelings), you can feel more comfortable and confident about saying what you really mean.

- Recommend a more suitable, substitute action. If you would like to avoid the slice of homemade cake that your mother-in-law is offering, try, 'Thanks, it looks lovely, but not right now. Instead, I'd really like another piece of that delicious fruit.' In this manner, you are taking control of the interaction, subtly shifting the conversation in a new, more healthy direction, away from further discussion of the cake towards a more appropriate food choice.

9.4 Medication taking and adjustment

Taking medication is a key self-care behaviour and most people with diabetes require at least one medication (often more than this) to control their blood glucose, blood pressure and cholesterol levels. Evidence suggests that only 30% of people with Type 2 diabetes obtain sufficient medication on prescription to take their medication 90% of the recommended time. For Type 1 diabetes only 72% of 15–25 year olds get sufficient insulin to meet their needs (Morris et al., 1997).

Activity 9.5 Insulin treatment and effective self-care

Suggested study time 15 minutes

Imagine you have just been told that the tablets you are taking for an illness are not sufficient any longer and you now need to start having injections. What are your initial feelings, questions and thoughts? Note these down.

Comment

When considering commencing insulin treatment, the main barrier to self-care is about the actual decision to self-inject. Many people with Type 2 diabetes delay starting insulin and recent studies have shown that the reasons for delay are usually based on inaccurate information and beliefs, as you read about in Chapter 8.

The common barriers to commencing insulin treatment can be summarised as follows:

- false beliefs about insulin such as it has to be injected into a vein or artery and the injections are very painful
- worries about extra expense and prescription needs
- concerns about having more hypos and less personal freedom
- the potential impact on social life and employment.

When comparing thoughts from people before and after starting insulin, several differences were found as shown in Table 9.5.

Table 9.6 People's views on insulin, before and after commencing treatment.

Thoughts before starting insulin	Thoughts after starting insulin
Insulin signifies disease progression	A natural progression
Insulin will make others perceive greater sickness	Gaining control (of life, eating, glycaemic levels)
Fear of needle injection	Best treatment at appropriate time
Insulin will be demanding to administer	Best option
Injecting insulin is painful	Feel really well, healthy, energetic
Difficult to inject the right amount at the right time	Pen devices are highly appreciated
My being on insulin causes my family and friends to be more concerned	

To support the person who needs to start insulin, it may be useful:

- for the health care professional to consider their own feelings about insulin and its burdens – some may see it as a failure
- to demystify insulin in primary care by encouraging GPs and practice nurses to care for people starting insulin therapy
- for health care professionals to talk about insulin from the beginning of the diagnosis and consider using a dummy injection of sterile water
- for the diabetes care team to recognise that starting people on insulin is not difficult – it just requires time and training
- for all concerned to recognise that starting insulin is not the only factor required to improve control – people need to learn how to adjust their lifestyles and other aspects of self-care
- to support people starting injections by arranging contact with people who already take insulin injections to help demonstrate how life will be now that they are taking insulin
- to use structured group education to help people explore their thoughts and feelings with others.

9.5 Self-monitoring

Many people with diabetes are asked to self-monitor their urine or blood glucose levels. These tests allow the person with diabetes and the health care team to make decisions about lifestyle changes and treatment. Unfortunately, recent evidence suggests that those who do test their blood glucose levels may not be better 'controlled' than those that do not! This result has led to a review of the barriers to effective testing (Coster et al., 2000). Polonsky has considered the reasons why people don't like testing their blood glucose levels as can be seen in Box 9.3.

Box 9.3 Ten reasons to hate blood glucose monitoring

1   Your meter makes you feel bad about yourself.

2   Monitoring seems pointless (because you believe there is nothing you can do about your blood glucose result anyway).

3   Checking your blood glucose reminds you that you have diabetes, which is something you'd probably rather not think about too much.

4   Your meter seems to control your life, telling you what you can and can't do.

5   Monitoring serves as an opportunity for your friends and family to bother you.

6   None of your health care providers ever does anything with the results anyway.

7   Checking blood glucose sometimes hurts.

8   Monitoring can be inconvenient.

9   Monitoring can be expensive.

10 Life is too busy and demanding to take the time for regular monitoring.

Activity 9.6 Imagine if...

Suggested study time 15 minutes

Imagine if you were taught how to use a screwdriver and were expected to tighten a screw into a piece of wood every day. How long would you keep it up? What questions would you have?

Comment

Many people are taught *how* to perform the test but are not always provided with an education programme that helps them know what to do with the results. There can often be very good reasons why people struggle to maintain their self-monitoring regimens as prescribed by their health care professional and these were considered in Box 9.3 (Polonsky, 1999). However with good support from the healthcare team, many of these issues can be resolved and appropriate self-care encouraged.

As you've probably realised, the emotional consequences of diabetes self-management are crucial, and it is to this that you turn next.

9.6 Emotions: awareness and management

You start by thinking about Angela's story (below) and how her emotions might affect her self-care.

Activity 9.7 Angela's story

Suggested study time 45 minutes

Read Case Study 9.1 and, where indicated, try to answer the questions asked about Angela's feelings and her self-care activities.

Comment

When diagnosed with diabetes, people may have difficulty accepting the fact that they have a chronic illness and the responsibilities that go with it; many are shocked and grieve at the loss of their health. Others may react with anger and frustration. Some may initially react with denial.

Not only is diabetes a demanding and burdensome condition, individuals are at risk of developing complications. Indeed, in the course of time, the majority of patients are faced with serious health problems and complications related to the diabetes. In addition, people with diabetes may be confronted with various social barriers (for example, taking out insurance, potential loss of their driving licence) and negative interactions with their environment. Diabetes self-management 'by the book' does not always pay and maintaining optimal control does not guarantee avoiding complications. Not achieving satisfactory glucose control, despite all good intentions and daily self-care efforts, can give rise to strong feelings of frustration, helplessness and ultimately 'diabetes burnout'. Hypoglycaemia can cause anxiety both in the person with diabetes and their partners.

Case Study 9.1

Angela is 49 years old, of Caribbean descent, and lives with her husband and two children. She has recently been diagnosed with Type 2 diabetes, following a recent check on her blood pressure. She has not experienced any symptoms but is not surprised as she has been overweight for many years and was constantly warned about the effects of her weight.

Now consider Angela's story again, five years later. How do you think Angela is feeling now?

Angela has now had Type 2 diabetes for 5 years. She is a busy wife and mother and has a part-time job as a nurse. She is now having to take nine different tablets for her diabetes, high blood pressure and high cholesterol. She also monitors her blood glucose level daily, and is trying to lose weight. She has not found it easy to find the time to do any exercise but tries to walk to the shops and back when she can. She is starting to forget to take her tablets.

Consider the next episode in Angela's story. How do you think Angela is feeling now? What effect will these feelings have on her ability to increase her self-care activities?

Angela has just returned from her annual review of her diabetes with her doctor. He has told her that her recent eye test for retinopathy is positive. She is starting to show signs of damage to the back of her eyes. He also told her that her kidney function is deteriorating. He advised her to improve her blood glucose level by remembering to take her tablets and improving her diet.

As you read in Chapter 8, diabetes can elicit strong emotional reactions; depression and diabetes-specific anxieties are common in people with diabetes. Not only are these emotions psychologically burdensome in themselves, they are likely to hamper a person's ability to self-manage their diabetes. Emotion management is an important and integral part of overall diabetes management.

9.7 Communication skills and the consultation

Although it may not be obvious, there is now increasing recognition that one of the key barriers to effective self-care is the health care system and, specifically, the health care professionals themselves. Effective communication skills are essential to every consultation between a health care professional and a patient (as discussed in Section 1.5).

● Why are communication skills essential for consultations between health care professionals and patients?

● Communication skills are essential for taking an accurate medical history, establishing a diagnosis and management plan, and enabling a patient to recall treatment decisions and to act on them.

There are many studies documenting the need for health care professionals to continually develop these skills. For instance, studies consistently show that health care professionals interrupt patient's responses to their questions, that patients and health care professionals often disagree (up to 50% in some studies) on the main presenting problem, that patients do not accurately recall treatment decisions and recommendations, and that patients consistently report wanting more and better quality information (Parkin and Skinner, 2003; Skinner et al., 2003).

Given the increasing prevalence of diabetes in people from minority ethnic backgrounds, communication and understanding between health care professionals and people with diabetes has become a more important issue. Many diabetes outpatient departments have Asian link workers or Asian support workers, who can facilitate communication between members of the health care team (Figure 9.4). It is not enough to have information leaflets translated into the Asian languages, such as Urdu or Punjabi. Some of the minority languages are only spoken and not read or written, and so information and support must be given verbally. Where translations are used, not only must they be accurate, they must also be culturally sensitive, given that some words are not salient or appropriate when translated. Greenhalgh et al. (1998) give a pertinent example of this in their work with British Bangladeshis: when translating from English to Bengali, for example, the Sylheti language has no expression for physical activity that has the same (positive) connotations that this concept has in English.

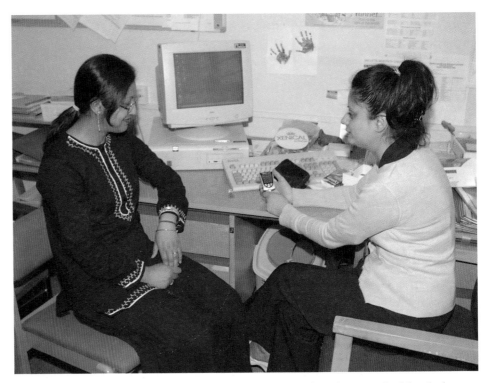

Figure 9.4   An Asian link worker (right) demonstrating the use of a blood glucose meter.

To recap, it is important to remember that the work of health care professionals is not limited to making a diagnosis, supplying information regarding health status and possible strategies for health maintenance or improvement. In addition, health care professionals need to assist each person in the processing of that information, setting of goals and incorporation of these negotiated strategies into their daily life. This is a process – the aim of which is to improve the patients' quality of physical, mental and social life.

The key issues in professional–patient communication are:

- exploring and agreeing roles and responsibilities
- agreeing agendas
- actively listening to the patient
- encouraging the patient to explore their thoughts and feelings
- communicating understanding
- observing the cues from the patient
- exploring emotions elicited by the patient
- joint goal setting and care planning
- provision of information
- agreeing follow up.

Activity 9.8 Communication with health care professionals

Suggested study time 10 minutes

Think about a recent consultation or interaction that you had with a health care professional.

- Were all the above ten points met?
- Who spoke the most?
- Who made most of the recommendations?
- Who made the decisions?
- How much time were you given to discuss your concerns?
- Were all your questions answered?

Comment

Many of us tend towards being passive when in the 'vulnerable' role of being a patient. We may assume that all we have to do is let the professional know what the problem is and then take their advice. We may try hard to listen to what is being said, but often after the session will remember all the questions that we wanted to ask but did not, due to lack of time, forgetting them, not getting an opportunity or when we did try to ask, not being responded to. We may walk away from the consultation believing that we have listened well to the instructions and know what to do but soon realise that we have missed some important issues. We may also experience a sense of 'not wanting to bother the doctor/nurse as they are such busy people'. We also may find that when we do follow the instructions that we have been given, the results or effects are not what we expected.

For many years it was assumed that health care professionals and their patients worked in harmony. The patient went along to the doctor or nurse for medication and advice on how to treat their condition and believed that all they had to do was follow the expert advice of the health care professional and their condition would be treated or cured. It was usually believed that the professional was responsible for the management of the condition and that the role of the patient was to follow the instructions. As conditions such as diabetes became more widespread, where the day-to-day decision making was in the hands of the patient, previous assumptions were questioned and conflicts between health care professionals and patients were identified.

A common behaviour in the consultation is to provide the person with diabetes with reliable and accurate information. However, this is often only partial pieces of information, or only information the health care professional thinks is important for the patient to know. They may even inadvertently misinform patients (for example, 'you have only got borderline diabetes'). It is also easy to bombard patients with too much information, present information in a complex and confusing manner and give information that the person with diabetes feels is irrelevant, all of which results in them disengaging and prevents them remembering or using the information. As one middle-aged man said, 'they have told me a lot of things, but not one of them has answered my questions'.

To prevent these problems, information provision can be broken down into distinct questions that the health care professional should be asking.

Why am I giving information?

Answering this question enables the health care professional to give the most appropriate information at the correct time. If the answer to this question is related to their own professional or personal needs then it is likely that the information is not appropriate (e.g. the doctor needs to teach the patient how their pancreas works for them to be able to manage their diabetes). However, if the information is in response to the patient's needs (e.g. the patient has asked for information, the patient seems unclear or confused, it will enable the patient to have *new* insights) then it is appropriate to provide information.

What does the patient already know?

Health care professionals are not the only source of information available to people with diabetes. Other important sources include partners, family, TV soaps and dramas, documentaries, friends and the general media including the internet. People do not necessarily remember what they have been told and may misunderstand what they have been told, or do not value the opinion of the provider of the information, even if they are a so-called expert. Furthermore, health care professionals do not always give consistent information and they frequently contradict one another. So before providing any information health care professionals should find out what the patient already knows or believes. Listening to patients express their knowledge also helps the health care professional gauge how to convey new information to them.

What information do I need to provide?

The answers to the first two questions tell the health care professional what information they need to provide. However, it is important to remember that information is only of use if it leads to understanding. It is essential to try to develop the patient's ability to manage their own diabetes. The result of these considerations is that the basic principles of diabetes care should be provided, rather than details. Unfortunately for many aspects of self-management there are no clear right or wrong answers, for example, injection regimens, dietary systems (counting the types and quantities of carbohydrate consumed, glycaemic index, etc.). Yet most health care professionals tend to form an opinion about what is best. All these opinions can be offered to people with diabetes, but they should be balanced with correct factual information about other options.

Has the individual understood what I have told them?

Once the information has been provided to the patient, health care professionals should not move on until they are sure the patient has heard, remembered and understood the information. This can be done by asking them to explain the information to the health care professional, or by asking them to think about the information and explain what this new insight gives them in understanding their diabetes management. This strategy also helps the person with diabetes to develop greater understanding and helps develop problem-solving skills. Just as importantly, this processing helps to embed the knowledge in their memory and leads to better retention and easier recall.

9.8 Qualities of effective communication

We communicate in many ways and on several levels at the same time – by word, intonation, facial expression, body language, by our actions and even by the way we dress or furnish our rooms. It is important, in order for patients to feel safe and able to express themselves honestly, that what health care professionals say and do conveys, amongst other things, empathy, hope and acceptance and that they are genuine and honest. It is also important that they are *congruous*. By this we mean that their communication by one method, for example, speech, is in accordance with their communication in other ways, for example, body language or intonation. These aspects are considered in more detail.

Empathy

To show **empathy** means that the health care professional – with professional distance, but with reason and feeling – understands the experiences, values, thoughts and feelings of the person with diabetes. When the person's way of living and the choices they make are understood, their actions become more logical and comprehensible. When this understanding is conveyed to the person they feel more secure, and feel noticed and acknowledged. By sharing this basic understanding of the person's situation, health care professionals also share a common ground for their continued work.

Empathy should not be confused with sympathy or liking (you do not have to like what you see). The health care professional is just trying to understand why the person with diabetes is acting, feeling and thinking in the way they are. Furthermore, to show empathy does not mean to pity or feel sorry for that person but simply to try and understand 'what it is like to walk in their shoes'.

Health care professionals show that they want to understand when they:

- listen actively
- ask open-ended questions
- give time for the patient to reflect on questions
- ask questions to get more detailed information
- tell the patient when there is something they do not understand.

Health care professionals show that they have understood when they:

- clarify, restate, paraphrase or summarise what they have heard from the patient
- reflect the patient's feelings.

Communicating hope

At the same time as the seriousness of diabetes and the complications that can follow are conveyed, it is also important to convey the message of hope that these complications can be avoided or delayed. This is no easy task! In order to convey hope health care professionals must believe in the patient's own resources to deal with self-care, that they can learn and change. A few can take giant leaps but the majority need to develop at a slower pace. Many patients do not believe that they can meet the demands that self-care makes on them. Perhaps they have tried unsuccessfully a number of times to lose weight. They have enthusiastically started an exercise programme but have given up when problems appear. Many patients express an 'all or nothing' mentality – that one should, when one has diabetes, live healthily in everything one does, whereas in reality a slight adjustment in mealtime patterns, or a weight reduction of 3 kilos may be all that is needed to see an improved blood glucose value. With the 'all or nothing' approach, it is easy to ignore all information regarding healthy living and not pay heed to the effect that small steps may have.

Health care professionals communicate hope when they:

- show empathy
- explain why the patient is the most important member of the health care team
- encourage the patient to discuss what they can do
- ask them what kind of support they need.

Acceptance

All people with diabetes have the right to demand that they be accepted as they are. By showing that they are accepted, a climate is created that makes it possible for the patient to open up and reflect on their situation and their way of dealing with their diabetes. In exactly the same way as with empathy, health care professionals do not need to like what they see or agree with the choices the patient makes. It is the patient's life and the choices are theirs – the health care professional's job is not to judge or assess but to make it easier for the patient to make informed decisions regarding their self-care within the life that they have chosen.

Health care professionals show acceptance when they:

- clarify, restate, paraphrase or summarise what they have heard from the patient as facts – that is without valuing what they have heard
- reflect the patient's feelings showing that they accept them
- let the patient's understanding of their situation (which, by now, is also the health care professional's understanding) be the starting point for the health care professional's continued work.

Genuineness

If health care professionals believe that each person is unique and that they have to listen to the person's story in order to understand them, they will convey this genuine interest. Then the patient feels noticed as an individual and perceives that their thoughts and opinions are important contributions to the task that they and the health care professional are to work on together.

If the health care professional thinks they know what the patient's problem is because they have met hundreds of patients like them, or they have experience of the same problem themselves, they will not be listening with genuine interest, and most patients will notice this immediately.

People show genuineness when they:

- ask questions out of interest, not as a routine
- listen actively
- use open questions
- give people time to reflect on questions.

Congruity

We are congruous when our communication by one method is in accordance with our communication in other ways (see above).

Health care professionals are not congruous if they say that diabetes is a serious illness but do not, at the same time, express their concern for a patient with a very high blood glucose level. They do not act congruously if they, after having explained the importance of doing blood glucose tests, do not ask to see the patient's test book. If the health care professional is convinced of the dangers of smoking and always asks about smoking history, they are being congruous.

Health care professionals are congruous if they:

- look serious when they show their concern about a patient's high blood glucose values
- always follow up on changes the patient has decided on
- ask the patient to tell them about something and when they do, listen carefully.

9.8.1 Group education

The use of group education or group intervention as a method of assisting people to self-care effectively, is becoming increasingly popular. The evidence so far from the DESMOND Collaborative suggests that this method can:

- be a more efficient use of resources
- provide more contact time for patients with health care professionals
- improve metabolic outcomes
- improve knowledge transfer
- improve health beliefs and attitudes towards self-care
- improve coping skills.

Some groups appear to be more successful than others and this may be due to the skills of the group facilitator. If the facilitator 'lectures' most of the time it may not be helpful in assisting people with diabetes to reflect on their current barriers to effective self-management. The qualities of effective communication discussed here are important and can shed some light on the success (or otherwise) of group education.

9.9 Summary of Chapter 9

This chapter has been concerned with diabetes self-management, and how it can be facilitated and supported by the health care professionals in the diabetes care team. You have considered the concept of self-management and have worked through some 'truths' about people and their responses to health and self-care. You then thought about empowerment, compliance and concordance and how these concepts differ. Barriers to self-care, and in particular the challenges of dietary management, have also been a focus of this chapter. You also considered emotions and their management during diagnosis and subsequent adaptation to diabetes. Finally, you have learned about communication skills and their importance during consultations or other interactions between members of the diabetes care team.

Questions for Chapter 9

Question 9.1 (Learning Outcomes 9.2 and 9.4)

Who is responsible for the care of the person with diabetes?

Question 9.2 (Learning Outcomes 9.2, 9.3 and 9.5)

What are the elements of effective self-management?

Question 9.3 (Learning Outcome 9.3)

Explain the terms 'compliance' and 'concordance'.

Question 9.4 (Learning Outcomes 9.3, 9.5 and 9.6)

Describe an empowerment model of diabetes care.

Question 9.5 (Learning Outcome 9.4)

What are the key strategies that can help people manage their dietary self-care?

Question 9.6 (Learning Outcomes 9.5 and 9.6)

How can good communication be achieved in the health care professional–patient relationship?

References

Anderson, R. M. and Funnell, M. M. (2000) 'Compliance and adherence are dysfunctional concepts in diabetes care', *Diabetes Educator*, **26** (4), pp. 597–604.

Anderson, R. M. and Funnell, M. M. (2001) *The Art of Empowerment*, Alexandria, American Diabetes Association.

Coster, S., Gulliford, M. C., Seed, P. T., Powrie, J. K. and Swaminathan, R. (2000) 'Monitoring blood glucose control in diabetes mellitus: a systematic review', *Health Technology Assessment*, **4** (12).

DESMOND Collaborative (2004) *DESMOND Newly Diagnosed Module: Educator Manual*, 2nd edn, Leicester, DESMOND Collaborative, pp. 5–7.

Greenhalgh, T., Helman, C. and Chowdhury, A. M. (1998) 'Health beliefs and folk models of diabetes in British Bangladeshis: a qualitative study', *British Medical Journal*, **316**, pp. 978–983.

Medicines Partnership (2005) *What is concordance* [online] Available from: http://www.concordance.org/about-us/concordance (Accessed June 2005).

Morris, A. D., Boyle, D. I. R., McMahon, A. D., Greene, S. A., MacDonald, T. M. and Newton, R. W. (1997) 'Adherence to insulin treatment, glycemic control and ketoacidosis in insulin-dependent diabetes mellitus', *Lancet*, **350**, pp. 1505–1510.

NHS UK Transplant (2005) [online] Available from: http://www.uktransplant.org.uk (Accessed June 2005).

Page, P., Verstraete, D. G., Robb, J. R. and Etzwiler, D. D. (1981) 'Patient recall of self-care recommendations in diabetes', *Diabetes Care*, **4** (1), pp. 96–98.

Parkin, T. and Skinner, T. C. (2003) 'Discrepancies between patient and professionals' recall and perception of an outpatient consultation', *Diabetic Medicine*, **20** (11), pp. 909–914.

Polonsky, W. H. (1999) *Diabetes Burnout*, Alexandria, American Diabetes Association.

Schlundt, D. G., Rea, M. R., Kiline, S. S. and Pichert, J. W. (1994) 'Situational obstacles to dietary adherence for adults with diabetes', *Journal of the American Dietetic Association*, **94**, pp. 874–876.

Skinner, T. C., Mehrshahi, R., Gregorry, R. and Jackson, S. (2003) 'Who remembers what happened in the consultation? Comparing patient and doctor recall with the video evidence', *Diabetologia*, **46** (Suppl. 2), p. 246.

LIVING WITH DIABETES

10.1 Introduction

As you have been reading, in diabetes care the emphasis is frequently on the biological or medical aspects of the condition. This emphasis is reinforced by the nature of diabetes management, which includes assessment and treatment of a number of aspects that contribute to the complexity of diabetes. The person with diabetes is expected to attend a GP surgery or hospital clinic to see a range of health care professionals about a number of topics. The doctor may ask for measurements of blood glucose, HbA_{1c}, blood pressure, lipids and weight on several occasions in a year. In addition, each year the patient has their annual review to assess the possible development of complications. This entails, as described in Chapter 5, examination of the eyes, a test of urine for microalbuminuria and an assessment of the nerves and vascular state of the feet. As a result of some of these examinations, a range of treatments may be required. The diabetes specialist nurse may facilitate much of the above assessment and treatment and, in addition, has a specific role in education and psychosocial support. The dietitian has a specific role in assessing and helping patients with dietary change. The podiatrist specifically assesses and educates patients regarding foot care but also treats patients whose feet are vulnerable. All of these roles overlap to a certain extent and health care professionals share responsibility for education in all aspects of diabetes self-management.

You should not be surprised that there is such an emphasis on the physical aspects of diabetes; as you now know, there is great complexity to this condition. Health care professionals know that the development of complications leads to further tests and treatments that can have profound implications on every aspect of a person's life. The aims of the tests and treatments are to achieve targets which research has shown can prevent the chronic and disabling ill-health that can result from the complications of diabetes.

Chapter 9 introduced the idea of how consultation and communication can help the person with diabetes to self-manage effectively. This chapter builds on this notion to look at specific aspects of life that might be affected by having diabetes.

10.2 Culture

One of the dilemmas that health care professionals often have is acknowledging that people with diabetes have a choice when it comes to treatments. 'Aha,' they might say, 'if they knew what we know then they would take advice'. Unfortunately it isn't as simple as that. People respond differently and one reason for this may be cultural influences. It is, therefore, very important for health care professionals to understand culture and cultural influences. Cultural influences may be assumed if clothes or language reveal that the individual is from a certain background, religion or country. However, just because a person is wearing certain clothes, it does not mean they automatically have particular religious or cultural beliefs. If the cultural influence is to do with beliefs and values, difficulties can arise if the aims and objectives of the health care professional differ from those of the person with diabetes.

Activity 10.1 Mrs Ahmed and her doctor

Suggested study time 30 minutes

Before progressing on to the next section, consider some of the possible responses of a health care professional in relation to the life of Mrs Ahmed, who has Type 2 diabetes. Make some brief notes on what you think might happen in a consultation between Mrs Ahmed and her doctor.

Mrs Ahmed is originally from India. She is very overweight with a BMI over 30, a blood glucose level that puts her at risk of developing long-term complications and she also has high blood pressure. Mrs Ahmed has a large family. She spends the day cooking enormous meals that involve a substantial amount of oil. For Mrs Ahmed, it is important to provide for her family in this way. Her weight is a sign that she is a good wife and mother and to lose weight may signal poor family provision or even ill health. She ventures out of the house only to shop and is busy with family-related activities for most of the day.

Comment

Everyone has a **culture**, which is defined by beliefs and behaviours that are shared among a group of people. A person can have a cultural origin but in addition can be influenced by other social groups to which they belong which may be based on religion, gender, sexual orientation or class. Culture is defined by how a person experiences their world with others.

The consultation between Mrs Ahmed and her doctor might include the doctor realising that family status and weight are important issues in Mrs Ahmed's way of life, even though they might be at odds with the doctor's understanding of the management of diabetes by reducing weight and eating low-fat, low-sugar foods. If this is the case, the doctor and Mrs Ahmed might have a conversation about how to work together towards the best control of her diabetes. The doctor might include other family members if Mrs Ahmed wishes it, so they can support her in any changes she decides to make. On the other hand, a doctor who only sees Mrs Ahmed as being overweight and having poorly controlled diabetes might make inappropriate suggestions or demands about what she should do, regardless of her lifestyle. As you read in Chapter 9, this type of consultation is unlikely to lead to any changes in Mrs Ahmed's situation. You might have made some reference to these two possibilities in your notes.

10.2.1 Finding out about someone's culture

It is common to think of cultural considerations only in relation to people from certain ethnic backgrounds. However, every one of us has a culture that influences the way we live our life. One way of understanding someone's culture is to ask open questions that invite the individual to talk about their family life and work (if relevant) and to include questions that relate to beliefs about health and illness, for example, 'What remedies do you use at home regarding your health?' and 'Can you tell me more about the way you think about and prepare food?' (Figure 10.1) (Open questions were discussed in Section 1.5.3.)

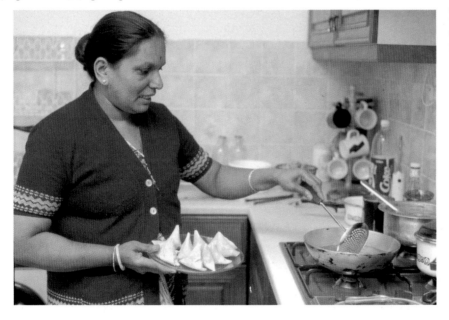

Figure 10.1 In some cultures, meals and preparing food have greater importance than in others.

Activity 10.2 Finding out about culture

Suggested study time 30 minutes

Describe the types of open question you could use to find out more about someone and what is important to them in terms of family life, health and illness.

Comment

One of the aims of diabetes care in relation to cultural influence is to understand how different people may respond and to help the individual to consider how to make the most of the health care system. The question 'What would be helpful to you in managing your diabetes?' is useful as it enables the person to prioritise their needs, rather than have instructions dictated to them. It is much more likely that people will stick to a decision or a plan they have made themselves than one that is imposed upon them.

In relation to types of open questions, one of our course team suggested, 'What is an average day like for you?' or 'If you had to make a list of the things that were important to you in life, what would be the top three?' as questions they would ask.

Another suggested asking, 'On a scale of one to ten in increasing importance, what score would you give your health?' or 'What advice would you give to someone like yourself about managing their diabetes?'

One of the important aspects of open questions such as these is listening to the answers carefully. In a book called *The Art of Empowerment*, which contains stories from diabetes educators about how they enable people to be successful in living with diabetes, the authors write:

> 'we've learned that educators need to ask good questions and listen well to discover these elements in their patients' stories.'

> (Anderson and Funnell, 2001)

The 'elements' that they refer to include psychological, clinical, financial, cultural, spiritual and social dimensions, all of which influence the way people live with diabetes.

As you have read, finding out about people's social and cultural circumstances is vital if self-care is to be optimised. Within these circumstances are some very specific aspects of life with diabetes that are also affected by legal requirements that are outside the individual's control. It is to these that you turn next.

10.3 Driving

It is a legal requirement for people with Type 1 diabetes (who are injecting insulin or using an insulin pump) and people with Type 2 diabetes who are either on tablets or tablets and insulin, or insulin alone, to inform the Driver and Vehicle Licensing Agency (DVLA) of their condition. People with diabetes treated by diet alone do not need to inform the DVLA (Diabetes UK, 2004). People on tablets will have an unrestricted licence but will be requested to inform the DVLA again if they start to use insulin. People taking insulin need to have their licence reviewed at least every three years and this is done automatically when the DVLA send a renewal form to the person to complete. The form is called 'DIAB 1' (see Figure 10.2; DVLA, 2005) and includes a section for the person to give permission for the DVLA to contact their medical advisor, so that if necessary, the DVLA can ask either the GP or hospital consultant to supply a medical report.

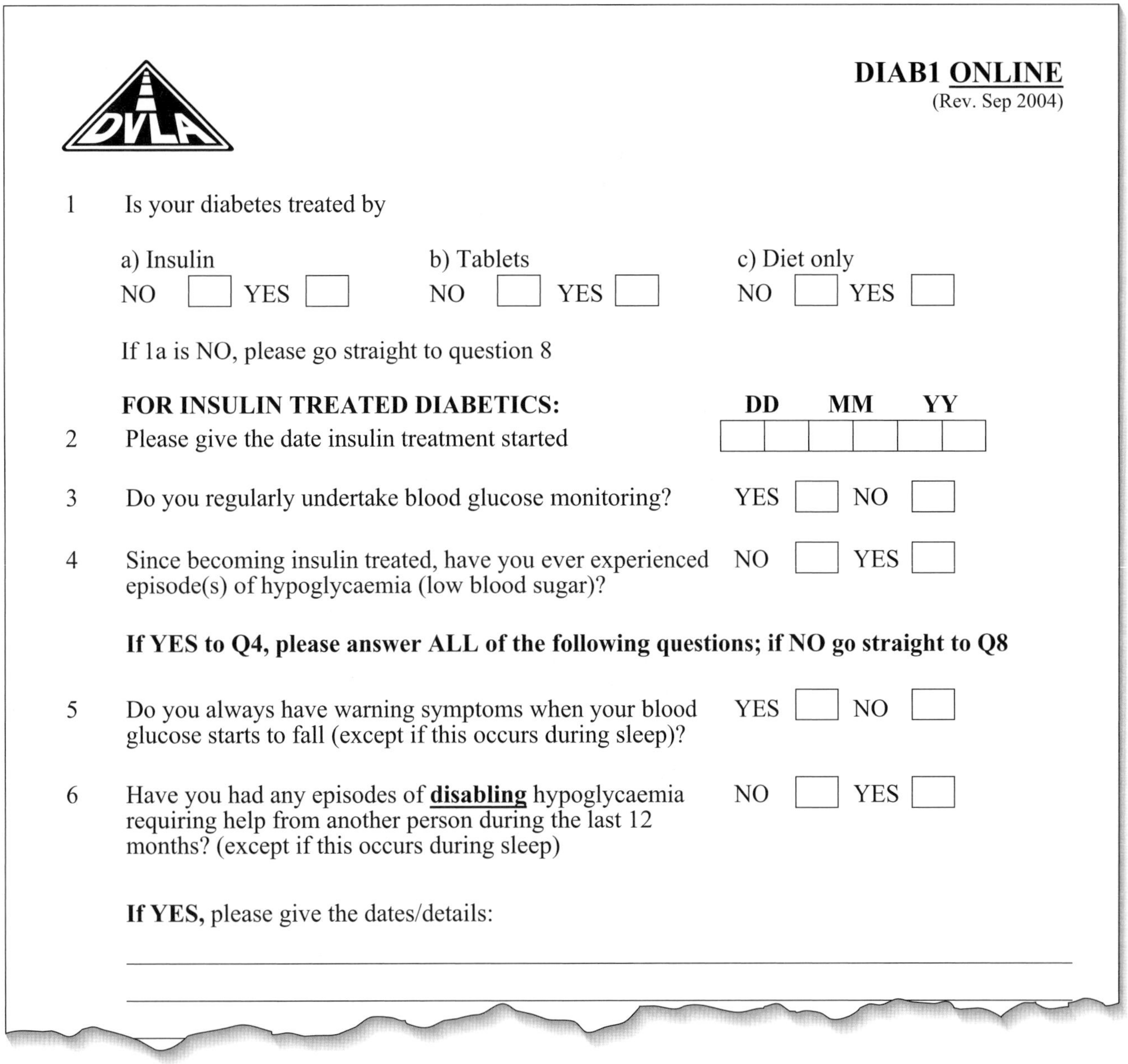

DIAB1 ONLINE
(Rev. Sep 2004)

1   Is your diabetes treated by

a) Insulin   b) Tablets   c) Diet only
NO [ ] YES [ ]   NO [ ] YES [ ]   NO [ ] YES [ ]

If 1a is NO, please go straight to question 8

FOR INSULIN TREATED DIABETICS: **DD   MM   YY**
2   Please give the date insulin treatment started   [ ][ ][ ][ ][ ][ ]

3   Do you regularly undertake blood glucose monitoring?   YES [ ]   NO [ ]

4   Since becoming insulin treated, have you ever experienced   NO [ ]   YES [ ]
     episode(s) of hypoglycaemia (low blood sugar)?

If YES to Q4, please answer ALL of the following questions; if NO go straight to Q8

5   Do you always have warning symptoms when your blood   YES [ ]   NO [ ]
     glucose starts to fall (except if this occurs during sleep)?

6   Have you had any episodes of **disabling** hypoglycaemia   NO [ ]   YES [ ]
     requiring help from another person during the last 12
     months? (except if this occurs during sleep)

     If YES, please give the dates/details:

     _____

Figure 10.2 Part of the form 'DIAB 1' from the DVLA.

Areas of concern that lead the DVLA to request a medical report are if the
individual reports that they experience hypoglycaemia without warning symptoms
or have a reduced visual acuity to an extent that makes their eyesight too poor to
drive (this may be due to diabetic eye disease). Another reason is if the person has
significant peripheral neuropathy causing reduced sensation in their feet, as this
could make use of foot pedals unreliable and consequently make driving very
dangerous.

The DVLA can restrict driving licences to one, two or three years, depending on
the information they receive from the person themselves or the doctor. They can
also revoke a driving licence, either temporarily or permanently.

Diabetes treated with insulin may also lead to restrictions on the kind of vehicle you can drive. Usually vehicles should weigh less than 3.5 tonnes and have fewer than eight seats. Some taxi companies will not take on drivers who need insulin but others will, subject to a regular medical report from the driver's doctor.

Passenger carrying vehicle (PCV) and large goods vehicle (LGV) licences cannot be held by anyone taking insulin, for either Type 1 or Type 2 diabetes, and at present this is an absolute ban. You can hold a licence of this type if you take tablets and/or are following a healthy eating and physical activity plan as treatment for diabetes.

Reading about all these regulations can make your head spin – it is easy to see how confusion arises and how often people with diabetes who need to report their condition to the DVLA do not do so. Work through the following activity to think about these issues further.

Activity 10.3 The implications of restrictions

Suggested study time 25 minutes

Make some notes on how restrictions on driving could impact on someone's life.

Comment

You may have thought of some of the following.

A person's driving licence might be essential for their livelihood so that, for example, losing an LGV licence might also mean losing a job as a lorry driver. A person's self-worth is often defined by their work and losing that work can be a blow to self-esteem. There is also the aspect of feeling rejected or less of a person or provider if you are unable to work due to your health. Someone who is used to being independent might resent feeling as though they are more in need of help to work or socialise than previously. There are also other implications of not being able to drive; for example, who runs the children to school in the morning? Who does the shopping? How does one have a social life (or attend the diabetes clinic), especially if living in an area where there is little public transport?

On the other hand, some people see their diabetes as actually enhancing their ability to do their job or find it an encouragement to aim for something different as a result. People often cite how reliable, punctual or attentive to detail they can be because of having to take care of their diabetes and how they turn it into an advantage rather than a difficulty.

10.4 Insurance

Unfortunately people with diabetes may either have their insurance premiums increased as a result of having diabetes or be excluded altogether from certain policies. This is because insurance companies consider people with diabetes to be at higher risk of ill-health, especially with regard to future complications.

10.4.1 Car insurance

It is necessary for the person with diabetes to inform their car insurance provider once diagnosis is made. Depending on treatment (i.e. healthy eating and physical activity, tablets or insulin), this may lead to a change in premium. Failure to report the diagnosis of diabetes or a change in treatment is considered as not providing the company with 'material facts' and may lead to the policy being cancelled.

Diabetes UK, who have campaigned for better insurance arrangements for people with diabetes, have noted that companies may refuse to quote if:

*   the DVLA has issued a restricted licence
*   diabetes has been diagnosed within the last 3 years
*   diabetes is controlled by insulin
*   there is a history of hypoglycaemia
*   there is a history of any accident where diabetes may have been implicated.

Diabetes UK reports that discrimination has been reduced since the introduction of the Disability Discrimination Act 1995.

10.4.2 Travel insurance

It is vital that people with diabetes take out adequate travel insurance when travelling abroad. However, the standard travel insurance offered when purchasing a holiday or travel may be limited and often does not cover pre-existing conditions such as diabetes. The insurance company needs to be aware of the diagnosis and treatment, and the person taking out the insurance needs to be aware of the features of the scheme by reading the small print! For example, a minimum of £500 000 should be available for European travel and £1 000 000 elsewhere in the world (in 2005). Insurance should cover air ambulance and medical repatriation as well as medication and hospital care abroad.

Diabetes UK has an insurance broker who specialises in all aspects of insurance for people with diabetes and who can be contacted through Diabetes UK (the link is available from the course website). Case Study 10.1 illustrates how important it is to have travel insurance when you have diabetes.

Case Study 10.1

Sandra was excited about her first holiday abroad to Spain. She was 18 and travelling with a group of friends of around the same age. The holiday was for 2 weeks and during that time she found the tendency was to turn night into day. She slept all morning and got up in the early afternoon and sunbathed on the beach until early evening when she would have her main meal. She would then go out to clubs where she would drink lots of alcohol and dance for several hours. She found it difficult to organise her insulin injections around her different mealtimes and sleeping schedule. She missed several injections as a result of the change in her routine and because she was worried about becoming hypo.

A few days into her holiday she had an episode of vomiting which she thought might be due to a bug she had picked up. She missed out her insulin injection that night. The vomiting seemed to get worse and worried friends contacted the local doctor who diagnosed ketoacidosis and arranged for her to be admitted to hospital.

Sandra was insured and the cost of her 5-day stay in hospital and delayed trip home was paid for by the insurance company. The popular holiday destinations are unfortunately used to this kind of scenario and as a result have developed an expertise in dealing with diabetes emergencies.

Activity 10.4 Lifestyle changes on holiday

Suggested study time 45 minutes

Lifestyle can change dramatically when on holiday. Make a list of the changes that have to be accounted for when managing diabetes on holiday.

Comment

Our course team included the following on their lists of changes:

- different mealtimes and types of food available
- more or less activity than usual
- crossing time zones and jet-lag
- changes in sleeping patterns
- holiday upset stomach or other illness
- driving regulations in different countries
- sunstroke
- effect of more alcohol
- medical terminology in different languages and names of medicines available
- access to medical help.

All of these factors affect diabetes and its control; for example, an illness makes the blood glucose level go up and extra activity makes it go down. There may be stricter or more lenient rules about driving when you have diabetes or it can be more difficult to see a doctor if you need one. Some people think they can have a holiday from their diabetes as well as from their everyday routine, but if anything, diabetes needs to be more carefully thought about when away from home.

10.5 Employment

Many people fear that if they mention their diabetes on a job application form or at interview they will be discriminated against. The Disability Discrimination Act 1995 extends to diabetes and supports the individual if they believe they have been discriminated against on the grounds of having diabetes, providing there is reasonable evidence.

In general, people with diabetes can work as well as anyone else. There are some special considerations in relation to the need to eat regularly if someone is on insulin treatment or sulphonylurea tablets, which can cause hypoglycaemia if not balanced with food. Also, shift work or changing work hours require adjustments to treatment in order to maintain control. In the past, such working patterns were considered inappropriate when you had diabetes, but today the large number of regimens for managing diabetes means that it is possible for people to tailor their care to suit their particular circumstances and maintain their diabetes control.

There are, however, some areas of employment that are considered out of bounds to people taking insulin. These include commercial pilots, the armed forces, offshore work, train driving and ambulance driving. Some forms of employment, for example staying in the police force after diagnosis, are subject to individual consideration. Many types of employment have ceased to have a blanket ban on people taking insulin as a result of campaigns by people or organisations such as Diabetes UK. One example of this is the fire service. In the past firefighters automatically lost their job if they developed insulin-treated diabetes. As a result of a successful campaign by a firefighter, who developed Type 1 diabetes in service, along with Diabetes UK, firefighters can continue to be employed subject to certain circumstances and medical reports. The International Register of Firefighters with Diabetes (IRFD) has been set up as a result. You can learn more about this by visiting the IRFD website Diabetes Discrimination in Employment, available as a link from the course website. Activity 10.5 helps you to consider these issues more closely.

Activity 10.5 Firefighting

Suggested study time 45 minutes

Read the story of Jack in Case Study 10.2. What would your role be in helping someone like Jack if you were (a) his brother or sister, (b) the fire-service counsellor or (c) his diabetes consultant?

Comment

Thinking about the people involved in Jack's life reinforces awareness of the need for support and networking to stop people becoming isolated in these circumstances. When people are isolated, they may have fewer opportunities for thinking practically about their situation or hearing what others think and can offer. So the main role of anyone involved with Jack would be to ensure he has opportunities to discuss his situation and options as much as possible, and to be positive about his opportunities as a young man who is still healthy, even though he has diabetes. Although for Jack, the break-up with his wife might be permanent, sometimes it is possible to be reconciled once the issues can be discussed and put into context. Belonging to organisations such as the fire service can be linked to self-image, so having to give it up can be perceived as a blow to masculinity, which may have affected his relationship with his wife. This highlights the importance of enabling Jack to keep in touch with the reality of what has happened to him and what the consequences might be.

Case Study 10.2

Jack was 24 when he was admitted to hospital with newly diagnosed Type 1 diabetes. He was a firefighter and the youngest member of his watch. Despite support from his colleagues he was suspended from duty and waited 2 years for his appeal. During this time he gained weight as his general fitness that he had previously maintained for his work deteriorated, and he became depressed. This put a strain on his marriage. He lost his appeal to be reinstated because his employers argued that during a fire the effort of firefighting might cause his blood glucose to drop and he might not be able to tell if he was hypoglycaemic as symptoms could be misinterpreted. Jack was devastated and as he withdrew from family and friends his marriage finally broke up.

This last activity demonstrates the importance of social support when there are difficulties in life. The next section focuses on family involvement in diabetes and whether this affects self-care.

10.6 Family

Many people believe that when they have a personal crisis or even when they have personal struggles, they should deal with it on their own. Likewise loved ones, including family and friends, often don't know how to help. Research has shown that people, including children and teenagers as well as adults, do better if they have the support of others. However, involvement of family and friends should be with the individual's permission and involvement should be realistic.

There are some cultures where family involvement is paramount. Greene (2004) found that in Italy, for example, family members made a person's diabetes their business too, with many family members accompanying a teenager to their outpatient clinic appointment. These researchers found that diabetes control tended to be better in such circumstances than in an equivalent town in the UK, where a young person was encouraged from a young age to manage their diabetes and appointments independently of their family.

Activity 10.6 Family involvement

Suggested study time 45 minutes

Make a list of the pros and cons of increased family involvement in a person's diabetes. Reflect on your own family situation and how involved your family might be or how much you would want them to be if you had diabetes.

Comment

'Sharing the load' is an obvious advantage of other people being involved in a person's diabetes. In many relationships, one partner is mainly responsible for shopping and food preparation, and this role means that they might do a lot of the thinking about what types and how much food the person with diabetes is served. On the other hand, some families become completely engrossed in diabetes and the whole routine revolves around it, which can be a disadvantage as it limits flexibility.

Some of our course team members said that they would want lots of help from their family and would rely on them for support to manage their diabetes. Others said they would not want to burden their families as they had a lot to cope with already. One person said that they would consider it interfering if their family wanted to get involved in their diabetes and they would want to get on with their treatment on their own, except perhaps when they were unwell. You might have come up with something different again. You can see from this that there is a great variety of ways in which families can be involved and it is important to find out how things work for an individual rather than making assumptions.

10.7 Sex, relationships and diabetes

With regard to personal relationships and sex, diabetes can affect close relationships in lots of different ways. For example, it can bring partners closer together as they tackle the situation jointly. In other cases, diabetes can come between a couple if the person with diabetes perceives the other as wanting to be over-involved or even nagging them about the condition. Often, having diabetes is dealt with in a relationship in the same way as the couple might deal with anything else, and this can be more or less successful.

Worry or concern about diabetes or its treatment can affect sex drive or desire for both men and women. Having diabetes can also influence a person's view of their attractiveness to their partner or potential partner and affect their sex drive in this way. Practical issues such as the increased chances of a hypo during sex can also affect people's enjoyment or interest in sex. Some people complain that sex cannot be spontaneous because of the need to avoid hypos when you are on insulin or sulphonylurea tablets. Another very real issue for men is erectile dysfunction (Section 6.6.2). This can happen either temporarily or more permanently and can dramatically affect a relationship. Successful treatment is available if the man wants it, but the experience of losing erections can have a profound effect with associated psychological repercussions. Erectile dysfunction needs to be dealt with sensitively by professionals or counsellors with a special interest.

10.8 The demands of treatment

Having diabetes means that you may have to do tests and injections and/or take one or more tablets every day. Some people with Type 2 diabetes may need to take more than five different sorts of tablet at different times during the day to control the blood glucose level, blood pressure and cholesterol, for example. People with Type 1 diabetes may have to inject insulin and take tablets as well. It is difficult to remember to do all of these things every day. Research in Scotland (Donnan et al., 2002) has shown that many people do not collect enough prescriptions for the number of tablets or the amount of insulin or tests they are prescribed over a year. The more tablets people are prescribed per day, the harder it is for them to remember to take them all. In general people remember to take a tablet if it is a once-daily prescription. However, if they need to take tablets more frequently, or more than one tablet, the likelihood of their remembering to take them is reduced. This is not behaviour peculiar to having diabetes – it is difficult for anyone to remember to take tablets a number of times a day, even if it is for a limited time, such as a course of antibiotics. Diabetes medication (tablets and insulin) must be taken every day of life, so it would be unrealistic to expect people to do it perfectly every day. However, knowing that it is easy to forget means that you can work out ways of reminding yourself. Walker and Rodgers (2004) give some practical tips on how to remember to take tablets, which include suggestions such as keeping tablet packets by the kettle, or setting a small alarm for the time needed, or keeping a supply of tablets in a day bag or in the car, so that they can be accessed when out of the house. The hard part of taking tablets for diabetes is that often people do not feel unwell with or without the tablets, so there are few 'cues' to remind people to take them.

As you read at the beginning of this chapter, the other demand on day-to-day life with diabetes is the need to attend for medical care regularly. In general, people need to have an annual check up, as described in Chapter 5. In addition to this, they would usually have a further consultation during the year and maybe more if they needed to have blood pressure checks, podiatry appointments or retinal screening. All this is important in preventing complications but can be very time consuming. As with other sorts of routine appointments, such as at the dentist or optician, people sometimes forget to attend, especially if they feel well. Some people feel stigmatised by the need to attend specialist clinics; others feel reassured by the check-ups because it means they can find out if anything has changed since their last appointment. It is certainly true that people who regularly attend their appointments have the best chance of any problems being detected and treated at an early stage, especially because many of the complications of diabetes are 'silent' and only cause physical symptoms when they are far advanced. This is particularly true of kidney and eye disease, which often seem to people to come on overnight, although their build up is actually over years.

In addition to the need to attend clinics and appointments regularly, the person with diabetes also needs to ensure that they have continuous supplies of their medication and testing strips. This entails ordering and collecting prescriptions at the appropriate times. We have already talked about how difficult it can be to remember to take medication, but an added chore is to make sure it is there in the first place. Fortunately, most people with diabetes that is being treated with medication get *all* their medicines free. People can apply for a prescription charge exemption by completing a form which they send to the local health trust. However, the exemption does not apply to people who manage their diabetes by healthy eating or physical exercise, so these people may need to pay for their prescriptions for medication such as blood pressure or cholesterol tablets and blood glucose testing equipment, unless they are exempt from prescription charges for another reason.

Prescribers are sometimes reluctant to prescribe large quantities of medication at one time and may not be allowed to do this by their local health organisation, for example the primary care trust. Therefore, obtaining supplies even on repeat prescriptions can be a time-consuming and frustrating aspect of having diabetes.

Activity 10.7 What care to expect

Suggested study time 1 hour

Read Offprint 10.1 'What diabetes care to expect' from Diabetes UK (2003). Make a list of all the tests and investigations that you would need to have every year if you had diabetes. Think about the ones that would make you most anxious and how you would feel while you were waiting for the results.

Comment

In the booklet there is an annual review checklist that includes the following:

- physical checks: blood pressure, weight, legs and feet, the back of the eyes, injection sites
- blood tests: blood glucose, HbA_{1c}, kidney function, blood lipids
- discussion: about day-to-day life and the effect diabetes is having, specific difficulties or concerns about managing diabetes, questions about developments in diabetes or other aspects.

As we have said, some people find the check-ups reassuring; others find they make them very anxious. For many people, there are certain aspects of the check-ups that they dislike more than others. The course team asked some people with diabetes what they thought: one person said it was the eye examination they got worked up about as they were fearful of going blind; another said they didn't like the discussion aspect, as they always felt they were going to be told off. Yet another person said they dreaded going for their 'MOT' (as they called it), but they always came away pleased that they had been given a clean bill of health.

10.9 Pregnancy

In Section 4.7 you looked briefly at the medical management of diabetes in pregnancy. Women with diabetes are as able to become pregnant as those without diabetes, as having diabetes does not make conceiving more difficult. However, it is particularly important for diabetes to be well controlled before and at the time of conception as if the blood glucose level is too high during the first eight weeks of pregnancy (that is, often before a women knows she is pregnant), it can affect the development of the baby's main organs which occurs during this time. For the rest of pregnancy it is equally important for diabetes to be well controlled because a continuous high blood glucose level can make the baby grow too large, and prevent their lungs from developing properly. The effect of this is that at the end of the pregnancy, delivery is very difficult and the baby may need to have intensive care to enable them to breathe properly. These problems can be prevented by planning a pregnancy and making sure that the blood glucose level is kept within very strict limits for the majority of the pregnancy. In practice, this means a lot of hard work for the person concerned, including

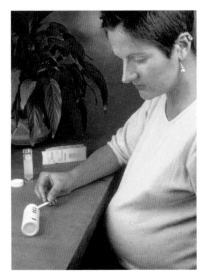

Figure 10.3 Regular monitoring of urine is essential in pregnancy.

regular monitoring of urine (Figure 10.3) and blood glucose. However, most women are highly motivated to manage their diabetes for the sake of their baby and many say that the best diabetes control they have ever had was during pregnancy! A personal account of pregnancy and diabetes can be found at Diabetes UK (2000).

Good diabetes care from specialists is an important factor in enabling a woman with diabetes to have a successful pregnancy. An obstetric/diabetes team would typically include a consultant in diabetes, an obstetrician, a midwife, diabetes specialist nurse and dietitian, plus support staff such as health care assistants and diabetes care technicians. Frequent appointments at the obstetric/diabetes clinic are needed, at least fortnightly, as the baby's growth and development as well as the woman's diabetes control need to be monitored and any concerns and practical issues need to be addressed. Challenges in pregnancy with diabetes include the following.

- The need for more insulin as pregnancy progresses – as the baby grows, the hormones in the placenta oppose the action of insulin, so making more insulin necessary.

- A woman needs to learn to increase her own doses in response to an increase in blood glucose level, or start to do this more promptly than usual.

- Hypos can be more frequent both because of the strict control of diabetes and because, in particular during the first 3 months, some women find they have fewer or different warning signs, which can be quite frightening, although hypos do not harm an unborn baby.

- Finally, a woman with Type 2 diabetes may well need to start insulin instead of tablets before or at the time of becoming pregnant, as most tablets for diabetes cannot be used in pregnancy. This might mean an extra learning experience which takes time, and it is not guaranteed that she will come off insulin at the end of her pregnancy as her diabetes may need insulin to control it afterwards, too.

- Recall from Section 2.5.3 whether there are other issues in relation to diabetes and pregnancy.

- As you read in Section 2.5.3 there is a type of diabetes which appears for the first time during pregnancy. Gestational diabetes occurs in women who are already susceptible to diabetes, but is brought to the fore by the insulin resistance caused by pregnancy.

Women who are found to have gestational diabetes (it usually appears from the 28th week onwards) need to have exactly the same care and control as women who already have diabetes. The difference is that after the baby is born, the woman's blood glucose level usually returns to normal. However, it is very important to ensure that someone who has had gestational diabetes is properly followed up with routine blood tests (at least every 3 years), as they have a high risk of developing it again in a future pregnancy and of having Type 2 diabetes in the future. Women who have gestational diabetes can reduce this risk by keeping their weight within normal limits and by exercising regularly to improve their insulin sensitivity. Health care workers can help by ensuring that women know what the risks are and what steps they can take to reduce them. Diabetes UK has an informative magazine about pregnancy called *Pregnancy and diabetes* (Figure 10.4) that can be obtained via their website.

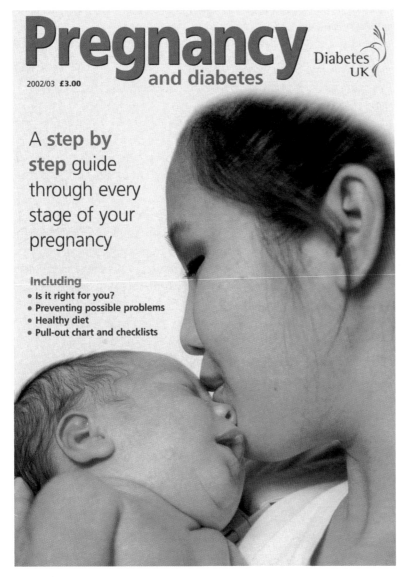

Figure 10.4 *Pregnancy and diabetes*, available from Diabetes UK.

10.10 Lifestyle and diabetes

People with diabetes are no different from anyone else, with varying social activities and other lifestyle preferences, and in general there are no restrictions on their choice of activities. It is true, however, that the risks of certain behaviours are greater when added to having diabetes. For example, the effects of being overweight or of heavy smoking on circulation and blood pressure can add to the effects that diabetes already has on its own. Conversely, the benefits of physical activity and healthy eating can also be greater when you have diabetes, since your risks of high cholesterol and high blood pressure are already high. However, people with diabetes are no less able to live perfectly healthy lives than anyone else and need the same kind of encouragement and motivational support as people without diabetes. One factor that is important in diabetes is the knowledge about how to manage the condition in different circumstances. Education about diabetes that is non-judgmental but informative about practical aspects – what someone can *do* in a given situation – works best. For example, it is likely that at some point in their life, a young person will be tempted to try smoking, heavy drinking or drugs and the fact they have diabetes will not necessarily prevent them from being tempted. This may also coincide with a move away from home, perhaps to university or college where a young person is likely to be exposed to a different lifestyle and less family involvement. What is helpful is information on how they can manage their diabetes at the same time. So while a blanket 'don't do it' is unlikely to be successful, giving them the information they need to be safe might minimise the risks of these behaviours. Engaging in health risky behaviours is not limited to young people, of course, and many older people already have lifestyles that may not allow their diabetes to be well controlled when they are first diagnosed. The education process in this situation can involve a great deal of 'unlearning' about food and drink, physical activity and smoking, often challenging long-held beliefs. The process of education can take time, and it is important that people have access to the widest variety and the most up-to-date information possible. There are many opportunities that can be offered, from local discussions and education sessions, to national organisations, websites and internet support groups. Sometimes people complain about never meeting anyone else with diabetes, so creating opportunities to do this can encourage people to learn from each others' successes.

There are a few key messages that health care workers can reinforce at each opportunity as they can make the difference between a safe and a dangerous situation. These include:

- if you have Type 1 diabetes, *never* stop taking your insulin as it is essential for life
- if you are a woman with diabetes, avoid becoming pregnant by accident if your diabetes is not very well controlled
- if you feel as though you are hypoglycaemic, do a blood test to check as waiting can lead to it becoming much worse and harder to treat by yourself
- don't drink alcohol on an empty stomach if you are on insulin or sulphonylurea tablets, because alcohol can block the liver's normal response to low blood glucose and so delay recovery from a hypo.

Many people with diabetes undertake demanding sports or 'extreme' activities. This may be in response to having diabetes and a desire to prove that the activity can be done; others may develop diabetes when they are already engaging in these activities. Sir Steven Redgrave (Figure 10.5a) and Billie Jean King (Figure 10.5b) are just two of many high-performing sports people with diabetes. Whatever the circumstances, it is perfectly possible to achieve demanding feats, although the need for careful training and preparation is no different if you have diabetes than if you haven't. The effect of these activities on diabetes, and vice versa, needs to be considered when planning how to manage blood glucose levels safely. Diabetes UK has an information leaflet and also runs training sessions and provides support for people who want to take part in activities such as marathon running and mountain climbing, which also fundraise for the organisation (see the course website for links).

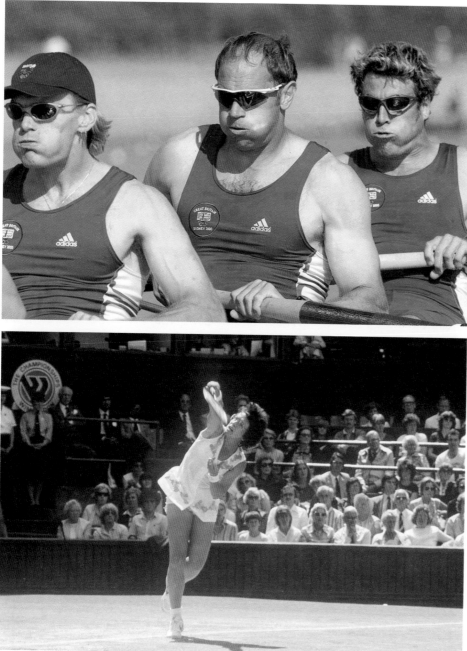

Figure 10.5 (a) Sir Steven Redgrave (centre); (b) Billie Jean King.

(a)

(b)

10.11 Living with long-term complications of diabetes

Some of the effects of diabetes can be severe. You have seen in earlier chapters that retinopathy can lead to reduced sight or blindness, nephropathy can mean that kidney function is limited or may need to be replaced by dialysis, and peripheral neuropathy can lead to amputation. In addition, the risk of heart disease (angina, heart failure or heart attacks) is greater in people with Type 2 diabetes and can severely limit a person's activities. Depression is also common in people who have diabetes. How do people manage in these circumstances?

There are a number of strategies. First, people affected need a lot of support and practical help, not only by diabetes services and from their families and friends, but also from agencies such as meals on wheels, community nursing services and disability organisations such as the Royal National Institute for the Blind or the National Kidney Federation (links are available from the course website). Second, the financial burden on people is increased as they may no longer be able to work even though they are of working age, and they may have increased costs such as transport to and from necessary appointments, for devices they need, alterations to their home or buying medical equipment. Third, the impact on quality of life can be severe. Research has shown that people affected by the complications of diabetes have a significantly decreased quality of life than those without complications. This might seem obvious, but it is an important consideration in terms of the impact of social isolation and depression on people. It can be seen as a downward spiral, where a person may not take care of themselves and their diabetes because they are feeling low.

Activity 10.8 The effects of complications

Suggested study time 45 minutes

Make notes on the possible effects of the long-term complications of diabetes on a person's daily life in Table 10.1 below. We have completed a couple to get you started.

Table 10.1 The effects of complications.

Complication of diabetes	Effect on day-to-day life
Retinopathy causes reduced vision	Not able to drive any longer – need to depend on others or public transport
Peripheral neuropathy causes a foot ulcer	Need to keep weight off the affected foot – reducing mobility; regular appointments with podiatrist; district nurses need to visit at home, restricting options for going out

Comment

The effects that diabetes complications have on someone's day-to-day life vary according to the severity of their condition and the help they get at home or at work. Another factor may be how much control they have over their diabetes or whether they think that diabetes 'controls' them. In completing Table 10.1 you might have gone back to have a look at earlier chapters, particularly Chapters 5 and 6 or had a look at statements 10–12 of the diabetes NSF.

10.12 Living with someone who has diabetes

Finally in this chapter you look at what it is like to live with someone who has diabetes. Often such people are informally called 'carers' and can be parents, wives, husbands, partners or housemates. It can be hard to see someone you care about having the extra burden of managing their diabetes and it can also cause some friction for adult partners if the other person doesn't want or need any help or support. Parents have the responsibility of looking after their child's diabetes even when they find it upsetting, and living with a teenager with diabetes can bring extra stress. The stress or worry doesn't suddenly stop if the son or daughter decides to leave home, e.g. to go to university. Many people, however, find a routine that works for them and the level of involvement will be varied. Those living with someone with diabetes often say they feel they do not receive the same information as people with the condition do, even though they may need it just as much to aid their understanding. Some partners are responsible for all the domestic arrangements, including food and cooking, so need to know as much, if not more than, the person with diabetes. For this reason, many publications now are aimed at people living with someone who has diabetes and organisations such as Diabetes UK and support networks such as Diabetes Insight also recognise the need for other people to be involved. Diabetes is a 24-hour-a-day condition, and many partners, friends and parents need to get involved in emergency care too, such as during night time hypos or if something goes wrong on holiday. This points to the need for them to be well informed and education sessions and information needs to be targeted at these people. Carers can get fed up and frustrated too, about the effect of diabetes on their own lives and their relationship with the person with diabetes. The opportunity to share their feelings and experiences with others in a similar position is often welcome.

10.13 Summary of Chapter 10

You have come to the end of your study of *Diabetes care*; we hope you have enjoyed the course and that you have found it informative and thought provoking.

In this final chapter you have looked at aspects of living with diabetes every day, the challenges it presents and ways of dealing with them. You have seen how cultural influences may impact on diabetes care and how all those involved must avoid making assumptions about each other. You've also read about the possible effects of diabetes on employment opportunities. In the workplace the barriers are gradually coming down for people who are managing their diabetes successfully. We have also seen how demanding diabetes care can be and that support from other people can help to ease the burden if that is what the person with diabetes wants. Medical care is a necessity with diabetes and even more so in some situations, such as pregnancy, and health service staff need to recognise that some people can be very anxious about the results of tests and investigations. Long-term complications need to be coped with and adapting to living with these complications can mean many changes to day-to-day life. Those closest to people with diabetes can also be thought of as 'living with diabetes' and their role is often central to the success of managing the condition.

We'll leave the final word to Joe, who has had Type 1 diabetes since he was a child, now for 43 years. He says of living with diabetes:

> 'diabetes is a marathon, not a sprint…what I need from people is help to stay in the race.'

Questions for Chapter 10

Question 10.1 (Learning Outcome 10.2)

Give two examples of questions you could ask to find out more about what an individual thinks about having diabetes and how it can fit into their life.

Question 10.2 (Learning Outcome 10.3)

What are the requirements to inform the DVLA for people with diabetes who: (a) manage their diabetes by healthy eating and physical activity; (b) manage their diabetes using tablets; (c) use insulin to manage their diabetes? What are the implications for the person with diabetes in each case?

Question 10.3 (Learning Outcome 10.4)

Give three examples of jobs that are not open to people with diabetes taking insulin treatment.

Question 10.4 (Learning Outcomes 10.4 and 10.6)

Describe three ways in which you could make information available to people with diabetes and to people living with a person who has diabetes.

Question 10.5 (Learning Outcome 10.5)

Describe some of the ways in which diabetes can affect relationships.

Question 10.6 (Learning Outcome 10.6)

What are some of the challenges that people with diabetes face every day?

REFERENCES

Anderson, R. M. and Funnell, M. M. (2001) *The Art of Empowerment*, Alexandria, American Diabetes Association.

Diabetes UK (2000) *Balance. Trimester one (weeks 0-16): The early days* [online] Available from: http://www.diabetes.org.uk/balance/187/187preg.htm (Accessed June 2005).

Diabetes UK (2003) *What diabetes care to expect* [online] Available from: http://www.diabetes.org.uk/manage/what.htm (Accessed June 2005).

Diabetes UK (2004) *Driving and diabetes* [online] Available from: http://www.diabetes.org.uk/infocentre/inform/downloads/Drive04.doc (Accessed June 2005).

Donnan, P. T., MacDonald, T. M. and Morris, A. D. (2002) 'Adherence to prescribed oral hypoglycaemic medication in a population of patients with Type 2 diabetes: a retrospective cohort study', *Diabetic Medicine*, **19**, pp. 279–284.

DVLA (2005) DIAB 1 [online] Available from: http://www.dvla.gov.uk/ (Accessed May 2005)

Greene, A. (2004) *A social anthropological study of diabetes control in young people in Scotland and Italy.* Personal communication.

National Kidney Federation [online] Available at http://www.kidney.org.uk (Accessed June 2005).

Royal National Institute for the Blind [online] Available at http://www.rnib.org.uk (Accessed June 2005).

The International Register of Firefighters with Diabetes (2005) [online] Available from: http://www.irfd.org (Accessed June 2005).

Walker, R. and Rodgers, J. (2004) *Diabetes: a Practical Guide to Managing your Health*, London, Dorling Kindersley.

ANSWERS TO QUESTIONS

Question 1.1

Mr Patel may react in many different ways. He may be relieved at the diagnosis, having suspected something much worse and, if the treatment makes him feel better, he may be very positive about the diagnosis. The changes he has to make to his lifestyle and how difficult he finds them will also affect how he feels about being told he has diabetes. The fact that he knows someone with diabetes may provide reassurance, but his cousin has had some problems so this may cause Mr Patel great anxiety. Mr Patel's family may have similar feelings. If Mrs Patel is responsible for meals, she may be concerned about the changes in diet and how to achieve them. They may both worry that their children will be affected. Sometimes people have a lot of worries about diabetes and some of these may be based on incorrect information. Anxiety and fear may lead to tensions within the family. Mr Patel may be worried about his job or how his diabetes will fit in with his cultural beliefs and values. It is important to remember that individuals react in different ways depending on their circumstances.

Question 1.2

The GP is the doctor in the community, who looks after all the family's health needs, not just their diabetes. The practice nurse works in the GP's surgery. This nurse has often undertaken additional training in diabetes care and so can run diabetes clinics in which she can give advice and provide care to people with diabetes. The diabetes specialist nurse works solely in the field of diabetes care and is available to give advice and support, and to teach people with diabetes. The podiatrist provides advice and treatment for the prevention and management of foot problems. The dietitian specialises in nutritional advice, and the retinal screening technician takes photos of the back of the eye to pick up any changes caused by diabetes. Mr and Mrs Patel are the centre of this team and need to convey information to the team so that they can all work together in providing the best care for Mr Patel.

Question 1.3

Good team work can be achieved by each team member:
1 knowing his or her own responsibilities
2 valuing the contribution of the others
3 communicating effectively within the team, both verbally and through written or computerised records.

Question 1.4

The benefits of good communication are:
- the person with diabetes can discuss his/her individual needs and problems and this should result in care which is acceptable and appropriate to the individual. This means that the person is more likely to feel satisfied and to follow the advice given;
- the person with diabetes understands the advice given, and feels confident with the team, since they listen to his concerns and answer questions;

- every member of the team knows what is happening and they can all work together. Where there is poor communication, mistakes can be made or inappropriate care and advice given.

Question 1.5

The nurse might ask Mr Patel further questions. She could observe his non-verbal communication, which might indicate he was worried. If Mr Patel did not speak English, she might use an interpreter. She could also look at his medical notes.

Mr Patel could also ask questions. He could take a family member with him for support or to speak on his behalf. He might want to write down the answers he is given or ask for an information leaflet. He might want to access the internet for further information.

Question 1.6

'I expect you know about all about this, don't you?' is a *leading question*. Mr Meek is likely to say yes he does know, otherwise he will feel rather stupid, after all Jane has just said he ought to know.

'Have you got your record with you?' is a *closed question*. Mr Meek could just say no. Some people do not need any encouragement to talk, and given a chance will tell you their life history. But people who are shy or nervous may just answer a closed question with a plain yes or no and may not tell you the important things.

'How are you?' is an *open question* and gives Mr Meek the opportunity to say how he really feels. However, you may have thought that this phrase is used as a greeting and often people do not listen to the answer. If you really want to know how someone is you may need to rephrase the question or ask it again later.

Question 1.7

Confidentiality means that personal information about a person should be kept private. For example, in Mr Patel's case, this means that no one outside the team caring for him should be told he has diabetes unless he gives permission. This includes his family, manager and colleagues at work and his friends.

Question 1.8

You could have noted any three of the points listed below:

- talking to the person with diabetes and finding out their specific needs and problems
- negotiating with the individual their care plan
- informing the person with diabetes and gaining their consent
- maintaining accurate records
- good communication within the team
- staff should undertake regular updating and should not carry out procedures for which they have not been trained
- any problems and errors should be reported so that lessons can be learnt from them

- risk assessment of the plan of treatment and care
- measures to prevent infection: good hand washing techniques, use of sterile equipment, aseptic technique, use of sharps boxes
- safe storage of drugs and hazardous substances.

Question 1.9

Some infections such as hepatitis B and HIV are transmitted through blood and other body fluids, so that if people accidentally stab themselves with a used needle they could develop these illnesses. Needle stick injuries can be prevented by:

- taking care when handling sharp equipment
- not re-sheathing used needles or lancets, except where there is no appropriate method of safe disposal
- using a sharps box or other safe container to store used needles, etc.

Question 2.1

Diabetes is diagnosed by measuring the plasma glucose level. If the level is 11.1 mmol/l or more on a random sample then the person has diabetes, when symptoms are present. If no symptoms are present the plasma glucose level needs to be abnormal on two separate occasions. A fasting plasma glucose level of 7.0 mmol/l is also used to make a diagnosis of diabetes. Occasionally an oral glucose tolerance test will be used to make the diagnosis.

The type of diabetes is diagnosed by clinical symptoms and signs. People with Type 1 diabetes have often lost a lot of weight and may have ketones in the urine at the time of diagnosis. In contrast, people with Type 2 diabetes may not be diagnosed for quite some time despite their elevated plasma glucose levels. In Type 2 diabetes it is rare to have ketones in the urine. Being thirsty or getting up at night to pass urine may be associated with getting older, not only with having diabetes.

Question 2.2

The completed table is shown in Table 2.2.

Table 2.2 Answer to Question 2.2.

Criterion	Type 1 diabetes	Type 2 diabetes
Age at onset	Can occur at any age, but more commonly in children and young adults	More common in older people, but can occur in younger people
Treatment	Insulin is the only therapy available	Diet alone, diet and tablets and/or insulin can be used
Presence of ketones	Ketones occur if the blood glucose level becomes high	Ketones uncommon
Cause	Complete lack of insulin	Combination of not enough insulin and/or resistance to its actions

Question 2.3

Insulin is the most important hormone in the development of diabetes.

People with Type 1 diabetes do not produce any insulin at all. They cannot lower their blood glucose level without injecting insulin. They use insulin injections to keep their blood glucose level normal.

People with Type 2 diabetes produce insulin, but not enough to lower their blood glucose level to normal and they may be resistant to the action of insulin.

Question 2.4

You may inherit a condition-causing gene from *one* parent only and will also have the condition even though the gene from the other parent is normal. This is known as autosomal dominant inheritance. This is different from autosomal recessive inheritance when you must inherit the condition-causing gene from *both* parents to have the condition yourself. Diabetes is thought to be a multifactorial condition, where many different genes may be important.

Question 2.5

The following factors are all important in deciding the risk of someone developing diabetes:

- ethnicity
- obesity
- lack of exercise
- family history of diabetes
- increasing age
- previous gestational diabetes.

Question 2.6

Obesity is defined as greatly elevated body mass index, to an extent which is associated with serious increased risk to health.

The body mass index (BMI) indicates whether an adult is a healthy weight for their height. To calculate BMI divide the weight (in kg) by the height (in metres) multiplied by itself:

$$BMI = \frac{\text{weight (kg)}}{\text{height} \times \text{height (m}^2)}$$

A BMI value greater than 30 kg/m² indicates obesity.

Question 3.1

Examples of groups or organisations involved in providing diabetes care include Diabetes UK and local Workforce Development Confederations or Directorates. (Further examples are given in Section 3.2.1.) You will have found information on their roles if you visited their websites.

Question 3.2

National Service Frameworks (NSFs) are government plans to ensure equality in the delivery of a high-quality service. The NSF for diabetes set a 10-year target for the delivery of 12 standards of care and good practice for diabetes (see Figure 3.2 and Chapter 1, Table 1.1).

Question 3.3

Your answer to this question is likely to be a personal one. Perhaps you chose 'Detection and management of long-term complications' because you have never had an annual review or you have never had your feet examined by a podiatrist. You may want to approach your diabetes team and see if they have a plan to improve the situation. You may have chosen 'Identification of people with Type 2 diabetes' because your diabetes clinic often sees people who have been diagnosed with diabetes as a result of being treated for another condition and not because they were aware of any symptoms or risk factors. Perhaps local people at risk could be identified and screened at regular intervals? Perhaps you selected 'Prevention of diabetes' because whether you are a person with diabetes, someone who works in a diabetes clinic or just an interested party, you may feel that Type 2 diabetes in particular could be preventable if the wider population received better information and education about lifestyle changes for health reasons.

Question 3.4

You may have chosen any of the roles listed in Section 1.3 of Chapter 1 or mentioned in Sections 3.2 and 3.4 of this chapter. Regardless of the examples you chose, all of these people work as part of the same team – the diabetes team – and this gives them all something in common. Depending on the examples chosen, other similarities and differences include the levels of qualifications or training of the individual and whether they work in a primary or secondary care environment. We are sure you thought of others that are equally relevant.

Question 3.5

The word 'empowerment' probably means different things to different people. In this chapter we have placed emphasis on helping people to help themselves by being involved in their own care. This means that people take more control of their care, both for themselves as an individual, and also for others by being involved in determining local services and priorities. An empowerment approach to care takes psychological and social factors, as well as medical ones, into account.

In an empowering relationship you would probably expect to find at least some of the following, as described by Hiscock and colleagues (2001, p. 25):

A friendly, warm, and 'equal' approach to the patient

A willingness to understand the impact of diabetes on other aspects of the individual's life and lifestyle

A 'partnership approach' to treating the condition

A willingness to make time to discuss issues and answer questions

A proactive approach to making referrals to other health care professionals.

Question 4.1

There are several different treatment options for someone with Type 2 diabetes, but fewer options for someone with Type 1 diabetes. People with Type 1 diabetes need to start insulin injections straight after being diagnosed. There are specific features of someone presenting with diabetes that help you decide whether a person with Type 1 diabetes needs urgent treatment: ketonuria and a high blood glucose level suggest that treatment needs to be given with urgency. If there is also heavy breathing, with abdominal pain and vomiting then the person should be treated as a medical emergency. There are different types of insulin available and treatment recommendations are dependent on the person's specific needs.

People with Type 2 diabetes can be treated with different classes of drug; they may also have insulin. Treatment recommendations depend on factors such as weight (obesity), age, kidney function, etc. There are both contraindications and side-effects of drugs which must be taken into account. Before undertaking medication, changes in diet and exercise can be explored to see if they can help in treatment.

Question 4.2

Quick-acting insulins, such as Actrapid®, need to be injected 20–30 minutes before a meal and last for several hours. The very quick-acting insulins, such as Humalog®, can be injected with a meal and have a very rapid onset.

Question 4.3

Diet and exercise can be used to help manage Type 2 diabetes in the following ways:

- Exercise aids weight loss. It also increases sensitivity to insulin and helps to lower the blood glucose level.
- Losing weight and taking exercise also helps to lower blood pressure and cholesterol.
- Weight loss will make someone more sensitive to their own insulin. Therefore any insulin that the person makes will be used more effectively. This helps to lower the blood glucose level.
- Eating a healthy diet and avoiding lots of refined sugar is also helpful as the glucose level after a meal will not go as high as it might after eating very sugary foods.

Question 4.4

The drug of choice for people with Type 2 diabetes who are overweight is metformin. This drug is used because it lowers the blood glucose level without the side-effect of weight gain.

Question 4.5

There is no widely accepted evidence that aromatherapy has any effects on diabetes. However, it may have benefits by making the person feel better in general.

Question 4.6

The reason that people with diabetes often receive treatment for their blood pressure and cholesterol is because one of the long-term aims in helping people manage their diabetes is to reduce complications relating to diabetes. If blood pressure and cholesterol are high, lowering them will help to reduce both microvascular and macrovascular complications associated with diabetes.

Question 5.1

Various investigations take place during an annual review. They include reviewing blood glucose control, measuring levels of HbA_{1c} and ketones in the blood and determining the lipid profile. Blood pressure is measured and the BMI is determined along with waist measurement. Lifestyle, including diet history, smoking and exercise is discussed.

Various members of the diabetes team are involved in the annual review, for example the diabetologist, dietitian, and diabetes care technician.

Question 5.2

The tests that contribute to the checks for risk of coronary heart disease are: blood pressure, blood lipid profile, smoking history, lifestyle, BMI and waist measurement.

Question 5.3

There are several possible reasons why Mrs Smith's HbA_{1c} level is high. Her meter could be faulty, she may not be using it correctly, she may be using the wrong strips or they could be out of date or damaged. She may be testing infrequently and only when she knows her tests will be satisfactory. She may be only testing at a certain time of day and missing high results at other parts of the day. There could be an abnormality with her haemoglobin which is giving a high HbA_{1c}, or there may be a problem with the laboratory equipment (these last two reasons are very unusual).

Question 5.4

HbA_{1c} measures the amount of haemoglobin in the blood that has been changed or glycated by the prevailing blood glucose concentration over the previous two to three months. If the blood glucose has been within normal limits for most of the time, the HbA_{1c} is likely to be normal. If the blood glucose has usually been higher than normal, then a greater percentage of haemoglobin will have been in contact with glucose and therefore glycated. The HbA_{1c} will therefore be higher than normal. If the blood glucose has been lower than normal (because the person with diabetes has had a lot of episodes of hypoglycaemia or low blood glucose) then the HbA_{1c} value will be lower than normal. Unfortunately, if the blood glucose has been equally high and low, then a normal HbA_{1c} may be the result. This is why the patient's own home blood testing record is important.

Question 5.5

Ketones may be found in the urine and blood of people with Type 1 diabetes who have insufficient insulin in their blood to control their blood glucose level and prevent the breakdown of body fats into ketones. Ketones can also be found in small quantities in the urine of people who have been fasting for a prolonged period of time.

Question 5.6

The equation to calculate BMI is as given in Chapter 2

$$BMI = \frac{weight\ (kg)}{height \times height\ (m^2)}$$

Jane has a BMI of $\dfrac{70\ kg}{(1.75 \times 1.75)\ m^2} = 22.9\ kg/m^2$

Nina has a BMI of $\dfrac{70\ kg}{(1.52 \times 1.52)\ m^2} = 30.3\ kg/m^2$.

A BMI greater than 25 kg/m² is a risk factor for CHD, so Nina has a higher risk than Jane.

Question 6.1

The common long-term complications of diabetes include nephropathy, neuropathy, retinopathy, cataracts, glaucoma, erectile dysfunction, heart attacks, angina, strokes, transient ischaemic attacks, hypertension, foot ulcers, amputation.

Question 6.2

High blood glucose, hypertension, abnormal blood lipids, smoking and obesity all increase the risk of developing atheroma which is significant in the development of macrovascular complications.

High blood glucose and hypertension are also significant in the development of microvascular complications. It is important that these risk factors are picked up early and advice given so that the risk of developing complications is minimised.

Question 6.3

Three types of eye disease associated with diabetes: cataracts (clouding of the lens); glaucoma (increased pressure in the eye potentially causing optic nerve damage); and retinopathy (changes in the blood vessels of the retina affecting vision in the later stages).

Question 6.4

Diabetic nephropathy refers to damage to the filtering units (nephrons) of the kidney that allows protein to be filtered out of the blood and into the urine. One of these proteins is albumin, and microalbuminuria is the term used when it is found in the urine. In the later stages this seriously affects the way the kidneys function and they are no longer able to regulate the water and electrolyte balance of the body or to remove waste. Substances such as creatinine accumulate in the blood, and urea and electrolyte levels become abnormal.

Question 6.5

Cardiovascular disease is associated with the presence of atheroma in the large arteries of the body, and having diabetes predisposes people to atheroma. Cardiovascular disease appears as angina, heart attacks, transient ischaemic attacks, strokes and poor circulation to the feet and legs.

Question 6.6

Diabetic neuropathy refers to the changes in the nerves outside the brain and spinal cord, that occur because of microvascular disease. There are three types of peripheral nerves: motor, sensory and autonomic. Autonomic neuropathy can result in erectile dysfunction, low blood pressure, chronic diarrhoea, urinary incontinence, abnormal heart rhythms, and difficulty in controlling body temperature. Sensory neuropathy results in pain or numbness, usually of the feet. It is common to have pain even though sensory nerves may have been lost. The sensory neuropathy symptoms may include pricking, tingling, burning, aching or needle-like pain. These are all signs of increased nerve activity that occurs in the remaining damaged or healing nerves. The last category of diabetic neuropathy, motor neuropathy, results in muscle wasting and joint changes.

Question 6.7

Sensory neuropathy will result in the failure to be aware of injuries or pain. Motor neuropathy can affect the muscles leading to an abnormally shaped foot; this can then result in high-pressure points on the walking surfaces of the foot. The build up of atheroma in the blood vessels leads to a poor blood supply. All of these factors mean that the person with diabetes is more prone to ulcers on their feet that are then very slow to heal, they may become infected and gangrene may result.

Question 6.8

Mr Evans should seek an urgent appointment with the podiatrist for treatment of the foot ulcer. He can prevent further damage by:
- wearing correctly fitted shoes
- not going barefoot
- checking his shoes for stones, etc. before putting them on
- washing his feet daily and inspecting them for signs of injury or asking someone else to inspect them
- maintaining good diabetes control.

Question 6.9

The following tests, measurements and examinations are carried out at the annual review to identify the long-term complications of diabetes:
- blood pressure
- urine test for microalbuminuria and blood tests for electrolyte and creatinine levels
- retinal screening and visual acuity
- foot examination and tests for sensation.

Question 7.1

The answer to this can be found in the description of Mrs James in Case Study 7.1. The most obvious signs and symptoms are tiredness, thirst and polyuria. A blood glucose reading would be above the normal limit. In Type 1 diabetes, hyperglycaemia may be accompanied by the development of ketones in the urine and breath, and that can be measured in the blood or urine. There may be loss of weight, particularly in people with Type 1 diabetes.

Question 7.2

Anybody with diabetes is at risk from developing hyperglycaemia if the diabetes is not controlled sufficiently with diet and medication. Short periods of hyperglycaemia occur in people who have forgotten their medication, been given too small a dose of insulin, eaten too much starchy food, taken less exercise than usual, or during periods of illness and stress.

Question 7.3

As the glucose level rises in the blood (above about 10 mmol/l) the kidneys start to produce large amounts of urine as glucose is removed from the body. The loss of large amounts of fluid as urine causes dehydration. This causes thirst, which is the body's mechanism for increasing fluid replacement. Insulin has an important function in the conversion of glucose into energy. If the hyperglycaemia is due to insufficient insulin, then glucose is not converted into energy, which causes tiredness.

Question 7.4

The person with Type 1 diabetes would make sure they gave themselves the correct dose of insulin, and that their insulin delivery device was working correctly. They would eat starchy food regularly. They may decide to eat more food or take less insulin if they have been exercising recently. If they had been drinking alcohol, they might decide to monitor their blood glucose more carefully, and may need to have some extra carbohydrate to counteract the hypoglycaemic effects of excess alcohol.

Question 7.5

Diet lemonade does not contain glucose so it is not an appropriate treatment for hypoglycaemia. Although a sandwich contains carbohydrate, and is broken down into glucose in the gut, this takes at least an hour and so is not very suitable as a treatment. However, a starchy snack should be consumed when the hypoglycaemia has been successfully treated with quick-acting carbohydrate.

Question 7.6

James should monitor his blood glucose regularly, at least four-hourly. He may have to take extra doses of insulin but certainly should not stop his insulin. He should try to drink plenty of sugar-free fluids to prevent dehydration. If he can, he should test for the presence of ketones in his urine or blood, which may be a sign that he needs medical help.

Question 8.1

The four strategies that can be used to enhance self-efficacy are mastery experience, modelling, social persuasion and emotional regulation (Section 8.2.3).

Question 8.2

The two means by which depression may influence diabetes control are firstly through behaviour, for example via people's diet and physical activity (exercise). Depression can also affect diabetes control through physiological mechanisms, for example the amount of cortisol in the body affects the blood glucose level.

Question 8.3

The categories of belief that make up an individual's personal model of diabetes are: what it is (identity), what caused it (cause), how long it will last (duration), what effect it will have (consequences), and what can be done about it (treatment effectiveness).

Question 8.4

The six steps to giving a diagnosis of diabetes to someone are:

1   elicit patient views

2   prompt that serious news is to be given

3   give the news without jargon

4   elicit reactions to encourage emotional expression

5   give reassurance and hope

6   explain, support and answer questions.

Further details are given in Box 8.1.

Question 9.1

The responsibility for the care of the person with diabetes ultimately lies with the person themselves, although the team must offer support.

Question 9.2

The elements of effective self-management consist of dietary changes, physical activity, blood glucose monitoring and taking medication.

Questions 9.3

'Compliance' can be explained as the act of following treatment recommendations. 'Concordance' can be explained as a process of prescribing and taking medication based on partnership.

Question 9.4

An empowerment model of diabetes care can be described as one where care is patient-led, with shared expertise between the health care professionals and the person with diabetes and where the person with diabetes is viewed as the problem solver and care giver.

Question 9.5

The key strategies for managing dietary self-care, are: (1) develop a plan, (2) modify the environment, (3) get perspective, (4) structured cheating, (5) new not old, (6) address boredom and (7) assertive strategies (see Section 9.3).

Question 9.6

Good communication can be achieved in the health care professional–patient relationship by focusing on the ten key issues in professional–patient communication:

- exploring and agreeing roles and responsibilities
- agreeing agendas
- actively listening to the patient
- encouraging the patient to explore their thoughts and feelings
- communicating understanding
- observing the cues from the patient
- exploring emotions elicited by the patient
- joint goal setting and care planning
- provision of information
- agreeing follow up.

Question 10.1

Examples of questions you could ask include: 'How do you think you got diabetes?' 'What do you think will change about your life now you have diabetes?' 'What parts of having diabetes might be particularly difficult for you?' In general, any open questions that involve the person's thoughts, feelings or beliefs will help to reveal their personal perspective on living with diabetes.

Question 10.2

(a) People are not required to inform the DVLA. The DVLA requires anyone to inform them if they use (b) tablets or (c) insulin to manage their diabetes. Once the DVLA has been informed, people on tablets have an unrestricted licence but are requested to inform the DVLA again if they start to use insulin. People on insulin treatment are issued with a licence restricted to one, two or three years, depending on the answers an individual gives to the questionnaire DIAB 1 and a report from their doctor that the DVLA may also request.

Question 10.3

Jobs that are not open to people using insulin treatment include: the armed forces; commercial pilot; ambulance or train driving; offshore platform work.

Question 10.4

There are many ways in which information about diabetes can be made available including: having material available in diabetes clinics, health centres and libraries; publicising websites; giving out information about local support groups.

Question 10.5

Diabetes can have an impact on relationships within the family, for example when close family members want increased involvement, sometimes against the wishes of the person with diabetes. Sexual relationships can also be affected, but diabetes can also bring couples closer as they face situations together.

Question 10.6

The challenges of living with diabetes every day include: never having a holiday from the management of diabetes; having to remember to do tests, take medication and obtain prescriptions; attending appointments; needing to be extra careful before and during pregnancy; facing the judgement of others regarding work; possibly having to accept help even though you don't want to; the threat of complications.

ACKNOWLEDGEMENTS

Grateful acknowledgement is made to the following sources for permission to reproduce material within this product.

Cover

Cover image and title page © Mike Dodd.

Figures

Figures 1.2, 1.3, 1.7, 1.11 Mike Ford and Dave Muscroft/The Open University; *Figure 1.6* Dr John Brackenbury/Science Photo Library; *Figure 1.8* Baillie, L. (2005) *Developing Practical Nursing Skills* 2nd edn, Arnold, A member of the Hodder Headline Group; *Figure 1.9* Seewoodhary, R. and Stevens, S. (1999) 'Transmission and Control of infection in Opthalmic Practice', *Community Eye Health*, Vol 11, No 30 1999. © Community Eye Health Journal, International Centre for Eye Health, London; *Figure 1.10* Courtesy of Tracy Finnegan; *Figure 2.2* Vander, A. J., Sherman, J. H. and Luciano, D. S. (2001) *Human Physiology, The Mechanisms of Body Function*, 8th international edition, copyright © 2001, 1998, 1994, 1990, 1985, 1980, 1975, 1970 by McGraw-Hill Inc; *Figure 2.6* Blackwell Science Ltd; *Figure 3.1* Mike Levers/The Open University; *Figures 3.2 and 3.3* Crown copyright material is reproduced under Class Licence Number C01W0000065 with the permission of the Controller of HMSO and the Queen's Printer for Scotland.*Figure 4.1* www.trafford.nhs.uk/diabetes/therapeuticguidance. Crown copyright material is reproduced under Class Figure Licence Number C01W0000065 with the permission of the Controller of HMSO and the Queen's Printer for Scotland; *Figure 4.8* Balance of Good Health, reproduced by permission of the Health Education Authority; *Figure 4.9* http://www.nhlbi.nih.gov/guidelines/obesity/bmi_tbl.htm; *Figures 5.1, 5.4 right and left, 5.6a, 5.6b, 5.7b, 5.8 and 5.10* Mike Ford and DaveMustcroft/The Open University; *Figure 5.2* Ed Young/Science Photo Library; *Figure 5.3* Courtesy of Tracy Finnegan; *Figure 5.4 middle, 5.5, 5.6c: 5.9a, 5.9b, 5.12a, 5.12b and 5.12c* Mike Levers/The Open University; *Figure 5.11a* Yoav Levy/photolibrary.com; *Figure 5.11b* van Wynsberghe, D., Noback, C. R. and Carola, R. (1995) *Human Anatomy and Physiology*, 3rd edn, McGraw-Hill Inc;*Figure 6.3, 6.4a, 6.4b and 6.4c* Courtesy of Dr Renee Page; *Figure 6.5a, 6.6, 6.9, 6.10a, 6.10b and 6.10c* Mike Ford and Dave Muscroft/The Open University; *Figure 6.5b* Mile Levers/The Open University; *Figure 6.8* Science Photo Library; *Figure 6.11* Courtesy of Duncan Banks; *Figure 6.13a* John Callan/Shout Picture Library; *Figure 7.1* Diabetes UK; *Figure 7.2* Courtesy of Duncan Banks; *Figure 7.3 and 7.5* Mile Levers/The Open University; *Figure 7.4a* Courtesy of Tracy Finnegan; *Figure 8.1* Courtesy of Heather Holden; *Figure 9.1* © The DESMOND collaborative; *Figure 9.2* Medicines Partnership; *Figure 9.3* Chad Ehlers/Alamy; *Figure 9.4* © Courtesy of Duncan Banks/The Open University; *Figure 10.1* Sally and Richard Greenhill; *Figure 10.2* Crown Copyright © Driver and Vehicle Licensing Agency Swansea SA6 7JL; *Figure 10.3* Science Photo Library; *Figure 10.4* © Diabetes UK 2000; *Figures 10.5a, 10.5b* Empics Ltd.

Tables

Table 1.1 National Service Framework for Diabetes Standards, Department of Health, HMSO, © Crown copyright 2005; *Table 4.1* © Diabetes UK; *Table 9.1* American Diabetes Association; *Table 9.5* Schlundt, D. et al. (1994) 'Situational obstacles to dietary adherence for adults with diabetes' *Journal of the American Dietetic Association*, August 1994, Volume 94, no 8. Copyright © 1994 by The American Dietetic Association.

Box

Box 8.2 © Psychiatric Research Unit, WHO Collaborating Center for Medical Health, Frederiksborg General Hospital, DK-3400 Hilerod.

Every effort has been made to contact copyright holders. If any have been inadvertently overlooked the publishers will be pleased to make the necessary arrangements at the first opportunity.

INDEX

Glossary terms and their page references are printed in bold. Entries in italics indicate items mainly, or wholly, in a figure or table.

A

Accident and Emergency units 77, 82

active listening 13

acupressure 95

acupuncture 95

adherence 207, 208, 209

adrenalin 156, 166

African–Caribbean people, propensity for diabetes 46, 49, 50, 179

airborne spread 21

Alberti, Professor Sir George 55

alcohol consumption 87, 106, 107, 248

    and hypoglycaemia 163, 165

    in pregnancy 96

    recommendations *212, 213, 214*

alcohol rub *22*

α cells 31, 39

alpha-glucosidase inhibitors 90, 93

amino acids 31–2, *39*

angina 105, 148, **149**, 249

annual review 58, 67, 104, 106–8, 124, 244

    blood pressure 120

    coronary heart disease 150

    diabetes care technician *60*

    eye examinations 7, 129, 134–5, 136–7, 245

    foot examination 143, 245

antidepressants 68, 199

aorta 148

aqueous humour 131, 135

aromatherapy 95

aseptic technique 24, 25

Asian link workers 14, **59**, 223, *224*

Asian people, propensity for diabetes 46, 49, 50, 51, 55

aspirin 99

atheroma 119, 142, 149

atrium 148

Audit Commission 4

autoimmune disease 44, 74

autonomic nerves 140

autonomic neuropathy 105, **140**

autosomal dominant conditions 50

autosomal recessive conditions 50

B

background retinopathy 132, 134

Balance of Good Health *86*

balanced diet 85, 86–7, 96, 107, 247

beliefs

    about diabetes 177–82

    about self 186–90

    about treatment 182–5

β cells 31–2, 162

    antibodies destroying 44

biguanides 90–1, 92, 99, 100, 160, 161

biosynthetically 78

bladder 137, 138

blood glucose level 30

    brain 38, 39

    complementary therapies 95

    controlling 2, *62*, 68, 76–7, 87, 108, 158–9

    diabetes complications 98, 130, 234

    and diet 8, 32–4, 35, 157, 160, 166, 179–80

    effect on eyes 130–1, 134, 136

    effect of stress 156, 158

    and exercise 34–5, 89, 90, 160, 166, 179–80, 248

    fat tissues' effect on 36, *37*, 38, *39*, 156, 166

    glycaemic index 87, *88*

    insulin's effect on 38, 43

    liver's effect on 34, *37*, 38, *39*, 156, 166

    lowering therapies 77, 84, 90–5, 99, 100, 204, 243

    meters 40, 107, 110–11, 113, 118, 221, *224*

    monitoring 40, 44–5, 47–8, 58–9, 99–100, 108–13, 220–1, 233

    record keeping 12, 13, 107

skeletal muscles' effect on 34, *37*, 38, *39*, 156, 166

    see also glucose; hyperglycaemia; hypoglycaemia

blood glucose meters 40, 107, **110**–11, 113, 118, 221, *224*

blood pressure 48, 57, 59, **119**

    controlling *62*, 97, 98–9, 100, 147, 204, 243

    and coronary heart disease 147, 149

    hypertension 98, 106, 119, 122, 129, 147, 149

    kidneys' effect on 138

    monitoring 100, 119–22, 123, 149, 244

blood spillage 114, 115

blood tests

    blood glucose meters 40, 107, 110–11, 113, 118, 221, *224*

    equipment 114–16

    finger prick tests 23, 40, 44, 97, 99, 100, *112*

    phlebotomist 7, 8, 10

    plasma glucose level 40, *41*, 43, 47, 74, 85, 113–14

    for renal damage 138, 139

    venous blood samples 113–16

    see also glycated haemoglobin levels

blood vessels

    atheroma 119, 142, 149

    macrovascular complications 42, 97, 106, 119, 130, 204

    retinal *131, 132*, 133

    see also cerebrovascular accident; cerebrovascular disease; microvascular complications

blurred vision 83, 135–6, *170*

BNF *see* British National Formulary

body mass index (BMI) 38, 49, **51**, 52, 59, 234

    calculating 87, *88*, 122, *123*

bovine (beef) insulin 78

bracelet, medical alert *164*, 168

brain
    blood glucose level 38, 39
    see also cerebrovascular accident
breast feeding, diabetes risk factor 51
British National Formulary (BNF) 94, 98

C

car insurance 239
carbohydrates 30
    alpha-glucosidase inhibitors 90, 93
    balanced diet 86
    breaking down 32, *33*, 36
    hypoglycaemia 162, 164, 165, 166, 167, 168
cardiovascular disease, diabetes risk factors 57, 147
    see also coronary heart disease
care
    children 56, 58, *62*, 180–1
    cost of 4
    diabetes team 6–11, 16–17, 25, 55–60, 129
    diabetic emergencies *63*
    education groups 56–7, 69
    framework for 61–4
    local diabetes networks *64, 65,* 245, 251
    local needs 69–70
    new roles 60–1
    settings 64–5
    see also annual review; National Service Framework for Diabetes
cataracts 134, **135**
CBT *see* cognitive behavioural therapy
cells 31
    glucose uptake 36, *39*, 43
central obesity 122
cerebrovascular accident (CVA) (or stroke) 4, 6, 97, 105, 119, 130, **149**
cerebrovascular disease (CVD) 105, 106, **149**
chain of infection *23*
Changing Workforce Programme 61
CHD *see* coronary heart disease
children
    diabetes clinics 56, *62*

hospital treatment 56, 58, *63*, 64
    inherited abnormalities 50
    managing diabetes 56, 58, *62*, 180–1
    pen devices *81*
cholesterol 98
    blood cholesterol level 59, 100, 118–19
    plasma cholesterol level 40
    reducing 98–9, 104, 118, 147, 222, 243
    see also lipids
chromosomes 49–50
chronic 42
Clinical Action Teams 63
closed questions 13
closed vacuum system 114, 115
CODE-2 UK 4
cognitive behavioural therapy (CBT) 199
communication skills 1, 107
    acceptance 228
    communicating hope 227–8
    communication barriers 14–15
    communication in teams 10–15, 17, 25
    congruity 227, 229
    and the consultation 223–6, 234
    effective 227–9
    empathy 227, 228
    genuineness 228
    listening and questioning 12–13
    negotiation 13, *14*
    non-verbal communication 11–12
    qualities of effective 227–9
    in teams 11
complementary therapies 95–6
compliance 207, 208, 209, 210, 211, 229
complications (of diabetes)
    cardiovascular disease 147
    cerebrovascular disease 97, 105, 106, 119, 130, 149
    clinical care *62, 63*, 68
    coronary heart disease 149
    detection and management *63*, 76, 104–6, 108, 129, 134–9, 143–4, 150
    foot disorders 105, 128, 130, 142–7, 150, 179
    onset of 127–9, 196, 233, 244, 249–50, 252

preventing 97–9, 103, 124, 233, 244
    risk factors 85, 103, 104, 105–6, 123, 157, 234
    see also eye disease; kidney disease; macrovascular; microvascular
concordance 207, **210–11**, 229
confidentiality 17–19, 25
congruity 227, 229
contraindications 91, 92, 93, 94, 96, 98, 100
cornea 131
coronary heart disease (CHD) 105, 106, **149**
    angina 105, 148, 249
    aspirin 99
    atheroma 119, 142, 149
    and depression 196
    Framingham CHD risk score 123
    myocardial infarction 4, 149, 249
    risk reduction 97, 99, 118, 119, 122, 123, 147
    screening 150
    structure of the heart 148
    and tablet therapy 91, 92
    Type 2 diabetes 119, 122, 123, 249
    see also cardiovascular disease
cortisol 156, 196
counsellors 57, 141
creatinine 139
cross infection 21, 25
culture 234–6, 251
CVA *see* cerebrovascular accident
CVD *see* cerebrovascular disease
cystic fibrosis 49, 50

D

DAFNE (Dose Adjustment for Normal Eating) 20, **69**
DAWN Study 183–5
DCCT *see* Diabetes Control and Complications Trial
DCT *see* diabetes care technician
defining diabetes 29–30
Delivery Strategy for the NSF for Diabetes 61, *62*
Department of Health 61, *64*
depression 7, 68, 105, 249
    and diabetes 196–9
    diagnosing 197–8

effects of 196, *197*, 242

treating 199

DESMOND (Diabetes Education and Self-Management for Ongoing and Newly Diagnosed) Collaborative **69**, 205, 206–7, 229

dextrose tablets 164, 166, 168

DIAB1 form 236, *237*

diabetes care team 6–9

diabetes care technician (DCT) 9, 57, 60, 61, 108, 246

diabetes clinic staff 9, 58–9

diabetes clinics 6, 7, 58–9, *62*, 64, 74, 104, 137

Diabetes Control and Complications Trial (DCCT) 108, 113, 119, 131, 157

diabetes insipidus 30

diabetes mellitus 30

    beliefs about 177–82

    conveying the diagnosis 191–6

    diagnosing 40–2, 52, *74*, 75

    gestational 48, 51, *63*, 97, 157, 246

    GPs' attitude to 183–5

    impact of 2–6

    incidence 2, 4, 49, 50, 55, 65, 105, 204

    managing 73

    rare forms 49

    risk factors 42, 47, 50–2, *62*, 105–8, 123, 157, 204

    undiagnosed diabetes 48, 49

    WHO definition 41, 44

    see also Type 1 diabetes; Type 2 diabetes

diabetes specialist nurses (DSN) 8, 60

    annual review 7, 129, 233

    children 58

    educational role 82, 139, 159

    pregnancy 59, 97, 246

Diabetes UK 45, 58, 61, 69, 81, 159

    DESMOND Collaborative 69, 205

    employment 241

    hypoglycaemia 162, 164

    incidence of diabetes 2

    insurance 239

    local care services 65, 245, 251

    physical training 248

    pregnancy 246, 247

diabetic dyslipidaemia 106, **118**, 119, 122, 149

diabetic foods 87

diabetic ketoacidosis (DKA) *see* ketoacidosis

diabetic nephropathy 105, 108, 130, 137, 138–9, 249

    see also kidney disease

diabetic neuropathy 130, 140–2, 143–4, 149

diabetic retinopathy 105–6, 108, 129, **130**, 132–4, 222, 249, *250*

    see also eye disease

diabetologist 8, 58, 59, 82, 184

    annual review 7, *129*

diagnosis

    conveying the diagnosis 191–6

    depression 197–8

    diabetes 40–2, 52, *74*, 75

    Type 1 diabetes 44–5, 47, 75, 76

    Type 2 diabetes 47–8, 74, 76, 84–5

dialysis 138, 249

diastolic pressure 120

diet

    advice on 8, 56–7, 58, 76, 83, 106, 108

    balanced diet 85, 86–7, 96, 107, 247

    compliance 208

    cultural factors 234, *235*

    dietary management 214–19, 229

    effect on blood glucose level 8, 32–4, 35, 157, 160, 166, 179–80

    glycaemic index 20, 87, *88*

    recommendations *212, 213*

    Type 2 diabetes 46, 48, 104, 129

dietitian 7, **8**, 233, 246

    educational role 57, 58, 68, 85, 87, *107*

direct contact 21–2

Disability Discrimination Act 1995 239, 240

DKA *see* ketoacidosis

Driver and Vehicle Licensing Agency (DVLA) 19, 164

    licence restrictions 236–8, 239

driving, diabetes and 18, 19, 83, 85, 90, 252

    car insurance 239

    hypoglycaemia 162, 164, 237, 239

    licence restrictions 236–8, 239

drugs

    alpha-glucosidase inhibitors 90, 93

    antidepressants 199

    biguanides 90–1, 92, 99, 100, 160, 161

    blood pressure control 98, 119, 149, 222, 243

    cholesterol-lowering 98, 104, 118, 222, 243

    erectile dysfunction 141

    post-prandial regulators 90, 93, 162

    safety 25

    sulphonylureas 90, 92, 93, 161, 162, 163, 240

    thiazolidinediones 90, 92

    see also contraindications

DSN *see* diabetes specialist nurses

DVLA *see* Driver and Vehicle Licensing Agency

dyslipidaemia *see* diabetic dyslipidaemia

E

ECG (electrocardiograph) 150

education for self-management 203–5

    barriers to self-care 212–14

    communication skills 223–9, 234

    compliance 207, 208, 209, 210, 211, 229

    concordance 207, 210–11, 229

    diabetic specialist nurses' role 8, 82, 139, 159

    dietary management 214–19, 229

    emotions, awareness and management of 221–3, 229

    empowering patients 207–11, 229

    group education 57, 58–9, 61, 69, 229

    health care professionals' responsibilities 205–7, 208, 210–11, 233, 248

    self-monitoring 220–1, 226

education groups 57, 58–9, 61, 69, 229

electrolytes 138, 139

emergency treatment *63*

emotional regulation 186, 190

emotions

    awareness and management 221–3, 229

    psychological aspects of diabetes 14, 190–6, 199

empathy 227, 228

employment, diabetes and 2, 240–2, 251–2

empowering patients *62*, 66–7, 100, 207–11, 229

empowerment **66**, 208–9

empowerment model of care 209

end-stage renal failure 138, 150

endocrine glands 31

endocrine hormones 31

enzymes 32

epidemiology 42

erectile dysfunction 140–2, 243

excretion 138

exercise

benefits 89, 128, 247, 248

and blood glucose level 34–5, 89, 90, 160, 166, 179–80, 248

controlling blood pressure 98, 149

recommendations *212, 213, 214*

Type 2 diabetes 46, 48, 51, 75, 89

Expert Patients Programme 61

eye, structure of 131–2

eye disease, diabetes complications 57, 68, 97, 128, 244

blurred vision 83, 135–6, *170*

cataracts 134, 135

dilating drops 16, 134, 135

eye examinations 7, 8, 16, 134–5, 136–7, 244, 245

glaucoma 135

incidence 130

laser treatment 134

sight loss 4, 129, 130, 136, 150, 249

see also diabetic retinopathy

F

family, diabetes and 18, 19, 242–3, 251

family history of diabetes 46, 48–9, 50, 52, *74*, 179, 191

fasting 34, 36, 38

plasma glucose levels *41, 42*, 47, 74, 85

fat tissue

glucose stored in 36, *37*, 38, *39*, 156, 166

insulin resistance 46

lipohypertrophy 83

fatigue 3–4, 43, 58, 76, 105, *170*

fats in food

balanced diet *86*, 87

breaking down 32, *33*, 36

fatty acids 32, **36**, *37, 46*

fibrates 98, 118

finger prick tests 23, 40, 44, 97, 99, 100, *112*

firefighters, diabetes and 241–2

fluid loss 43

foods

breakdown of *33*

diabetic 87

glycaemic index 87, *88*

types 32, *33*

see also carbohydrates; diet; fats in food; proteins

foot care advice 144–6, 147

foot disorders

amputations 4, 147, 150, 179, 249

annual examinations 143–4, 147, 233, 244, 245

foot care 144–6, 147

gangrene 130, 142

ingrown toenails 57, 58, 145

peripheral neuropathy 105, 128, 130, 142

peripheral vascular disease 105

ulcers 7, 128, 142, 146, 147

footwear, suitable 7, 144, 145, 147

fovea 131, 132

Framingham CHD risk score 123

fructose 33

G

gangrene 130, 142

general practitioner (GP) 9

annual review 106, 124, 129, 233

attitudes to diabetes 183–5

diabetes care 4, 29–30, 57, 59, *64*, 67–9, 91, 98, 123, 183–5

diagnosing diabetes 45, 47–8, 74, 75, 85, 154

hospital referrals 56, 58, 74

see also health care professionals

genes 44

abnormalities 49, 50

description 49–50

Type 2 diabetes 46

gestational diabetes 48, 51, *63*, 97, 157, 246

GI *see* glycaemic index

glaucoma 135

glibenclamide 162, 163

gliclazide 92, 161, 162

GlucaGen® 169

glucagon 31, **39**, 166, 167, 169

glucocorticoids 156

glucose 30

food ingredient 33

function 31, 35

insulin's effects on 36, 38, *39*, 43

metabolism 35–6, *37*

oral glucose tolerance test 42–3, 48, 97

plasma glucose level 40, *41*, 43, 47, 74, 85, 113–14

production 32

renal threshold 113

stored in fat tissue 36, *37*, 38, *39*, 156

stored in liver 34, *37*, 38, *39*, 156

stored in skeletal muscles 34, *37*, 38, *39*, 156

tolerance testing 41–2, 48

2-hour glucose test 42

urine, levels in 43, 47–8, 58–9, 74, 100, 109, 113, 155

see also blood glucose level

glycaemic index (GI) 20, **87**, *88*

glycated haemoglobin (HbA$_{1c}$) levels 97, 100, 109, **116**–18, 123–4, 155, 245

glycogen 34, *37, 39, 46*

gut *31*, 32

alpha-glucosidase inhibitors 90, 93

H

haemorrhages, retinal 132, 133–4

hand hygiene 21, *22*, 23

hard exudates, retinal 132, *133*

HbA$_{1c}$ *see* glycated haemoglobin levels

HDL-cholesterol 118

see also lipids

health care professionals

communicating with patients 10–15, 25, 223–9, 234

conveying the diagnosis 191–6

responsibilities 205–7, 208, 210–11, 233, 248

see also individual professions

health centres, diabetes care 7, 9, 56, 58–9, 64, 65

heart, structure of 148

heart disease *see* coronary heart disease

high-density lipoprotein (HDL) 118

holidays 239, 240

hormones 30, **31**

    cortisol 156, 196, *197*

    excess 49

    glucagon 31, 39, 166, 167, 169

    produced in fat tissue 36

    stress hormones 156, 158, *197*

hospitals

    diabetes clinics 6, 7, 58–9, *62*, 64, 74, 104, 119, 137

    GP referrals 56, 58, 74

    standards of care 4, *63*

hygiene 21–5

hyperglycaemia 34, 43, 122

    causes 153–7

    and depression 197–8

    effects 37, 105–6, 154–5, 156–7, 169

    exercise and 35

    in pregnancy 155, 157, 245–6

    preventing 157–9

    recognising 159

    symptoms 159–60, *170*

    treating 160–1

    see also blood glucose level

hypertension 98, 106, 119, 122, 129, 147, 149

    see also blood pressure

hypoglycaemia (hypos) **34**, 117

    causes 164–6

    complementary therapies 95

    and driving 162, 164, 237, 239

    effects 161, 163

    exercise and 35

    fear of 163, 181–2, 219

    hypoglycaemic awareness 164

    patient education 58, 83

    in pregnancy 165, 246

    preventing 164, 166, 240

    recognising 167

    symptoms 83, 161, 162, 163, 167, *170*

    treating 167–9

    see also blood glucose level

hypos *see* hypoglycaemia

Hypostop 169

I

identification, carrying of 164, 168

impaired fasting glycaemia (IFG) 42

impaired glucose tolerance (IGT) 42, 48, 91

incidence 44

    increasing 2, 4, 49, 55, 105, 204

    Type 2 diabetes 50, 65

indirect contact 23

infections

    chain of *23*

    effects on diabetics 37, 155

    risk of 21–5

    urine infections 22, 139

informed consent 16, 25, 114

injections

    needles 79, 80, 81, 82, 112, 114, 115

    patient anxiety 77–8, 82, 219–20

    pen devices 57, 59, 81, 82, 83, 155, 183

    pumps 81, 83

    sites *79*, *80*, 83, 155, 165

    syringes 80, 82, 114, 115

    training in 57, 58, 59, 82

insulin 38

    abnormalities of 49

    absorption rates 83

    actions of *39*, 43

    dosage 79, 82, 84, 109, 118, 155, 158, 165, 166

    drugs interacting with 49

    glucose uptake 36, *39*, 43

    injecting 57, 58, 59, 77–8, 79–82

    intravenous infusion 58, 158

    in non-diabetics 40, *41*

    pen devices 57, 59, 81, 82, 83, 155, 183

    preconceptions about 183–4

    production 31, 32, 34, 35, 46

    resistance 38, *46*, 77, 156, 246

    self-care 219

    storage 25, 83

    and tablet therapy 90–3, 161, 243

    therapy 77–84

    training in administering 57, 58, 59, 219–20

    types of 78–9, 82, 158, 161, 162, 166

insulin resistance 38, *46*, 77, 156, 246

    reducing 90–2

insurance, diabetes and 238–40

iris **131**, 135

islets of Langerhans 31, *32*, 39

K

ketoacidosis (DKA) 36, 37, 43–5, 57, 117–18, 158–9, 169, 239

ketone bodies 36

ketones 36, *37*, 43, 117–18, 156, 157

ketonuria 36, 37, 58, *74*, 117–18, 156, 157, *170*

kidney, structure of 137–8

kidney disease, diabetes complications 4, 57, 68, 97, 244

    diabetic nephropathy 105, 108, 130, 137, 138–9, 249

    dialysis 138, 249

    end-stage renal failure 138, 150

    hypoglycaemia 165

    renal threshold 113

    tablet therapy 91, 93

    see also urine

King, Billie Jean 248, *249*

Kussmaul's respiration 159

L

LDL-cholesterol 118

    see also lipids

leading questions 13

learning facilitator 61

lens 131, 134, 135

lifestyle

    changing 85, 89, 90, 92, 98–9, 109, 129, 139, 182

    dietary management 214–19, 229

    holiday changes 239, 240

    self-care 212–14

link workers 14, 57, 223, *224*

lipids 77, **98**, 100, 204

    diabetic dyslipidaemia 106, 118, 119, 122, 149

    monitoring 118, 123, 245

    reducing in the blood 98–9

    see also cholesterol

lipohypertrophy 83

liver 31

    effect on blood glucose level 34, *37*, 38, *39*, 156, 166

insulin resistance 46
and tablet therapy 90, 91, 92, 93
living with diabetes 233–4
complications 249–51
culture 234–6, 251
demands of treatment 243–5, 252
employment 2, 240–2, 251–2
family 18, 19, 242–3, 251
insurance 238–40
lifestyle and diabetes 247–8, *249*
pregnancy 245–7, 252
sex and relationships 140–2, 243
see also driving; self-management
local care needs 69–70
local diabetes networks 58, *64*, 65, 245, 251
Local Implementation Teams 63
long-acting insulin 78, 79, 162, 166
low-density lipoprotein (LDL) 118
Lucozade® 33, 41, 87, 168

M

macrovascular 42
complications 97, 105, 106, 119, 130, 204
managing diabetes
children 56, 58, *62*, 180–1
see also medical management
mastery experience 186
maturity onset diabetes of the young (MODY) 46, 50, *74*
medical management 73
blood glucose control 2, 76–7, 208
complementary therapies 95–6
insulin therapy 77–84
monitoring 99–100, 108
non-insulin therapies 84–5
other therapies 97–9
pregnancy and diabetes 96–7
tablet therapy 90–5, 99, 100, 160
see also self-management
medium-acting insulin 78, 82, 162
metabolism 35, *37*
metformin 90–1, 92, 99, 100, 160, 161
microalbuminuria 139, 233
microaneurysms 132
microvascular complications **42**, 97, 105–6, 108, 136–7, 138–42, 150, 204

see also diabetic neuropathy; diabetic retinopathy
mid-stream specimen of urine (MSU) 139
minerals 32
mmol/l 34
modelling 186, 187
MODY *see* maturity onset diabetes of the young
monitoring
blood glucose level 108–17
ketone level 117–18
lipid levels 118–19
self-monitoring of glucose level 109–13, 123–4, 160–1, 220–1, 226
monofilament 143, 144
motor nerves 140
motor neuropathy 142
MSU *see* mid-stream specimen of urine
multidisciplinary teams 7, 25
multifactorial conditions 50
muscle 34–5
see also skeletal muscle
myocardial infarction 4, 149, 249
myocardium 148

N

National Clinical Director for Diabetes 63
National Diabetes Support Team 63
National Electronic Library for Health (NELH) 69
National Institute for Health and Clinical Excellence (NICE) 61, 81, 93, 117
National Service Framework for Diabetes (NSF) **5**, *62*, *63*, *64*, 65, 66, 69–70, 200
Delivery Strategy 61, 62
needle stick injuries 24
needles 79, 80, 81, 82, 112, 114, 115
negotiation in communication 13
NELH *see* National Electronic Library for Health
nephrons 137, 138
nephropathy *see* diabetic nephropathy
nerves
diabetic neuropathy 128, 130, 140–2, 143–4
see also microvascular complications

neuropathy *see* diabetic neuropathy
neurotip 143, 144
NICE *see* National Institute for Health and Clinical Excellence
nocturia 3, *74*, **75**
non-verbal communication 11–12
normal flora 21
NSF *see* National Service Framework for Diabetes
nurse practitioner 58

O

obesity 38, 52
body mass index 49, 51, 52, 59, 87, *88*, 122–3
central obesity 122
measuring 57
and tablet therapy 92
and Type 2 diabetes 46, 47, 48, 49, 51, 75, 90, 156
obstetricians 57
oestrogen 31
OGTT *see* oral glucose tolerance test
OHAs *see* oral hypoglycaemic agents
open question 13
optic disc 132
optic nerve 132, 135
optometrist 7, 9, 57, 129, 136, 137
oral glucose tolerance test (OGTT) 41–2, 48, 97
oral hypoglycaemic agents (OHAs) *see* tablet therapy
orthotist 7, 9
osmotic diuresis 154

P

pancreas 31
insulin production 32, 34, 35, 90
stimulating 90, 92, 93, 162
pancreatitis 49
patients 1
beliefs about diabetes 177–82
beliefs about self 186–90
beliefs about treatment 182–5, 219–20
communicating with health care professionals 10–15, 25, 223–9, 234
cultural factors 234–6, 251

diabetes information 29–30, 82, 84, 85, 124, 203, 206–7
education groups 57, 58–9, 61, 69, 229
empowering *62*, 66–7, 100, 207–11, 229
informed consent 16, 25, 114
receiving the diagnosis 191–6, 222
record keeping 12, 13, 17, 107
'sick day rules' 158, 159
see also self-management
PCTs *see* Primary Care Trusts
pen devices 57, 59, **81**, 82, 83, 155, 183
peripheral neuropathy 105, 128, 130, **140**, 142, 143–4, 237
peripheral vascular disease 105
pharmacist 7, **9**, 57, 59
phlebotomist 7, **8**, 9, 10
plasma 40
plasma cholesterol level 40
plasma glucose level 40, *41*, 43, 47, 74, 85, 113–14
podiatrist 7, **8**, 57, 59, 142–3, 233, 244
polyuria 105, 154
porcine (pig) insulin 78
post-prandial regulators 90, 93, 162
practice nurse 9, 57, 58, 85, 96, 98
annual review 106, 124, 129
pre-proliferative retinopathy 133
pregnancy 48
diabetes care in 57, 59, *63*, 96–7, 245–7, 252
gestational diabetes 48, 51, *63*, 97, 157, 246
hyperglycaemia in 155, 157, 245–6
hypoglycaemia in 165, 246
and tablet therapy 92, 93, 246
primary care team **9**, 10, 25
Primary Care Trusts (PCTs) 63, *64*, 65, **110**
proliferative retinopathy 133
protein-deficient diabetes 49
proteins
balanced diet *86*, 87
breaking down 32, *33*
presence in urine 138–9
psychological aspects of diabetes
beliefs about diabetes 177–82

beliefs about self 186–90
beliefs about treatment 182–5
depression 7, 68, 105, 196–9, 242, 249
emotions 14, 190–6, 199
'parcel' case study 2, 173–6, 177, 190–1, 195–6, 199
psychologist 7, **9**, 57
pulmonary artery 148
pumps 81, 83
pupil 131, 135

Q
quick-acting insulin 78, 158, 161, 166

R
random glucose test **41**, 47, 48, 74
record keeping 16–19, 120
Redgrave, Sir Steven 2, 248, *249*
reflexology 95
renal damage 139
see also kidney disease
renal threshold 113
repaglinide 93, 162
retina 131, 132–3
retinal screening 7, 8, 134–5, 244
see also diabetes complications; eye disease
retinal screening technician 7, **8**
retinopathy *see* diabetic retinopathy
risk assessment 20
risk of developing Type 2 diabetes 42, 47, 50–1, 52
reduction *62*
see also family history of diabetes
risk factors for diabetic complications 103, 105–6, 107–8, 157
assessing risk 103
awareness 127–9
reduction 100, 123, 204
Royal National Institute for the Blind 136, 250

S
'safe clip' 112
safety
and drugs 25

risk assessment 20
risk of infection 21–5
safe treatment 19–20, 25
salt, limiting intake 87, 98, *212*, *213*, *214*, 217
screening
for CHD 150
for complications of diabetes 127–50
for eye disease 136
for nephropathy 138–9
secondary care 10, 25
selective serotonin reuptake inhibitors (SSRIs) 199
self-efficacy 186, 187, 190, 217, 218
self-management 182, 199, 203
barriers to 212–14
behaviour change 204–5, 209–11
beliefs about self 186–90
communicating with health care professionals 25, 223–9, 234
compliance 207, 208, 209, 210, 211, 229
concordance 207, 210–11, 229
dietary management 179, 214–19, 229
emotions 221–3, 229
group education 57, 58–9, 61, 69, 229
health care professionals' responsibilities 6, 205–7, 208, 210–11, 233, 248
medication taking and adjustment 219–20, 243–4
record keeping 12, 13, 17, 107
see also living with diabetes
self-monitoring
of blood glucose 109–13, 123–4, 160–1, 220–1, 226
of urine glucose 113
sensory nerves 140
sex and relationships 243
erectile dysfunction 140–2
Sexual Dysfunction Association 141
SHA *see* Strategic Health Authorities
sharps disposal boxes 24, 25, 82, 112, 115
short-acting insulin 78, 162
'sick day rules' 158, 159
sight loss 4, 129, 130, 136, 150, 249
see also eye disease

skeletal muscles 34
  effect on blood glucose level *37*, 38, *39*, 156, 166
  insulin resistance 46
Skills for Health 61
small intestine 32
SMART goals **187**, 188, 216
smoking 106, 107, 108, 136, *212*, *213*, *214*, 247
Snellen Chart *134*
social persuasion 186, 187–90
sphygmomanometers *119*, 120, *121*, 149
SSRIs *see* selective serotonin reuptake inhibitors
Standards for NSF 5
statins 98, 118
steroids 156
stomach *31*, *32*
Strategic Health Authorities (SHA) 61, 63, *64*, 65
stress, effect on blood glucose level 156, 158
strokes *see* cerebrovascular accident
subcutaneously 79
sulphonylureas 90, 92, 93, 161, 162, 163, 240
symptoms *74*
  depression 68, 105, 197–8
  excessive urine 3, 30, 43–5, 58, 74, 105, 154, *170*
  fatigue 3–4, 43, 58, 76, 105, *170*
  genital itching 105
  hyperglycaemia 159–60, *170*
  hypoglycaemia 83, 161, 162, 163, 167, *170*
  thirst 3, 30, 43, 44, 45, 58, 74, 105, 154, *170*
  weight loss 43, 44, 58, 74, 105, *170*
syringes 80, 82, 114, 115
systolic pressure 120

T

tablet therapy 104, 179, 222
  alpha-glucosidase inhibitors 90, 93
  biguanides 90–1, 92, 99, 100, 160, 161
  contraindications 91, 92, 93, 94, 96
  effects 90, 92, 93, 162, 240
  GPs over-reliance on 183, 184

and insulin 90–3, 161, 243
  post-prandial regulators 90, 93, 162
  and pregnancy 92, 93, 246
  problems with 94–5, 158
  remembering to take 243–4
  sulphonylureas 90, 92, 93, 161, 162, 163, 240
  thiazolidinediones 90, 92
team work 10–11
testosterone 31
thiazolidinediones 90, 92
thirst, symptom of diabetes 3, 30, 43–5, 58, 74, 105, 154, *170*
thyroid
  disease 44
  hormone 31
TIA *see* transient ischaemic attacks
tourniquets 114, 115
traditional model of care 209
transient ischaemic attacks (TIA) 149
translators 14, 57, 104, 223
travel insurance 239–40
treatment
  beliefs about 182–5
  children 56, 58, *63*, 64, 180–1
  demands of 243–5, 252
  hyperglycaemia 160–1
  hypoglycaemia 167–9
  informed consent 16, 25, 114
  safety 19–20, 25
  Type 1 diabetes 67–9, 77, 78–9, 82, 208, 243
  Type 2 diabetes 46, 48, 65, 77, 90–5, 96, 104, 243
triglycerides 118
tuning fork 143, 144
2-hour glucose test *42*
Type 1 diabetes 3, 29, **43**–4
  beliefs about 180–1
  complications 128–9
  diagnosing 44–5, 47, 75, 76
  ketone testing 118, 156
  pregnancy 96

  risk factors 51, *74*, 108, 157
  treatment 67–9, 77, 78–9, 82, 208, 243
  Type 2, comparison with 47, 52, 104
Type 2 diabetes 3, 29, **45**
  beliefs about 181–2
  complications 129, 234, 249
  conveying the diagnosis 191, 193–4, 195
  coronary heart disease 119, 122, 123, 249
  and depression 197
  diagnosing 47–8, 74, 76, 84–5
  and diet 46, 48, 104, 129
  and exercise 46, 48, 51, 75, 89
  gestational diabetes 48, 51, *63*, 97, 157, 246
  GPs lack of knowledge 183–4
  incidence 49, 50, 65
  maturity onset diabetes of the young 46, 50, *74*
  and obesity 46, 47, 48, 49, 51, 75, 90, 156
  pregnancy 96, 246
  risk factors 50–1, 52, *62*, 75, 123, 157
  treatment 46, 48, 65, 77, 90–5, 96, 104, 243
  Type 1, comparison with 47, 52, 104
  undiagnosed 2, 49, *62*, 154–5, 159, 180

U

U & Es 139
UK Prospective Diseases Study (UKPDS) 108, 109, 113, 119, 131, 147, 157
ulcers 7, 128, 142, 146, 147
urea 138
ureter 137
urinalysis 57, **58**, 59, 99–100, 138–9, 233
urine
  excess production 3, 30, 43–5, 56, 74, 105, 154, *170*
  glucose levels 43, 47–8, 56, 57, 74, 100, 109, 113, 155
  infections 22, 139
  ketonuria 36, 37, 56, *74*, 117–18, 156, 157, *170*
  microalbinuria 139, 233
  nocturia 3, *74*, 75
  testing strips 43, 45, 118, 139
  urinalysis 57, 58, 59, 99–100, 138–9, 233
  see also kidney disease

V

venepuncture 114, 115

venous blood sample 113–16

ventricle 148

very quick-acting insulin 78, 79

viruses, diabetes risk factor 51

visual acuity testing 134

visual cortex 132

vitamins 32

vitreous humour 132

vomiting 43

W

WDC *see* Workforce Development
  Confederations

WDD *see* Workforce Development Directorates

waist measurements 122, 123

weight loss 43, 44, 58, 74, 105, *170*

    controlling blood pressure 98

    from exercise 89

    hypoglycaemia 165, *170*

Workforce Development Confederations (WDC) 61

Workforce Development Directorates   (WDD) 61

World Health Organization

    definition of diabetes 41, 44

    incidence of diabetes 2

    WHO 5 Well-Being Measure *198*